Challenges and Advances in Airway Management

Guest Editor

SHARON ELIZABETH MACE, MD, FACEP, FAAP

EMERGENCY MEDICINE CLINICS OF NORTH AMERICA

www.emed.theclinics.com

Consulting Editor

AMAL MATTU, MD

November 2008 • Volume 26 • Number 4

SAUNDERS an imprint of ELSEVIER, Inc.

W.B. SAUNDERS COMPANY

A Division of Elsevier Inc.

1600 John F. Kennedy Boulevard ● Suite 1800 ● Philadelphia, Pennsylvania 19103-2899

http://www.theclinics.com

EMERGENCY MEDICINE CLINICS OF NORTH AMERICA Volume 26, Number 4
November 2008 ISSN 0733-8627, ISBN-13: 978-1-4377-0438-9, ISBN-10: 1-4377-0438-7

Editor: Patrick Manley

Emergency Medicine Clinics of North America (ISSN 0733-8627) is published quarterly by Elsevier Inc., 360 Park Avenue South, New York, NY, 10010-1710. Months of issue are February, May, August, and November. Business and Editorial Offices: 1600 John F. Kennedy Boulevard, Suite 1800, Philadelphia, PA 19103-2899. Customer Service Office: 6277 Sea Harbor Drive, Orlando, FL 32887-4800. Periodicals postage paid at New York, NY, and additional mailing offices. Subscription prices are $118.00 per year (US students), $229.00 per year (US individuals), $373.00 per year (US institutions), $167.00 per year (international students), $328.00 per year (international individuals), $450.00 per year (international institutions), $167.00 per year (Canadian students), $282.00 per year (Canadian individuals), and $450.00 per year (Canadian institutions). International air speed delivery is included in all *Clinics'* subscription prices. All prices are subject to change without notice. **POSTMASTER:** Send address changes to *Emergency Medicine Clinics of North America*, Elsevier Periodicals Customer Service, 11830 Westline Industrial Drive, St. Louis, MO 63146. Customer Service (orders, claims, online, change of address): Elsevier Periodicals Customer Service, 11830 Westline Industrial Drive, St. Louis, MO 63146. Tel: 1-800-654-2452 (U.S. and Canada); 314-453-7041 (outside U.S. and Canada). Fax: 314-453-5170. E-mail: journalscustomerservice-usa@elsevier.com (for print support); journalsonline support-usa@elsevier.com (for online support).

Reprints. For copies of 100 or more of articles in this publication, please contact the Commercial Reprints Department, Elsevier Inc., 360 Park Avenue South, New York, NY 10010-1710. Tel.: 212-633-3812; Fax: 212-462-1935; E-mail: reprints@elsevier.com.

Emergency Medicine Clinics of North America is covered in *MEDLINE/PubMed (Index Medicus), Current Contents/Clinical Medicine, EMBASE/Excerpta Medica, BIOSIS, SciSearch, CINAHL, ISI/BIOMED,* and *Research Alert.*

Printed in the United States of America.

Contributors

CONSULTING EDITOR

AMAL MATTU, MD, FAAEM, FACEP
Associate Professor and Program Director, Department of Emergency Medicine, University of Maryland School of Medicine, Baltimore, Maryland

GUEST EDITOR

SHARON ELIZABETH MACE, MD, FACEP, FAAP
Professor of Medicine, Department of Emergency Medicine, Cleveland Clinic Lerner College of Medicine of Case Western Reserve; Faculty, MetroHealth Medical Center, Emergency Medicine Residency; Director, Pediatric Education/Quality Improvement; Director, Observation Unit; Emergency Services Institute, Cleveland Clinic, Cleveland, Ohio

AUTHORS

ONSY AYAD, MD
Associate Medical Director of Pediatric Intensive Care Unit; Director of Pediatric Extracorporeal Membrane Oxygenation, Nationwide Children's Hospital; Assistant Professor of Pediatrics, The Ohio State University College of Medicine, Columbus, Ohio

ANI AYDIN, MD
Senior Resident in Emergency Medicine, Department of Emergency Medicine, NYU School of Medicine, New York, New York

ISABEL BARATA, MD
Director of Pediatric Emergency Medicine, North Shore University Hospital, Manhasset; Assistant Professor of Pediatrics, New York University School of Medicine, New York, New York

DAVID BURBULYS, MD, FACEP
Associate Clinical Professor of Medicine, David Geffen School of Medicine at UCLA, Department of Emergency Medicine, Harbor–UCLA Medical Center, Torrance, California

JAMES M. CALLAHAN, MD
Associate Professor of Clinical Pediatrics, University of Pennsylvania School of Medicine; Director of Medical Education, Division of Emergency Medicine, The Children's Hospital of Philadelphia, Philadelphia, Pennsylvania

ANN DIETRICH, MD, FAAP, FACEP
Professor of Pediatrics, The Ohio State University College of Medicine; Director of Risk Management and Quality Assurance, Section of Pediatric Emergency Medicine, Nationwide Children's Hospital, Columbus, Ohio

MARIANNE GAUSCHE-HILL, MD, FACEP, FAAP
Department of Emergency Medicine, Director of EMS and Pediatric Emergency Medicine Fellowships, Harbor-UCLA Medical Center; Professor of Medicine, David Geffen School of Medicine at UCLA, Torrance, California

RAN GOLDMAN, MD
Division Head and Medical Director, Division of Pediatric Emergency Medicine, BC Children's Hospital; Associate Professor, Department of Pediatrics, University of British Columbia; Senior Associate Clinician Scientist, Child & Family Research Institute (CFRI), Vancouver, British Columbia, Canada

MARK A. HOSTETLER, MD, MPH
Associate Professor, Department of Pediatrics, The University of Chicago, Pritzker School of Medicine, Chicago, Illinois

ORLANDO R. HUNG, MD, FRCPC
Professor, Department of Anesthesiology, Dalhousie University; Professor, Department of Pharmacology, Dalhousie University; Professor, Department of Surgery, Dalhousie University; Medical Director of Research, Department of Anesthesiology, Dalhousie University; Attending Neuroanesthesiologist, Department of Anesthesia, Dalhousie University, Capital District Health Authority, Halifax, Nova Scotia, Canada

NAZEEMA KHAN, MD
Joe DiMaggio Children's Hospital, Hollywood, Florida

KIANUSCH KIAI, MD
Associate Clinical Professor of Medicine, David Geffen School of Medicine at UCLA, Department of Anesthesiology, Ronald Regan Medical Center, Los Angeles, California

BARUCH KRAUSS, MD, EdM
Associate Professor of Pediatrics, Division of Emergency Medicine, Department of Pediatrics, Children's Hospital Boston, Harvard Medical School, Boston, Massachusetts

J. ADAM LAW, MD, FRCPC
Professor, Department of Anesthesiology, Dalhousie University; Professor, Department of Surgery, Dalhousie University; Attending Neuroanesthesiologist, Department of Anesthesia, Dalhousie University, Queen Elizabeth II Health Science Centre, Halifax, Nova Scotia, Canada

SHARON ELIZABETH MACE, MD, FACEP, FAAP
Professor of Medicine, Department of Emergency Medicine, Cleveland Clinic Lerner College of Medicine of Case Western Reserve; Faculty, MetroHealth Medical Center, Emergency Medicine Residency; Director, Pediatric Education/Quality Improvement; Director, Observation Unit; Emergency Services Institute, Cleveland Clinic, Cleveland, Ohio

ALAN P. MARCO, MD, MMM
University of Toledo College of Medicine, Toledo, Ohio

CATHERINE A. MARCO, MD
University of Toledo College of Medicine, Toledo, Ohio

JANE M. McGARVEY, MD
Attending Physician, Department of Emergency Medicine, Pennsylvania Hospital, Philadelphia, Pennsylvania

LESLIE MIHALOV, MD
Associate Medical Director, Nationwide Children's Hospital; Associate Professor of Pediatrics, The Ohio State University College of Medicine; Section Chief, Section of Pediatric Emergency Medicine, Nationwide Children's Hospital, Columbus, Ohio

MICHAEL F. MURPHY, MD, FRCPC
Professor and Chair, Department of Anesthesiology, Dalhousie University; Professor, Department of Emergency Medicine, Dalhousie University; Clinical Chief, Department of Anesthesia, Dalhousie University, Capital District Health Authority, Halifax, Nova Scotia, Canada

JOSHUA NAGLER, MD
Assistant Professor of Pediatrics, Division of Emergency Medicine, Department of Pediatrics, Children's Hospital Boston, Harvard Medical School, Boston, Massachusetts

CHARLES V. POLLACK, MA, MD, FACEP, FAAEM, FAHA
Chairman, Department of Emergency Medicine, Pennsylvania Hospital; Professor of Emergency Medicine, University of Pennsylvania School of Medicine, Philadelphia, Pennsylvania

ALEX ROGOVIK, MD, PhD
Assistant Director, Pediatric Research in Emergency Therapeutics (PRETx) Program, Division of Pediatric Emergency Medicine, BC Children's Hospital, Vancouver, British Columbia, Canada

GENEVIEVE SANTILLANES, MD
Pediatric Emergency Medicine Fellow, Departments of Emergency Medicine and Pediatrics, Harbor-UCLA Medical Center, Torrance, California

ADAM J. SINGER, MD, FACEP
Professor and Vice Chairman for Research, Department of Emergency Medicine, SUNY Stony Brook School of Medicine, Stony Brook, New York

BREENA TAIRA, MD
Research Fellow in Emergency Medicine, Department of Emergency Medicine, SUNY Stony Brook School of Medicine, Stony Brook, New York

DAVID C. TURELL, MD, FAAP
Staff Physician, Pediatric Urgent Care, Department of General Pediatrics, Children's Hospital, Cleveland Clinic, Cleveland, Ohio

Contents

Monitoring of Patients with Airway/Respiratory Disease

> Although the recognition of hypoxemia is greatly enhanced through the proper and informed use of the pulse oximeter, the device can never be relied on to take the place of the clinician at the bedside who makes sure that the data provided matches the clinical picture with which he or she is presented.

> Capnography provides continuous, dynamic assessment of the ventilatory status of patients. Carbon dioxide physiology and the technology utilized in end-tidal carbon dioxide monitor devices are reviewed. Clinical applications with regard to ventilation and airway management are discussed, including: verification of endotracheal tube placement, continuous monitoring of tube position, monitoring during procedural sedation and in the obtunded patient, and assessment of patients with respiratory illnesses. Current guidelines for use of capnography within emergency medicine are included. Potential future applications are also presented.

> A great deal of research has been conducted on the utility and usefulness of exhaled nitric oxide (NO) as a biomarker of airway inflammation and its role in the diagnosis of acute asthma exacerbations. This article reviews the pathophysiology of NO in asthma, evidence for the use of exhaled NO in acute asthma exacerbations, and the potential utility of devices available to emergency physicians for measuring exhaled NO.

which the lungs are ventilated with a low inspiratory volume and pressure, has been accepted progressively in critical care for adult, pediatric, and neonatal patients requiring mechanical ventilation and is one of the central components of current protective ventilatory strategies.

ECMO is an important tool to provide oxygen delivery and carbon dioxide removal in addition to cardiac support for patients with intractable reversible respiratory or cardiovascular collapse unresponsive to conventional treatment. Even though ECMO can be a life-saving modality, it is expensive and labor-intensive and carries a significant complication risk. Early recognition and prompt referral of patients who may benefit from ECMO in addition to careful patient selection, continuous communication between ECMO centers and their referral base, and meticulous care can improve the outcome of these critically ill patients who previously had no chance of survival.

The Difficult Airway

Pediatric airway problems are seen commonly in pediatric and general emergency departments, management of the pediatric airway is often stressful to providers. This article reviews the pediatric airway, highlighting the anatomic and physiologic differences between infant, pediatric and adult airways, and how these differences impact assessment and management of the pediatric airway.

Management of the airway is the first priority in any patient. Dealing with a difficult airway can be a challenge, whether or not it involves facemask ventilation, an intermediate airway device, laryngoscopy and intubation, or a surgical airway. Various scales predict which patient is likely to have a difficult airway. The goal of rapid sequence intubation (RSI) is to eliminate or mitigate untoward reflex responses to intubation. Although controversy has arisen regarding the various steps in RSI, it remains an essential component of emergency medicine practice.

RELATED INTEREST

Sleep Medicine Clinics, Volume 1, Issue 4, Pages 443–554 (December 2006)
Sleep-Related Breathing Disorders and Positive Airway Pressure Therapy in Adults
Max Hirshkowitz and Amir Sharafkhaneh, *Guest Editors*

THE CLINICS ARE NOW AVAILABLE ONLINE!

Access your subscription at:
www.theclinics.com

GOAL STATEMENT

The goal of *Emergency Medicine Clinics of North America* is to keep practicing physicians up to date with current clinical practice in emergency medicine by providing timely articles reviewing the state of the art in patient care.

ACCREDITATION

The *Emergency Medical Clinics of North America* is planned and implemented in accordance with the Essential Areas and Policies of the Accreditation Council for Continuing Medical Education (ACCME) through the joint sponsorship of the University of Virginia School of Medicine and Elsevier. The University of Virginia School of Medicine is accredited by the ACCME to provide continuing medical education for physicians.

The University of Virginia School of Medicine designates this educational activity for a maximum of *15 AMA PRA Category 1 Credits.*™ Physicians should only claim credit commensurate with the extent of their participation in the activity.

The Emergency Medicine Clinics of North America CME program is approved by the American College of Emergency Physicians for 60 hours of ACEP Category I Credit per year.

The American Medical Association has determined that physicians not licensed in the US who participate in this CME activity are eligible for *15 AMA PRA Category 1 Credits*™.

Credit can be earned by reading the text material, taking the CME examination online at http://www.theclinics.com/home/cme, and completing the evaluation. After taking the test, you will be required to review any and all incorrect answers. Following completion of the test and evaluation, your credit will be awarded and you may print your certificate.

FACULTY DISCLOSURE/CONFLICT OF INTEREST

The University of Virginia School of Medicine, as an ACCME accredited provider, endorses and strives to comply with the Accreditation Council for Continuing Medical Education (ACCME) Standards of Commercial Support, Commonwealth of Virginia statutes, University of Virginia policies and procedures, and associated federal and private regulations and guidelines on the need for disclosure and monitoring of proprietary and financial interests that may affect the scientific integrity and balance of content delivered in continuing medical education activities under our auspices.

The University of Virginia School of Medicine requires that all CME activities accredited through this institution be developed independently and be scientifically rigorous, balanced and objective in the presentation/discussion of its content, theories and practices.

All authors/editors participating in an accredited CME activity are expected to disclose to the readers relevant financial relationships with commercial entities occurring within the past 12 months (such as grants or research support, employee, consultant, stock holder, member of speakers bureau, etc.). The University of Virginia School of Medicine will employ appropriate mechanisms to resolve potential conflicts of interest to maintain the standards of fair and balanced education to the reader. Questions about specific strategies can be directed to the Office of Continuing Medical Education, University of Virginia School of Medicine, Charlottesville, Virginia.

The faculty and staff of the University of Virginia Office of Continuing Medical Education have no financial affiliations to disclose.

The authors/editors listed below have identified no professional or financial affiliations for themselves or their spouse/partner:
Onsy Ayad, MD; Isabel Barata, MD; David Burbulys, MD, FACEP; James M. Callahan, MD; Ann Dietrich, MD, FAAP, FACEP; Marianne Gausche-Hill, MD, FACEP, FAAP; Mark A. Hostetler, MD, MPH; Orlando R. Hung, MD, FRCPC; Nazeema Khan, MD; Kianusch Kiai, MD; Baruch Krauss, MD, EdM; J. Adam Law, MD, FRCPC; Sharon Elizabeth Mace, MD, FACEP, FAAP (Guest Editor); Patrick Manley (Acquisitions Editor); Alan P. Marco, MD, MMM; Catherine A. Marco, MD; Amal Mattu, MD, FAAEM, FACEP (Consulting Editor); Jane M. McGarvey, MD; Leslie Mihalov, MD; Joshua Nagler, MD; Charles V. Pollack, MA, MD, FACEP, FAAEM, FAHA; Alex Rogovik, MD, PhD; Genevieve Santillanes, MD; Adam J. Singer; MD, FACEP; Breena Taira, MD; David C. Turell, MD, FAAP; and Bill Woods, MD (Test Author).

The authors/editors listed below have identified the following professional or financial affiliations for themselves of their spouse/partner:
Ani Aydin, MD is employed by Bellevue Medical Center.
Ran Goldman, MD is an industry funded research/investigator for Gebaver Company.
Michael F. Murphy, MD, FRCPC serves on the Speakers Bureau for Covidien.

Disclosure of Discussion of Non-FDA Approved Uses for Pharmaceutical Products and/or Medical Devices.

The University of Virginia School of Medicine, as an ACCME provider, requires that all faculty presenters identify and disclose any off-label uses for pharmaceutical and medical device products. The University of Virginia School of Medicine recommends that each physician fully review all the available data on new products or procedures prior to clinical use.

TO ENROLL

To enroll in the Emergency Medicine Clinics of North America Continuing Medical Education program, call customer service at 1-800-654-2452 or visit us online at www.theclinics.com/home/cme. The CME program is available to subscribers for an additional fee of $195.00.

Foreword

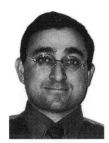

Amal Mattu, MD, FAAEM, FACEP
Consulting Editor

"The unofficial mantra of the specialty of emergency medicine is 'A-B-C: airway, breath sounds, circulation.'"[1] Though simplistic, this mantra emphasizes the appropriate priority for management of critically ill patients. From the very beginning in learning about emergency medicine, students and house officers learn that concerns about a patient's airway must precede all other issues. Loss of a patient's airway produces a more rapid transit to the morgue than any other condition. Consequently, proper training in management and protection of the airway is considered one of the most basic, yet critical, skills of any emergency physician. Virtually all emergency medicine training programs employ basic anesthesia rotations, skills labs utilizing fresh cadavers or simulation mannequins, advanced trauma airway rotations, and other assorted methods of airway training. Educational sessions in airway management are widely available for experienced emergency physicians as well—every year in the US and around the world, emergency medicine continuing medical education conferences offer numerous advanced lectures and training workshops in airway management. It would certainly be appropriate to amend the mantra of emergency medicine to A-A-A: airway, airway, airway! All other organ systems and concerns must usually take a backseat.

In this issue of *Emergency Medicine Clinics of North America*, Guest Editor Dr. Sharon Mace has assembled an outstanding group of physicians to provide an invaluable resource to update and advance our knowledge and skills in airway management. The articles are split into several sections, including methods of monitoring the airway, emerging therapies, and advanced intubation techniques. The authors address some of the basics in this issue, but the overall focus is on advanced modalities; consequently, there are multiple articles that focus on difficult and failed airways.

This issue represents an important contribution to education and clinical practice in emergency medicine. In itself, this issue constitutes a full reading curriculum for anyone that is beyond the *basics* of airway management and wants to advance to

Emerg Med Clin N Am 26 (2008) xv–xvi
doi:10.1016/j.emc.2008.10.003
0733-8627/08/$ – see front matter
emed.theclinics.com

a much higher level. This curriculum is certain to improve the care of our patients in the emergency department. Our thanks go to Dr. Mace and all of the authors in this outstanding issue.

Amal Mattu, MD, FAAEM, FACEP
Department of Emergency Medicine
University of Maryland School of Medicine
110 S. Paca Street, 6th Floor, Suite 100
Baltimore, MD 21201, USA

E-mail address:
amattu@smail.umaryland.edu (A. Mattu)

REFERENCE

1. Mattu A, Olshaker JS. Preface: Respiratory emergencies. Emerg Med Clin N Am 2003;21:xv–xvi.

Preface

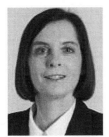

Sharon Elizabeth Mace, MD, FACEP, FAAP
Guest Editor

The assessment and treatment of every patient in emergency medicine begins with the "ABCs," or "Airway-Breathing-Circulation." This is true no matter what the patient's presenting complaint, age, or final diagnosis. The ABCs are the basis of all life support courses, whether Basic Life Support (BLS), Advanced Cardiac Life Support (ACLS), Pediatric Advanced Life Support (PALS), Neonatal Advanced Life Support (NALS), or Advanced Trauma Life Support (ATLS). This focus on the ABCs is often life-saving for our patients.

Of the ABCs, the first priority is to establish and maintain the airway. Our training programs, educational endeavors, and, more importantly, our clinical practice are all a reflection of this focus on and the importance of the airway. As the specialty of emergency medicine has progressed, our knowledge and skills have advanced far beyond basic airway management skills. Our physicians in-training are facile with the various devices and maneuvers that can aid the clinician in obtaining the definitive airway or intubation, and they are taught numerous advanced nonsurgical and surgical techniques for securing the airway.

The cornerstone of emergency medical care has been, is, and will continue to be management of the airway. This issue of *Emergency Medicine Clinics of North America* is a cutting-edge update of the current knowledge and advances in the assessment and management of the airway, as well as a discussion on the controversies surrounding the topic and a look at future trends. This issue is also intended to provide practical information and a useful approach with tips in airway assessment and management for the practicing emergency physician when confronted with a patient in respiratory distress/failure or in an arrest situation.

This issue begins with sections on pulse oximetry, capnography, and nitrous oxide that are designed to expand our knowledge regarding the monitoring of patients with respiratory disease, airway problems, or respiratory failure. Next, there is a review of emerging therapies: heliox, surfactant, ECMO, permissive hypercapnia, and noninvasive positive pressure ventilation that may affect our treatment of patients with airway and/or respiratory problems. There is discussion of the unique characteristics and, therefore, difficult airways of children and infants. This is followed by assessment of

Emerg Med Clin N Am 26 (2008) xvii–xviii
doi:10.1016/j.emc.2008.10.001
0733-8627/08/$ – see front matter **emed.theclinics.com**

the airway, with a focus on what constitutes a difficult or failed airway. When faced with the need to secure a definitive airway, especially a difficult airway, which maneuvers, retrograde intubation, devices, or drugs (eg, rapid sequence intubation or RSI) can assist us in successfully intubating a patient? Finally, should we encounter a situation with a failed airway, which measures can be used (eg, LMA or cricothyrotomy) to secure the airway, thereby, enabling oxygenation and ventilation of the patient?

Airway management is an integral part of emergency medicine practice, and emergency physicians are active in cutting-edge research related to the evaluation and treatment of patients with acute airway and/or respiratory problems. This issue of *Emergency Medicine Clinics of North America* has assembled current state-of-the-art knowledge on airway evaluation and treatment, enumerated controversies in airway management, and discussed future therapy. Emergency medicine physicians in any setting should find this issue valuable in their everyday practice.

I want to thank all of the authors, as well as Patrick Manley and the Elsevier staff and the Cleveland Clinic Center for Medical Art and Photography for their diligence in making this publication a reality. I also want to thank my family, friends, and colleagues for their love, support, and understanding that enabled this publication.

Sharon Elizabeth Mace, MD, FACEP, FAAP
Emergency Services Institute, E19
Cleveland Clinic
9500 Euclid Avenue
Cleveland, Ohio 44195

Cleveland Clinic Lerner College of Medicine of
Case Western Reserve, Cleveland, Ohio 44195

Observation Unit, Cleveland Clinic, 9500 Euclid
Avenue, Cleveland, Ohio 44195

Case Western Reserve University, Metro Health
Medical Center, 8500 Metro Health Drive
Cleveland, Ohio 44109

E-mail address:
maces@ccf.org (S.E. Mace)

Pulse Oximetry in Emergency Medicine

James M. Callahan, MD[a,b],*

KEYWORDS

• Pulse oximetry • Oxygenation • Hypoxia • Patient monitoring

In 1945, Comroe and Bothello[1] first reported on the inability of practitioners to recognize hypoxemia based on the presence of cyanosis until oxygen saturation reached dangerously low levels. Clinical cyanosis is not evident until there is at least 5 g/100 mL of desaturated hemoglobin. By this point, patients have arterial oxygen saturation rates around 80% or less depending on the concentration of hemoglobin in their blood. This is on the steepest part of the oxygen dissociation curve and puts the patient at risk of significant complications related to hypoxia. Since then, repeated attempts were made to develop methods and technologies to promote the early recognition of hypoxemia in patients.

In the early 1970s, significant progress was made in the development of reliable, relatively portable and affordable equipment, which made noninvasive monitoring of oxygen saturation possible in a variety of clinical settings. Pulse oximetry was quickly and widely accepted. A myriad of uses have been described in a wide variety of clinical settings. The value of pulse oximetry in patient care has been so great that pulse oximetry has been referred to as the "fifth vital sign"[2–4] and "...arguably the greatest advance in patient monitoring since electrocardiography."[5]

The emergency physician encounters pulse oximetry on a daily basis. It is imperative that the emergency physician has a firm understanding of the principles of how pulse oximetry works. Armed with this knowledge, the emergency physician is able to use this important technology appropriately, troubleshoot problems, and be aware of its limitations. This report reviews the history and principles underlying the development of pulse oximetry. Proper procedures for its application and use and indications for its use in emergency settings are discussed. Pitfalls and complications are highlighted and new advances reviewed. Pulse oximetry has become the fifth vital sign in many settings and many patient populations. The emergency physician must be ready to use this tool to its fullest potential.

[a] University of Pennsylvania School of Medicine, Philadelphia, PA, USA
[b] Division of Emergency Medicine, The Children's Hospital of Philadelphia, 34th Street and Civic Center Boulevard, Philadephia, PA, 19104, USA
* Division of Emergency Medicine, The Children's Hospital of Philadelphia, 34th Street and Civic Center Boulevard, Philadelphia, PA 19104
E-mail address: callahanj@email.chop.edu

Emerg Med Clin N Am 26 (2008) 869–879
doi:10.1016/j.emc.2008.08.006
0733-8627/08/$ – see front matter © 2008 Elsevier Inc. All rights reserved.

emed.theclinics.com

HISTORY AND PRINCIPLES

Attempts to develop noninvasive oximeters date back to the 1930s and 1940s when there was a special interest in being able to monitor oxygenation in pilots flying at high altitudes.[6] Early devices were not very portable, difficult to use, and did not accurately reflect arterial oxygen levels. Heating of tissues in which oximetry was to be measured contributed to improvements in accuracy of measurement when compared with actual blood oxygen saturation. In 1974, Aoyagi developed the first oximeters that used the pulsatile nature of blood flow in tissues to lead to a more accurate representation of arterial oxygen saturation levels.[7] This is the basis for the technology used in today's pulse oximeters.

Pulse oximeters use the principles of the Beer-Lambert Law, which states that the concentration of an absorbing substance in a solution is related to the intensity of light transmitted through that solution.[8] Pulse oximeters consist of two light-emitting diodes, one in the red range and one in the infrared range, and a detector. These are connected to a microprocessor that determines pulse oximetry (SpO_2) based on the relative amount of light transmitted through the tissue at these two wavelengths and an empirically derived algorithm of oxygen saturation levels based on the ratio of the transmitted light.

Oxygenated and deoxygenated hemoglobin absorb light at different wavelengths differently. Deoxygenated or "blue" blood absorbs light maximally in the red band, whereas oxygenated or "red" blood absorbs light maximally in the infrared band.[5,9,10] The pulse oximeter emits light at two wavelengths, 660 nm (red) and 940 nm (infrared). The emitter is placed so that it faces a detector through tissue that experiences the pulsatile flow of blood. The amount of light absorbed varies with each pulse, and the difference between the measurement of absorption at two points in the pulse wave will be caused by arterial blood alone.[5]

Approximately 600 individual measurements are made each second by rapidly switching the diodes on and off. The ratio of absorption of the two wavelengths of light are then compared with an algorithm in the microprocessor generated by empirically measuring the absorption in healthy volunteers at varying degrees of directly measured arterial oxygen saturation.[5,10] The display of the pulse oximeter usually includes values for the heart rate displayed as beats per minute as well as the oxygen saturation displayed as a percentage. The displayed value is usually an average based on the previous 3 to 6 seconds of recording.[5] Most models also show a plethysmographic representation of the arterial pulsation, which is useful in judging how accurately the device is detecting blood flow. This may be helpful in detecting problems in using the device.

Pulse oximeters need to be placed where the emitters and detectors face each other through approximately 5 to 10 mm of tissue that experiences pulsatile blood flow. The probes are most commonly placed on finger tips and ear lobes. Other sites where they may be applied include the bridge of the nose or nares, the cheek or tongue, and the toes in infants and small children. In neonates, especially low-birth-weight infants, they may be placed across the palms of the hand or soles of the feet.[11] It is important to be sure that the detector experiences minimal interference from ambient light and that the light from the emitter travels through tissue before reaching the detector. Failure to achieve these conditions can cause inaccurate pulse oximeter readings (see Pitfalls and Complications below).

APPLICATIONS IN EMERGENCY MEDICINE AND IMPACT ON CLINICAL CARE

Pulse oximetry is useful wherever hypoxemia could occur, and its detection would aid in the care of the patient. Pulse oximetry can also be helpful in monitoring the hemodynamic status of the patient. Multiple studies show its efficacy in detecting hypoxemia in a variety of patient populations and settings in emergency medicine. Other studies have shown a variety of other applications that provide other important information. In certain situations, regulatory and professional organizations mandate or strongly encourage its use.

Prehospital Care and use by Emergency Medical Services Personnel

Use of pulse oximetry in the prehospital setting has been prevalent for more than 20 years. Aughey and colleagues[12] showed that pulse oximetry performed in the field was accurate in the measurement of oxygen saturation when compared with co-oximetry measurement of saturation in arterial blood gas samples. Their sample showed outstanding correlation when the SpO_2 was $\geq 88\%$. They also showed excellent correlation between heart rates measured by pulse oximeter and electrocardiogram in a prehospital setting. Bota and Rowe showed that the sensitivity of physical examination by ambulance attendants for the recognition of hypoxemia in adult patients with serious complaints (many with chest pain or shortness of breath) was only 28%.[13] Even when oxygen was delivered, many patients remained hypoxemic. Pulse oximetry use in the prehospital setting has the potential to increase the recognition of hypoxemia and guide oxygen therapy.

However, Cydulka and colleagues[14] showed that paramedics were more likely than emergency medical technicians to use the pulse oximeter to guide the institution of oxygen therapy in hypoxic patients but that neither group used pulse oximetry to appropriately modify oxygen therapy in patients with SpO_2 $\geq 97\%$. Although pulse oximetry appears accurate in the prehospital setting, prehospital personnel should receive adequate instruction in the use of pulse oximetry, and modification of oxygen therapy could be better guided with its use.

During prehospital rapid sequence intubation (RSI), patients frequently experience desaturation.[15,16] Many times this, as well as bradycardia, is unrecognized by the personnel performing the intubation.[15] Use of pulse oximetry and attention to it in the development of preoxygenation strategies may be an important step in the development of prehospital RSI programs. The same group showed that the SpO_2 before intubation attempt was predictive of which patients would desaturate. In prehospital programs that use RSI, pulse oximetry and attention to it seem to be prerequisites for safety.

Use in Patient Triage

The use of pulse oximetry as a fifth vital sign in triage has been shown to significantly impact the care provided to a wide variety of patients. Recognition of hypoxemia is improved, patient care is more efficient, and appropriate care is instituted more rapidly when pulse oximetry is used in triage. The noninvasive nature of pulse oximetry allows for rapid, painless, and accurate evaluation of large numbers of patients.

In pediatric patients presenting to an emergency department (ED), clinical assessment had a sensitivity of only 33% and a negative predictive value of only 85% in determining hypoxia in pediatric patients.[17] In this same study, patient management was changed 91% of the time when the SpO_2 was known. Mower and colleagues[3] also showed that the use of pulse oximetry as a fifth vital sign in triage led to important changes in management in a small but significant number of patients, including changes in patient disposition. In pediatric patients with bronchiolitis, use of pulse oximetry in triage has been shown to decrease emergency department length of stay.[18] This study also showed that the presence of respiratory distress for predicting hypoxia had a sensitivity of only 74%.

The use of pulse oximetry as a fifth vital sign has also been shown to be useful in adult patients in triage. In adult patients, use of triage pulse oximetry was shown to lead to changes in triage classification in a small but significant number of patients[19] while another group showed that providing the triage SpO_2 to treating physicians led to significant changes (including changes in patient disposition) in the medical treatment of these adult patients.[20] The same group showed that similar changes, including changes in disposition, were found when pulse oximetry in triage was included in the care of geriatric patients presenting to emergency departments.[4] In all patients presenting to the emergency department with respiratory complaints or findings, it is clear that pulse oximetry should be used in their triage assessment.

Care of Critically Ill Patients in the Emergency Department

Continuous pulse oximetry is the standard of care in monitoring of patients in the ICU.[9] Care of critically ill patients in the ED is also aided by the use of continuous monitoring of the patient's SpO_2. Intubated patients and patients receiving mechanical ventilation require continuous pulse oximetry regardless of their location in the hospital. In the ED, as in other patient care settings, an abnormal SpO_2 is a sensitive and reliable sign of complications in these patients. In adult patients with respiratory distress, continuous pulse oximetry in the ED detected multiple episodes of clinically unrecognized hypoxemia as well as episodes of hypoxemia during several procedures including tracheal intubation, suctioning, and other treatments.[21]

Continuous pulse oximetry during ED intubation has been shown to decrease the frequency and duration of hypoxemia during emergency intubation attempts.[22] Pulse oximetry has also been shown to decrease use of arterial blood gas (ABG) testing in the ED in one study[23] and especially "unjustified ABG measurements" in another study.[24] This means that the use of an inexpensive, noninvasive, instantaneous and essentially painless technology has the ability to decrease ED charges, patient discomfort, and time to availability of essential clinical information.

Oximetry may be less prone to error and more accurate in the assessment of oxygenation in patients with cardiopulmonary disease when compared with ABG measurement.[5] ABG measurement requires correct technique. Practitioners who only rarely perform this procedure may not practice sufficient attention to detail to minimize error. In addition, the pain associated with the procedure may lead to a change in the patient's respiratory pattern and an increase in respiratory effort producing improved oxygenation, which is only transient. Clinicians may be misled by the results they obtain in this way.

Pulse oximetry has also been used to monitor adequacy of interventions during cardiopulmonary resuscitation. High-quality chest compressions often produce excellent pulse oximetry tracings in patients with a lack of spontaneous circulation. In a critical appraisal of use in this setting, the pulse oximeter proved beneficial in the management of primary respiratory arrest but less useful during external chest compressions. However, the availability of a pulse oximeter significantly altered the management in seven of 20 patients. Five of these 7 patients survived.[25]

Pulse Oximeters in Emergency Department Patient Assessment

Pulse oximeters that display pulsatile wave forms can be used to measure systolic blood pressure. Either the reappearance of the waveform with slow cuff deflation or the disappearance of the wave form with cuff inflation may be used. An average of these two measurements has been shown to have good agreement with blood pressures obtained by auscultation or blood pressures obtained by noninvasive measurement devices.[9]

Pulse oximetry wave forms have also been shown to be useful in the detection of pericardial effusions in children[26] and in assessing the degree of airways obstruction in patients with asthma[27,28] through the recognition of a pulsus paradoxus in the oximeter wave form. Frey and Butt showed in an ICU setting that pulse oximetry accurately reflected the pulsus paradoxus documented by invasive monitoring of patients.[29] Further development of the monitoring of pulsus paradoxus in this way may lead to improvements in the assessment and treatment of patients with asthma who present to the ED.[30,31]

Pulse oximetry has been shown to be predictive of the presence of pneumonia in elderly patients.[32] An SpO_2 less than 94% had a sensitivity of 80% and a specificity of 91% for the presence of pneumonia with a positive predictive value of 95%. Even more impressive was if there was a decrease of greater than 3% from the baseline value of the patient's SpO_2 there was a positive predictive value for the presence of pneumonia of 100%. Pulse oximetry has also been shown in children to be predictive of treatment failure in pediatric patients with severe pneumonia.[33]

Pulse oximetry has also been shown to be predictive of respiratory failure in patients with severe exacerbations of asthma. In children, SpO_2 levels of less than 90% to 92% are predictive of severe exacerbations and need for hospitalization and other additional therapies.[34,35] In adults, respiratory failure was rare in patients presenting with SpO_2 greater than 92%.[36] Above this level, the need for arterial blood gas monitoring could be safely avoided.

Sedation and Analgesia in the Emergency Department

Pulse oximetry is routine and mandatory in the monitoring of patients undergoing procedural sedation and analgesia in the ED. The American Academy of Pediatrics, American College of Emergency Physicians, American Society of Anesthesiologists, American Medical Association, and Joint Commission on the Accreditation of Healthcare Organizations all call for continuous pulse oximetry in patients receiving procedural sedation and analgesia in the ED or other settings.[37–42] Although the most important "monitor" for these patients is someone whose only role is to monitor and record the patient's vital signs, level of alertness, and respiratory effort, the pulse oximeter remains a vital piece of equipment that should be in place and watched carefully. Recognition of hypoxemia based on cyanosis is no better here than in any other setting. Most adverse events in this setting are related to a failure to adequately monitor and then rescue patients who have received these interventions.[43]

LIMITATIONS AND COMPLICATIONS

Pulse oximetry is an amazing technology that is invaluable in the everyday practice of emergency medicine. However, as with any technology, it is only as good as the practitioner who is using it. The emergency physician must be aware of the limitations of this technology and the complications associated with it. Unfortunately, many physicians have limited understanding of pulse oximetry.[9] One study found that less than 50% of physicians were aware that motion, arrhythmias, and things like nail polish could affect pulse oximetry readings.[44] Ultimately, the clinician must look at the patient, and if the pulse oximeter (or any other monitor) does not seem to be behaving in a way that is consistent with the clinical picture that is presented, the clinician must determine the cause of the discrepancy and act in a way that is in the best interest of the patient.

It is important to remember that pulse oximetry only reflects the state of oxygenation of the patient. It does not provide any information regarding the patient's ventilation, carbon dioxide level, or acid–base status. Especially when patients are receiving supplemental oxygen, they may have normal SpO_2 levels but be in respiratory failure with hypercapnia and respiratory acidosis. If information about ventilation is needed, capnography or blood gas measurements are needed. Likewise, if the acid–base status of the patient is in question, blood gas testing should be performed.

Pulse oximetry may be affected by physical factors, physiologic factors, and interference from substances that affect the transmission or absorption of light in the path of the oximeter's diode.

Physical Factors Affecting Pulse Oximetry

The pulse oximeter will only function if the transmitted light is detected by the detector, and there is an adequate change in the amount of light transmitted (because of the arterial pulsation in the tissue of that area of the body). Anything that interferes with this relationship will make the device susceptible to malfunction. If there is an inadequate pulse caused by decreased perfusion secondary to hypotension, hypothermia, or vasoconstriction, a satisfactory signal will not be detected, and no reading or a potentially inaccurate reading will be obtained.[5,7,9] Usually the pulse oximeter will display oxygen saturations that are falsely low in this setting. More worrisome is that poor perfusion will lead to a lack of a reading, and hypoxemia will go unrecognized until perfusion is improved or another means of determining the oxygenation status of the patient is used. Adult systolic blood pressures of less than 80 mm Hg have been associated with poor pulse oximetry performance.[7] The SpO_2 level displayed should only be assumed to be accurate when there is a high-quality plethysmographic tracing displayed on the monitor. Ideally, the display will show a pulse wave with a demonstrable dicrotic notch.

Patient movement can make it difficult for the detector to adequately "sense" light that is transmitted. Motion artifact is usually caused by motion of the probe relative to the patient's skin.[5] Sometimes, taping the pulse oximeter cable to the back of the extremity to which it is attached will minimize the amount of motion artifact. Having the patient rest their hand on a flat surface may also help.[5]

Ambient light may also interfere with pulse oximeters. Excessive exposure of the detector to ambient light may lead to inaccurate readings. In most cases of ambient light overexposure the SpO_2 level will tend toward 85% (the reading dictated by the algorithm in the microprocessor when the ratio of the absorbance of the two wavelengths of light is one) and therefore will be falsely low.[10] However, there have also been reports of falsely high readings when probes are exposed to high levels of ambient light, or probe displacement is not recognized and the probe is completely exposed to ambient light.[45,46] Making sure that the light from the diode is only sensed by the detector after it has passed through the tissue and that the detector is protected from ambient light is important. If light from the diode reaches the detector without passing through the tissues as is the case when probes are malpositioned or oversized, a *penumbra effect* may occur leading to a calculated saturation in the low 80s.[47] This will usually lead to an underestimation of the patient's SpO_2 level unless the patient is already hypoxemic.[11]

Physiologic Factors Affecting Pulse Oximetry

The major physiologic factor affecting pulse oximetry is the oxygen–hemoglobin dissociation curve. SpO_2 is an estimation of arterial oxygen saturation of hemoglobin (SaO_2), which is related to the partial pressure of oxygen in arterial blood (PaO_2). Because the oxygen–hemoglobin dissociation curve is sigmoidal in shape, at high PaO_2, or on the "flat part of the curve," large changes in PaO_2 level will lead to only minor changes in SpO_2 level. This is the major reason pulse oximetry is not the ideal technology for monitoring patients in whom hyperoxia is a major concern.

At lower levels of PaO_2, relatively small decreases in oxygen tension can lead to rapid decreases in oxygen saturation. It is therefore important to realize that a PaO_2 of 75 mm Hg usually is associated with an SpO_2 level of about 90%. However, an SpO_2 level of 80% usually is associated with a PaO_2 level of less than 50%. It is important to have a sense of the relationships between oxygen tension and saturation.

Substances that Interfere with Pulse Oximetry

Skin pigmentation is one factor that may affect the accuracy of pulse oximetry. In critically ill patients, readings that were more than 4% different from actual measured SaO_2 were found in 27% of black patients compared with only 11% of white patients.[9] Intravenous dyes such as methylene blue, indocyanine green, and indigo carmine can cause falsely low SpO_2 readings for up to 20 minutes after administration.[9]

Older pulse oximeters were prone to interference from nail polish.[7] However, newer work showed that even the nail polish colors that most affected the accuracy of the readings (black, purple, and dark blue) did not affect accuracy enough to be clinically significant.[48] The investigators also showed that rotation of the sensor probe by 90° did not completely eliminate the error in measurement. Despite these findings, the investigators state that removing nail polish might be helpful in some cases.

Abnormal Hemoglobins

Patients with abnormal hemoglobins are at risk of having inaccurate pulse oximetry results. Fetal hemoglobin does not seem to affect pulse oximetry.[7] Patients with sickle hemoglobin usually have readings similar to those with normal hemoglobin.[7] However, there have been reports of both falsely low and falsely high readings in patients with sickle cell disease.[7,49,50] These patients are at significant risk for pulmonary complications that are life threatening in addition to sepsis. In this population, oximetry data are extremely useful. In practice, it is very useful to keep a file of patients with sickle cell disease who use an ED and be sure part of the file is a baseline SpO_2 value obtained at a time when they are relatively well. Past medical records may be able to provide this information, and many patients with sickle cell disease or their families may be aware of this value. Significant deviations from their baseline SpO_2 level must be treated aggressively in terms of finding the etiology and in providing supplemental oxygen to decrease further complications.

Carboxyhemoglobin

Standard pulse oximeters that use only two wavelengths of light are prone to significant errors when abnormal hemoglobins are present. The most common causes of these types of errors are elevated levels of carboxyhemoglobin (COHb) and methemoglobin. COHb absorbs light in the red wavelength (eg, 660 nm) almost identically to oxyhemoglobin. Therefore, it is understandable how the standard pulse oximeter will interpret carboxyhemoglobin as oxyhemoglobin. This leads to a falsely elevated absorption ratio (red or oxygenated versus infrared or deoxygenated) that is sensed by the oximeter. Therefore, the reported SpO_2 level is an overestimation of the true SaO_2. This has been shown in several clinical studies, and, in fact, the pulse oximeter tends to overestimate the SaO_2 by the amount of COHb present except at extremely high levels of COHb.[51–53] In patients with suspected, known, or possible CO poisoning, it is important to directly measure CO levels as well as oxyhemoglobin levels by co-oximetry in addition to ABGs.[53] A new eight-wavelength pulse oximeter has been introduced that seems to accurately measure COHb and methemoglobin levels.[54]

Methemoglobin

Methemoglobin (MeHb) absorbs light equally well at both wavelengths used in standard pulse oximeters (660 nm and 940 nm). In the presence of MeHb, SpO_2, although somewhat reduced initially, overestimates actual SaO_2.[55,56] As the level of MeHb increases to 30% to 35%, the ratio of absorbance at the two wavelengths reaches a plateau and approximates one. At this ratio, the algorithm in the microprocessor gives a calculated SpO_2 value of 85%, and most pulse oximeters plateau at SpO_2 levels of 82% to 85%.[55,56] In light of MeHb levels by this time of 30% to 35%, this is a marked overestimation of actual SaO_2. Pulse oximetry must be interpreted with extreme caution in patients with known or suspected methemoglobinemia. The newer eight-wavelength oximeter seems to measure MeHb accurately as well and may represent a real advance in oximetry technology.[54]

Complications

Most complications related to pulse oximetry use are caused by a lack of understanding of the technology on the part of the clinician using the device. Recognition that the pulse oximeter only gives you information about oxygenation and not ventilation or acid–base status is often lacking or not thought about. A normal SpO_2 level provides a clinician with a false sense of security. Failure to consider the possibility of a dyshemoglobinemia may allow a patient with a seemingly acceptable SpO_2 level to actually remain hypoxic for a prolonged period of time. However, there have been actual complications related to pulse oximeters reported as well.

Digital injury has been reported when continuous pulse oximetry is used for prolonged periods especially in the setting of hypoperfusion or the use of vasopressor medications.[57] There have also been multiple reports of burns to digits and other body parts when non–magnetic resonance imaging (MRI) compatible pulse oximeter probes have been used in patients undergoing MRI scanning.[58,59] Ferrous portions of the probes become extremely hot in the setting of the scanner's electromagnetic field causing severe thermal injury.

NEW TECHNOLOGY

Newer pulse oximeters are more successful at dealing with several of the limitations that have plagued these devices since they first enjoyed widespread use 25 years ago. Motion causes fewer disturbances in pulse oximeter readings in newer models because of improved algorithms;[11] units have become smaller, lighter, and less expensive; and the development and clinical use of devices that measure COHb and MeHb will make oximetry even more useful in the ED setting.[11,54]

The development of reflectance oximeters, which do not rely on transmitted light but on reflected light, is underway. These are not yet reliable enough for clinical use but once perfected may address several other shortcomings of current oximeters. Other technologies are being developed that may be useful in assessing tissue oxygenation and brain oxygenation and perfusion.[11]

SUMMARY

Since first introduced into widespread clinical use 25 to 30 years ago, pulse oximeters have become so commonplace in clinical medicine that they are seen as providing an all-important "fifth vital sign." The pulse oximeter is a noninvasive, safe, essentially painless, and relatively inexpensive device that provides valuable and usually reliable clinical information rapidly. The value of oximetry is recognized by professional and regulatory organizations. It should be available in all settings in which emergency physicians care for patients and used frequently.

However, as with any technology, the device is only as good as the clinician who is using it. The emergency physician must have an understanding of the principles underlying the technology to understand its limitations and potential complications. Although the recognition of hypoxemia is greatly enhanced through the proper and informed use of the pulse oximeter, the device can never be relied on to take the place of the clinician at the bedside who makes sure that the data provided matches the clinical picture with which he or she is presented.

REFERENCES

1. Comroe JH Jr, Bothello S. The unreliability of cyanosis in the recognition of arterial anoxemia. Am J Med Sci 1947;214:1–6.
2. Neff TA. Routine oximetry: a fifth vital sign? Chest 1988;94:227.
3. Mower WR, Sachs C, Nicklin EL, et al. Pulse oximetry as a fifth pediatric vital sign. Pediatrics 1997;99:681–6.
4. Mower WR, Myers G, Nicklin EL, et al. Pulse oximetry as a fifth vital sign in emergency geriatric assessment. Acad Emerg Med 1998;5:858–65.
5. Hanning CD, Alexander-Williams JM. Fortnightly review: pulse oximetry: a practical review. BMJ 1995;311:367–70.
6. Severinghaus JW, Astrup PB. History of blood gas analysis. VI. Oximetry. J Clin Monit Comput 1986;2:270–88.
7. Mechem CC. Pulse oximetry. Up To Date 2007: Available at: http://www.uptodateon line.com/online/content/topic.do?topicKey=cc_medi/16589. Accessed April 11, 2008.
8. Sinex JE. Pulse oximetry: principles and limitations. Am J Emerg Med 1999;17: 59–67.
9. Jubran A. Pulse oximetry. Intensive Care Med 2004;30:2017–20.
10. Poets CF, Southall DP. Noninvasive monitoring of oxygenation in infants and children: practical considerations and areas of concern. Pediatrics 1994;93:737–46.
11. Marr J, Abramo TJ. Monitoring in critically ill children. In: Baren JM, Rothrock SG, Brennan JA, Brown L, editors. Pediatric emergency medicine. Philadelphia: Saunders Elsevier; 2008. p. 50–2.
12. Aughey K, Hess D, Eitel D, et al. An evaluation of pulse oximetry in prehospital care. Ann Emerg Med 1991;20:887–91.
13. Bota GW, Rowe BH. Continuous monitoring of oxygen saturation in prehospital patients with severe illness: the problem of unrecognized hypoxemia. J Emerg Med 1995;13:305–11.
14. Cydulka RK, Shade B, Emerman CL, et al. Prehospital pulse oximetry: useful or misused? Ann Emerg Med 1992;21:675–9.
15. Dunford JV, Davis DP, Ochs M, et al. Incidence of transient hypoxia and pulse rate reactivity during paramedic rapid sequence intubation. Ann Emerg Med 2003;42:721–8.
16. Davis DP, Hwang JQ, Dunford JV. Rate of decline in oxygen saturation at various pulse oximetry values with prehospital rapid sequence intubation. Prehosp Emerg Care 2008;12:46–51.

17. Manneker AJ, Petrack EM, Krug SE. Contribution of routine pulse oximetry to evaluation and management of patients with respiratory illness in a pediatric emergency department. Ann Emerg Med 1995;25:36–40.
18. Choi J, Claudius I. Decrease in emergency department length of stay as a result of triage pulse oximetry. Pediatr Emerg Care 2006;22:412–4.
19. Summers RL, Anders RM, Woodward LH, et al. Effect of routine pulse oximetry measurements on ED triage classification. Am J Emerg Med 1998;16:5–7.
20. Mower WR, Sachs C, Nicklin EL, et al. Effect of routine emergency department triage pulse oximetry screening on medical management. Chest 1995;108:1297–302.
21. Jones J, Heiselman D, Cannon L, et al. Continuous emergency department monitoring of arterial saturation in adult patients with respiratory distress. Ann Emerg Med 1988;17:463–8.
22. Mateer JR, Olson DW, Stueven HA, et al. Continuous pulse oximetry during emergency endotracheal intubation. Ann Emerg Med 1993;22:675–9.
23. Kellerman AL, Cofer CA, Joseph S, et al. Impact of portable pulse oximetry on arterial blood gas test ordering in an urban emergency department. Ann Emerg Med 1991;20:130–4.
24. Le Bourdelle's G, Estangnasie' P, Lenoir F, et al. Use of a pulse oximeter in an adult emergency department: impact on the number of arterial blood gas analyses ordered. Chest 1998;113:1042–7.
25. Spittal MJ. Evaluation of pulse oximetry during cardiopulmonary resuscitation. Anaesthesia 1993;48:701–3.
26. Tamburro RF, Ring JC, Womback K. Detection of pulsus paradoxus associated with large pericardial effusions in pediatric patients by analysis of the pulse-oximetry wave form. Pediatrics 2002;109:673–7.
27. Ryan CA. Detection of pulsus paradoxus by pulse oximetry [letter]. Am J Dis Child 1988;142:481–2.
28. Chadwick V, Peace S, Taylor B, et al. Continuous non-invasive assessment of pulsus paradoxus [letter]. Lancet 1992;339:495–6.
29. Frey B, Butt W. Pulse oximetry for assessment of pulsus paradoxus: a clinical study in children. Intensive Care Med 1998;24:242–6.
30. Rayner J, Trespalacios F, Machan J, et al. Continuous noninvasive measurement of pulsus paradoxus complements medical decision making in assessment of acute asthma severity. Chest 2006;130:754–65.
31. Arnold DA, Spiro DM, Desmond RA, et al. Estimation of airway obstruction using oximeter plethysmograph waveform data. Respir Res 2005;6:65. Available at: http://respiratory-research.com/content/6/1/65. Accessed June 9, 2008.
32. Kaye KS, Stalam M, Shershen WE, et al. Utility of pulse oximetry in diagnosing pneumonia in nursing home residents. Am J Med Sci 2002;324:237–42.
33. Fu LY, Ruthazer R, Wilson I, et al. Brief hospitalization and pulse oximetry for predicting amoxicillin treatment failure in children with severe pneumonia. Pediatrics 2006;118:e1822–30.
34. Boychuk R, Yamamoto L, DeMesa C, et al. Correlation of initial emergency department pulse oximetry values in asthma severity classes (steps) with the risk of hospitalization. Am J Emerg Med 2006;24:48–52.
35. Sole' D, Komatsu MK, Carvalho KVT, et al. Pulse oximetry in the evaluation of the severity of acute asthma and/or wheezing in children. J Asthma 1999;36:327–33.
36. Carruthers DM, Harrison BDW. Arterial blood gas analysis or oxygen saturation in the assessment of acute asthma. Thorax 1995;50:186–8.
37. Cote CJ, Wilson S, the Workgroup on Sedation, American Academy of Pediatrics and American Academy of Pediatric Dentistry. Guidelines for monitoring and

management of pediatric patients during and after sedation for diagnostic and therapeutic procedures: an update. Pediatrics 2006;118:2587–602.

38. Sacchetti A, Scharermeyer R, Gerardi M, et al. Pediatric sedation and analgesia. Ann Emerg Med 1994;23:237–50.
39. Godwin S, Caro D, Wolf S, et al. Clinical policy: procedural sedation and analgesia in the emergency department. Ann Emerg Med 2005;45:177–96.
40. Gross JB, Bailey PL, Connis RT, et al. Practice guidelines for sedation and analgesia by non-anesthesiologists. An updated report by the American society of anesthesiologists task force on sedation and analgesia by non – anesthesiologists. Anesthesiology 2002;96:1004–17.
41. Council on Scientific Affairs, American Medical Association. The use of pulse oximetry during conscious sedation. JAMA 1993;270:1463–8.
42. Commission on Accreditation of Healthcare Organizations. Accreditation Manual for Hospitals. St. Louis (MO): Mosby-Year Book, Inc.; 1993.
43. Cote CJ, Karl HW, Notterman DA, et al. Adverse sedation events in pediatrics: a critical incident analysis of contributory factors. Pediatrics 2000;105:805–14.
44. Howell M. Pulse oximetry: an audit of nursing and medical staff understanding. Br J Nurs 2002;11:191–7.
45. Costarino AT, Davis DA, Keon TP. Falsely normal saturation reading with the pulse oximeter. Anesthesiology 1987;67:830–1.
46. Poets CF, Seidenberg J, von der Hardt H. Failure of a pulse oximeter to detect sensor displacement. Lancet 1993;341:244.
47. Kelleher JF, Ruff RH. The penumbra effect: vasomotion–dependent pulse oximeter artifact due to probe malposition. Anesthesiology 1989;71:787–91.
48. Hinkelbein J, Genzwuerker H, Sogl R, et al. Effect of nail polish on oxygen saturation determined by pulse oximetry in critically ill patients. Resuscitation 2006; 72:82–91.
49. Lindberg LG, Lennmarken C, Vegors M. Pulse oximetry–clinical implications and recent technical developments. Acta Anaesthesiol Scand 1995;39:279–87.
50. Ortiz FO, Aldrich TK, Nagel RL, et al. Accuracy of pulse oximetry in sickle cell disease. Am J Respir Crit Care Med 1999;159:447–51.
51. Buckley RG, Aks SE, Esbom JL, et al. The pulse oximetry gap in carbon monoxide intoxication. Ann Emerg Med 1994;24:252–5.
52. Bozerman WP, Myers RAM, Barish RA. Confirmation of the pulse oximetry gap in carbon monoxide poisoning. Ann Emerg Med 1997;30:608–11.
53. Hampson NB. Pulse oximetry in severe carbon monoxide poisoning. Chest 1998; 114:1036–41.
54. Barker SJ, Curry J, Redford D, et al. Measurement of carboxyhemoglobin and methemoglobin by pulse oximetry: a human volunteer study. Anesthesiology 2006;105:892–7.
55. Barker SJ, Tremper KK, Hyatt J. Effects of methemoglobin on pulse oximetry and mixed venous oximetry. Anesthesiology 1989;70:112–7.
56. Wright RO, Lewander WJ, Woolf AD. Methemoglobinemia: etiology, pharmacology and clinical management. Ann Emerg Med 1999;34:646–56.
57. Wille J, Braams R, van Haren WH, et al. Pulse oximeter–induced digital injury: frequency rate and possible causative factors. Crit Care Med 2000;28:3555–7.
58. Shellock FG, Slimp GL. Severe burn of the finger caused by using a pulse oximeter during MR imaging. AJR Am J Roentgenol 1989;153:1105.
59. Dempsey MF, Condon B. Thermal injuries associated with MRI. Clin Radiol 2001; 56:457–65.

Capnography: A Valuable Tool for Airway Management

Joshua Nagler, MD*, Baruch Krauss, MD, EdM

KEYWORDS

- Capnography • End-tidal carbon dioxide • Ventilation
- Airway Management • Intubation

Capnography is the noninvasive measurement of the partial pressure of carbon dioxide (CO_2) from the airway during inspiration and expiration. Although capnography provides physiologic information on ventilation, perfusion, and metabolism, this article focuses on its utility as a real-time measure of ventilatory status, as this relates to airway management.

Although it only recently has become integrated into the practice of emergency medicine, principles essential to the development of capnography began to emerge more than 75 years ago. Initial physiologic studies demonstrating CO_2 waveforms as a means to measure airway dead space date as far back as 1928.[1] It was not until 1975, however, that the first collection of clinically obtained waveforms was published.[2] This work, coupled with concomitant technological advances including the introduction of mass spectroscopy, allowed for commercialization and more widespread use of modern capnography.

Since that time, capnography has become widely used in clinical medicine, initially within the practice of anesthesia.[3] Indications specific to emergency medicine first were published in 1985, and subsequent reviews in the literature described additional potential applications.[4–6] Growing supporting evidence has led to increased use of capnography within emergency departments (EDs), and position papers and guidelines from numerous professional societies now recommend or mandate its use.[7–9]

This article begins with a review of the terminology and technology of CO_2 monitoring, and a discussion of the relevant physiology and interpretation of the CO_2 waveform. The remainder of the article focuses on clinical indications for capnography related to ventilation and airway management, including use in intubated and nonintubated patients.

Division of Emergency Medicine, Department of Pediatrics, Children's Hospital Boston, Harvard Medical School, 300 Longwood Avenue, Boston, MA 02115, USA
* Corresponding author.
E-mail address: joshua.nagler@childrens.harvard.edu (J. Nagler).

Emerg Med Clin N Am 26 (2008) 881–897
doi:10.1016/j.emc.2008.08.005
0733-8627/08/$ – see front matter © 2008 Elsevier Inc. All rights reserved.

TERMINOLOGY

The maximum partial pressure of CO_2 obtained at the end of an exhaled breath is referred to as end–tidal CO_2 (EtCO$_2$). A capnometer reports the result as a numeric value. A capnograph adds a graphic display of a waveform representing expired CO_2 as a function of either volume or time, the latter being used most commonly in emergency medicine and emergency medical services (EMS). Such a waveform is referred to as the capnogram (**Fig. 1**). Capnography provides two distinct advantages over using numeric values alone. First, demonstration of a recognizable waveform provides validity for the measured EtCO$_2$ value, much as an appropriate tracing on a pulse oximeter assures providers that recorded oxygen saturation is real. Second, evaluation of the waveform can provide important information about underlying physiologic conditions and disease processes.[2,10,11]

TECHNOLOGY

The initial technology that brought capnography into widespread clinical use was mass spectrometry. Because of cost and complexity, however, this has not been used outside of the operating room. The more recent introduction of infrared spectroscopy has allowed for the development of capnographs, which are used in the ED and EMS settings.[12] Capnography based on infrared spectroscopy works on a similar principle as pulse oximetry. A beam of filtered infrared radiation is sent from a light source through a sample (exhaled air in the case of capnography) to a photodetector. Because CO_2 absorbs light at a very specific wavelength (4.26 µm), the amount of radiation that is absorbed can be measured, and the concentration of CO_2 in the sample is calculated. Capnographs using infrared technology may be hand-held, battery-powered, rugged units that work well in the prehospital and ED setting, or may be part of complete continuous bedside monitoring systems.

Capnographs can be differentiated further as mainstream or sidestream configurations, depending on the location of the photodetector or sensor. Mainstream units, also described as in-line, are designed for intubated patients and place the sensor directly on the hub of the endotracheal tube. Sidestream units continuously aspirate gas through microtubing to a sensor that is remote from the patient's airway within the monitor. These units can be used on intubated and nonintubated patients.

Although numeric values, trends, and waveforms provide valuable clinical information, the most commonly used CO_2 monitors in EDs are qualitative rather than

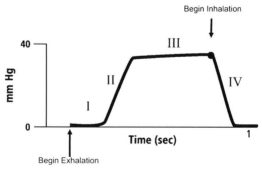

Fig. 1. The normal capnogram. (*From* Krauss B, Hess DR. Capnography for procedural sedation and analgesia in the emergency department. Ann Emerg Med 2007;50(2):174; with permission.)

quantitative.[13,14] Colorimetric end–tidal detectors, available for use in children and adults, contain indicator discs coated with material that reversibly reacts with CO_2 to produce hydrogen ions. The resultant change in pH causes the disc to change color, most commonly from purple to yellow, indicating a CO_2 concentration greater than 2%.[12] These single-use devices most frequently are used following intubation for the purpose of verifying endotracheal rather than esophageal tube placement, as will be discussed. They are designed to function for several hours following the initiation of their use, although color change may decrease over time. In addition, they can become occluded from secretions within closed airway circuits. Therefore, it is important that changing findings be interpreted carefully within clinical context.

CARBON DIOXIDE PHYSIOLOGY

Reviewing the production, transport, and elimination of carbon dioxide provides a framework for interpreting capnographic results, as alterations in any of these physiologic processes can effect $EtCO_2$.

CO_2 is produced in tissues as a by-product of aerobic metabolism. Therefore, any stimulus prompting increased metabolism will result in additional CO_2 production. This may include pathophysiologic conditions (eg, fever, sepsis, hyperthyroidism, trauma, and burns) and nonpathologic conditions (eg, exercise or increased intake of carbohydrates). Conversely, conditions associated with decreased metabolic needs (eg, hypothermia, hypothyroidism, sedation, and paralysis), will result in decreased CO_2 production.[15–17]

CO_2 diffuses passively out of cells into capillaries and then into circulation. Here, it is transported in three different forms. Most is transported as a bicarbonate ion (HCO_3^-), which forms following the combination of CO_2 and water, catalyzed by carbonic anhydrase. An additional 10% to 20% of CO_2 binds to the amino groups of proteins, most notably hemoglobin. When CO_2 is bound to hemoglobin, there is decreased affinity for oxygen, and vice versa. Therefore, as hemoglobin is oxygenated during passage through the pulmonary circulation, bound CO_2 is released allowing elimination in the lung. This is known as the Haldane effect.[17] The smallest fraction of CO_2 dissolves directly in plasma. Although this makes up only 5% to 10% of the CO_2 in circulation, it is a significantly greater amount than oxygen, which is approximately 20 times less soluble.[16]

Just as variation in CO_2 production can affect $EtCO_2$, so can alterations in circulation. Systemic circulatory collapse, such as in cardiac arrest, will result in decreased CO_2 delivery to the lungs and lower recorded $EtCO_2$ values, despite normal CO_2 production in the tissue.[18] Localized interruptions in pulmonary blood flow, such as with pulmonary embolism, also can decrease delivery of CO_2 for elimination, again resulting in lower $EtCO_2$ values.[19]

CO_2 is cleared through ventilation of the lungs. It crosses the blood–gas barrier comprised of the alveolar wall, interstitial fluid, and pulmonary capillary endothelium. Provided there is no pathology within these structures, CO_2 easily diffuses into the alveolar gas.

Minute ventilation refers to the volume of air moving in and out of the lungs in a given period of time, usually reported in liters per minute. The proportion of air that participates in gas exchange is referred to as alveolar ventilation, whereas the remainder comprises what is known as dead space ventilation. Dead space ventilation can be divided further into anatomic and physiologic. The volume of the airway, which serves to move air to those regions of the lung at which gas exchange actually occurs, is called anatomic dead space. It is always present and explains the small differential between arterial CO_2 concentration and $EtCO_2$ values. In healthy subjects, $EtCO_2$ is usually 2 to 5 mm Hg less than $PaCO_2$.[16] In contrast, physiologic dead space results from regions of the lung in which there is an imbalance between the ventilation and perfusion (ie, ventilation–perfusion [V/Q] mismatching). That is, those segments of lung that are relatively hypoperfused will have less CO_2 delivered, thus creating alveolar segments with little CO_2 to remove, thereby further contributing to dead space ventilation. Unlike anatomic dead space, physiologic dead space is reversible. Conversely, regions of the lung that are underventilated relative to their perfusion will have CO_2 delivered but not eliminated, also known as shunting. Because of poor ventilation, this CO_2 does not reach the capnograph, and the recorded $EtCO_2$ values from these areas again will be low. Therefore, the larger the relative proportion of the lung with V/Q mismatching, the lower the recorded $EtCO_2$ value will be, and the larger the gradient between the arterial CO_2 concentration and $EtCO_2$.[16]

PHYSIOLOGY OF THE WAVEFORM

Providing a graphic representation of the concentration of CO_2 over either time or volume creates a waveform. Here, the authors discuss only time-based capnograms.

A normal waveform has a trapezoidal appearance, comprised of four different phases of the respiratory cycle (see **Fig. 1**).[20] At the onset of exhalation, CO_2-poor atmospheric air at the sensor gives a baseline reading of zero (I). Shortly after exhalation begins and the air from anatomic dead space has cleared, synchronous release of alveolar air admixes with atmospheric air, and the $EtCO_2$ value rises rapidly (II). During the latter portion of exhalation, the concentration of CO_2 stabilizes, reflecting largely alveolar gas (III). The slight rise noted during this plateau phase results from dynamic elimination of CO_2 at the alveolar level, even during exhalation. The highest recorded value, at the end of expiration, is the $EtCO_2$, noted with a dot in **Fig. 1**. With inspiration, atmospheric air rushes by the sensor, and the concentration of CO_2 quickly falls back to zero (IV).

CLINICAL INDICATIONS FOR THE INTUBATED PATIENT
Confirming Endotracheal Intubation

There are numerous clinical indications for using capnography with regard to airway management. The most common of these is for confirmation of endotracheal intubation. The ability to distinguish between endotracheal and esophageal tube placement is crucial; failure to recognize and promptly correct a misplaced tube can be catastrophic. Studies have shown that 5% to 10% of intubation attempts in emergent settings result in esophageal tube placement, with even higher rates reported when performed on children or by prehospital personnel.[21–24] Multiple factors, including difficult intubating conditions, associated patient morbidity, inexperience of the provider managing the airway, and lack of rapid access to appropriate equipment may contribute to the high frequency of misplaced tubes.

Capnography provides a rapid, reliable, and practical method for differentiating endotracheal from esophageal tube placement (**Fig. 2**).[25] Although there are known limitations, capnographs, and in certain situations colorimetric end–tidal detectors, have been shown to be more accurate than conventional clinical signs or other diagnostic tests for confirming tube placement.

Direct visualization is a fundamental part of successful endotracheal intubation. The American College of Emergency Physicians (ACEP) notes that "direct visualization of the endotracheal tube passing through the vocal cords into the trachea constitutes firm evidence of correct tube placement."[9] This cannot be achieved in all cases,

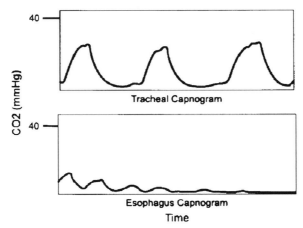

Fig. 2. Adult capnograms from a tracheal intubation (*top*) compared with an esophageal intubation (*lower*). (*From* Roberts WA, Maniscalco WM, Cohen AR, et al. The use of capnography for recognition of esophageal intubation in the neonatal intensive care unit. Pediatr Pulmonol 1995;19(5):263; with permission.)

however (eg, when the airway is occluded by blood, vomitus, or secretions, or when swelling, habitus, or anatomic anomalies prevent visualization of the glottic aperture). In addition, inexperienced practitioners may misidentify anatomic structures, or the tube may become dislodged. Therefore, it is recommended that tube position be verified by secondary means, even in circumstances where it has been witnessed to pass successfully through the cords.[7,9]

Auscultation frequently is used following intubation to confirm tube position. Bilateral breath sounds and absence of sounds over the epigastrum are consistent with an appropriately placed endotracheal tube. Practical experience, however, will echo reports in the literature describing cases where breath sounds were felt to be appreciated in patients who had esophageal intubations.[26,27] Extraneous noises during the management of critically ill patients in the prehospital or ED setting can make auscultation challenging. In addition, even under ideal circumstances, clinical findings can be misinterpreted. Airflow during positive pressure ventilation may sound different than in spontaneously breathing patients, and transmitted sounds can be misleading, particularly to inexperienced providers.[28]

Monitoring oxygen saturation is critical for intubated patients; however, following inadvertent esophageal intubation, there is potential for a significant lag time before hypoxia develops. In one animal model, nearly 50% of rats did not desaturate during the observed time period, and oxygen saturation was determined to be the least reliable method for detecting esophageal intubation in the study.[29] In a controlled human trial, preoxygenated patients did not desaturate for more than 30 seconds after esophageal intubation, and case reports highlight unrecognized esophageal intubations, with normal saturations lasting several minutes following tube placement.[27,30,31] Such potential delay precludes relying on pulse oximetry as a means for early detection of a missed intubation. Indeed, capnography uniformly has been shown to be superior to oximetry in this regard.[26]

Additional clinical and diagnostic methods for evaluating tube position also have been compared with capnography. Chest wall movement can be produced with tracheal and esophageal intubation, and tube condensation can be seen with more than 75$ of esophageal intubations, which means these signs may not be reliable.[26,32]

Fiberoptic bronchoscopy works well but is time consuming and not widely available in the ED, while transillumination using a lighted stylet has not been found to be consistently accurate.[28] Esophageal tube detectors have been shown to be valuable, particularly in cardiac arrest patients, but do not provide continuous, breath-to-breath information like capnography.[33] Although no single means is perfect in every circumstance, capnography has been reported to be the most reliable and practical means for determining correct tube position (**Fig. 3**).[26,28,29,31]

Based on the available evidence, tube position confirmation by capnography became the standard of care in anesthesia more than 20 years ago.[3] Revision of these original guidelines, and subsequent American Society of Anesthesiologists practice parameters have emphasized the importance of capnography in verifying endotracheal tube position.[34]

Similar position statements and recommendations from professional societies within emergency medicine also have emerged. A policy statement from the Emergency Medicine Journal includes the following, "Independent confirmation of correct tube placement by the use of devices that detect end–tidal carbon dioxide is mandatory for every endotracheal intubation performed in the emergency department."[35] The ACEP position paper on verification of endotracheal tube placement reads:

> "End–tidal CO_2 detection, either qualitative, quantitative, or continuous, is the most accurate and easily available method to monitor correct endotracheal tube position in patients who have adequate tissue perfusion."[9]

Finally, Advanced Cardiac Life Support guidelines from the American Heart Association (AHA) also endorse capnography noting, "Expired carbon dioxide detectors are very reliable in patients with perfusing rhythms and are recommended to confirm tube position in these patients."[7]

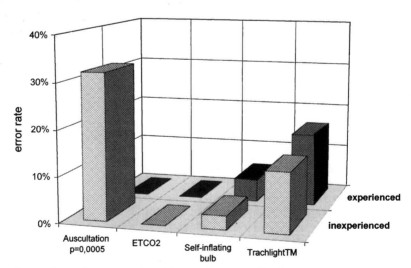

Fig. 3. Comparison of capnography with auscultation, self-inflating bulb (esophageal detector), and transillumination in verifying endotracheal tube placement. Comparison is made between attending physicians (experienced) and medical students (inexperienced). (*From* Knapp S, Kofler J, Stoiser B, et al. The assessment of four different methods to verify tracheal tube placement in the critical care setting. Anesth Analg 1999;88(4):768; with permission.)

Although clearly a useful tool in confirming tube placement, it is important to recognize those circumstances in which capnography may be less reliable. The AHA guidelines recognize the importance of perfusion when using capnography, as detection of CO_2 during exhalation is predicated on its delivery to the lungs for elimination. As a result, the specificity of capnography approaches 100% for tracheal placement of the endotracheal tube (ie, the presence of an appropriate waveform denotes tracheal intubation in patients with or without a pulse). The sensitivity for esophageal placement in cardiac arrest, however, is uncertain (ie, an absent waveform could be caused by esophageal intubation or tracheal intubation with poor pulmonary blood flow). Complete obstruction of the endotracheal tube, or a large air leak with admixture of atmospheric air also can give false-negative findings. In such circumstances, alternative means of verification must be implemented.

Conversely, false-positive results may be found when the tube tip is within the hypopharynx, where ventilation may be preserved sufficiently to record $EtCO_2$ yet the airway is not protected appropriately. In addition, because capnography is highly sensitive, studies have shown that CO_2 can be detected in an esophageal intubation if preceding aggressive bag–mask ventilation resulted in insufflation of the stomach with CO_2 containing air.[36] Animal studies also have demonstrated that recent consumption of large amounts of carbonated beverages also can produce false-positive findings.[37] In both circumstances, however, the concentration of CO_2 quickly diminishes over time, leading to a decline in the waveform or weakening of color change (see **Fig. 2**). Therefore, when using capnography to document tube position, it is recommended to monitor for changes over the initial 6 consecutive breaths.[12]

Despite substantial evidence supporting capnography as a means for confirmation of tube placement, as well as endorsement by numerous professional organizations, capnography still is not being used as often as it could be. A recent study found that colorimetric devices were available in only 77% of studied EDs, and less than one third of these sites had devices capable of continuous quantitative monitoring. Even within those institutions where the technology is available, more than half of providers reported that they rarely or never used it.[14] Further educational efforts are needed to encourage use of this technology and subsequent compliance with currently available guidelines.

Continuous Monitoring of Endotracheal Tube Position

Beyond initial tube placement, capnography also can provide an effective means to ensure that a tube remains in an acceptable position and functioning properly. Studies have shown that appropriately placed endotracheal tubes can migrate up to 5 cm and may become dislodged inadvertently as additional procedures are performed, or during patient transport.[38] In such circumstances, alteration or loss of the capnogram accompanied by a rapid decline in $EtCO_2$, or loss of color change on a colorimetric device should alert providers to the possibility of a dislodged or obstructed endotracheal tube.

Unrecognized misplaced intubation (UMI) is a term used to describe a tube in a location other than the trachea, unrecognized by the clinician. Regardless of whether this occurs at initial placement or following movement during patient care, the result is ineffective ventilation and oxygenation, and comparatively worse morbidity and mortality.[24,39] Studies investigating UMI rates vary; however, most report rates of 7% to 10% by both EMS personnel[40,41] and EM physicians,[23] although one recent study noted an alarming rate of 25% by paramedics.[24]

Data from prehospital intubations have demonstrated that continuous capnography can be effective in reducing UMI rates. A large review of intubations by EMS personnel showed that introduction of a systematic protocol resulted in a significantly lower esophageal intubation rate (0.3%), with the lowest incidence occurring after the introduction of capnography.[42] More recently, a prospective observational study found a significant difference in missed intubation rates for those EMS personnel using continuous end–tidal monitoring (0% esophageal intubations) versus those who were not (23% esophageal intubations).[43]

Continuous $EtCO_2$ monitoring for tube position is standard of care in anesthesia practice, both inside and outside the operating room.[3] Similarly, Intensive Care Society guidelines from Europe advocate for continuous capnography when transporting critically ill patients.[44] Emergency and prehospital medicine has perhaps even greater risk of UMI and inadvertent tube movement; therefore capnography ought to be used in the transport and care of these patients also.

CLINICAL INDICATIONS FOR THE NONINTUBATED PATIENT
Ventilatory Monitoring During Procedural Sedation and Analgesia

Management of pain and anxiety surrounding urgent and emergent procedures is a priority for EMS and in the ED. Consequently, procedural sedation and analgesia (PSA) have become integral to the practice of emergency medicine. Many PSA agents have the potential to cause respiratory depression and airway compromise. Early recognition and response to such potentially serious events is paramount. Detection traditionally has relied on continuous monitoring of heart rate, respiratory rate, and oxygen saturation. Pulse oximetry serves as a marker for oxygenation, while respiratory rate and clinical observation provide some information regarding ventilation. Capnography, however, offers a more precise and direct assessment of a patient's ventilatory status, and sidestream capnography allows for continuous monitoring of $EtCO_2$ in nonintubated patients by means of a nasal–oral cannula that samples CO_2 and simultaneously delivers low-flow oxygen. The resulting capnogram allows for continuous assessment of airway patency and respiratory pattern (**Fig. 4**).[20] As such, capnography can serve as an early warning system for prehypoxic respiratory depression in pharmacologically sedated patients.

Because many PSA agents affect respiratory drive with subsequent hypoventilation, a valid and sensitive tool would be expected to detect increases in $EtCO_2$ following their administration. Indeed, studies using numerous PSA agents have shown a transient but significant increase in $EtCO_2$, which returned to baseline following completion of the sedation.[45,46]

Such objective evidence of ventilatory changes can enhance conventional monitoring with pulse oximetry and clinical observation. That is, capnography appears to be more sensitive than clinical assessment or desaturation in detecting depressed respiratory effort. In a randomized trial of patients receiving fentanyl and midazolam, physicians identified respiratory depression in 73% of patients who experienced hypoxia, but failed to recognize it in any patient who did not become hypoxic.[47] Similarly, 10 of 39 (26%) patients undergoing PSA in another study population experienced 20-second periods of apnea. All cases were detected by capnography but none by clinical assessment alone.[48]

Empiric use of supplemental oxygen may decrease further the utility of pulse oximetry as an early warning system for respiratory compromise. Fu used an operating room setting to show that intubated patients receiving 25% or 30% FiO_2 did not desaturate during deliberate hypoventilation, whereas those being ventilated with room air under similar conditions did.[49] That is, when using oximetry monitoring alone, supplemental oxygen prevented recognition of known hypoventilation.

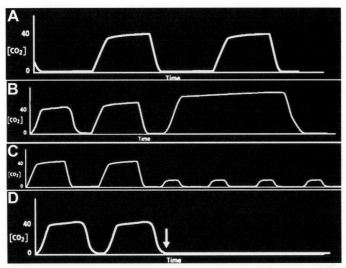

Fig. 4. Capnograms during PSA. (*A*) Normal waveform. (*B*) Patient with bradypneic hypoventilation, with normal tidal volume but slowed respiratory rate. (*C*) Hypopneic hypoventilation with decreased tidal volume resulting in increased dead space ventilation. (*D*) Loss of a waveform consistent with either complete laryngospasm or apnea. (*From* Krauss B, Hess DR. Capnography for procedural sedation and analgesia in the emergency department. Ann Emerg Med 2007;50(2):176–7; with permission.)

Trials regarding PSA outside the operating room also have demonstrated improved detection of adverse respiratory events using capnography. During PSA in a pediatric ICU, hypercarbia was found to be five times more common than hypoxia, and less than 25% of patients who had respiratory depression would have been detected using just pulse oximetry.[50] Similarly, a comparison of oximetry, capnography, and clinical observation using three different pharmacologic regimens in an ED showed that 75% of pediatric patients who had respiratory compromise were noted by EtCO$_2$ monitoring only.[51] Finally, a randomized, blinded, controlled pediatric trial also noted capnography was superior to clinical observation in detecting respiratory events. In this study, staff relying on clinical assessment but blinded to EtCO$_2$ monitoring reported hypoventilation in 3% of patients and did not identify any patients who had apnea. Capnographic data, however, suggested that ventilation was compromised in more than 50% of these cases, and nearly 25% fulfilled the predetermined criteria for apnea.[52]

Adult studies mirror these results. In one recent comparison, pulse oximetry detected only one third of study patients who met criteria for respiratory depression.[53] Similarly, a blinded, prospective trial was terminated before completion after interim safety analysis demonstrated convincing evidence that capnography provided clinically relevant advanced warning of hypoventilation during PSA. In this study, 70% of the patients who had an acute respiratory event had changes in the capnogram, occurring as early as 4 minutes before changes noted by oximetry or clinical observation.[54]

Although there is convincing evidence that capnography can provide a means for early detection of sedation-related hypoventilation, the clinical significance of these findings with regards to improving patient outcomes has not been shown. As such, current policy statements support rather than mandate use of capnography for PSA monitoring.[55–57]

Monitoring Ventilatory Status of the Unconscious or Obtunded Patient

The evidence supporting the use of capnography to monitor patients during PSA can be extrapolated more broadly to patients who have depressed mental status. Obtundation may result from intoxication, drug overdose, sepsis, central nervous system vascular events, trauma, or other neurologic insults. Capnographic assessment for hypoventilation or progressive respiratory depression in such patients can provide objective evidence and early warning for impending respiratory or airway compromise, and guide decisions regarding the need for further airway management.

Large case series have described successful use of capnography as a means for monitoring nonintubated patients at risk for respiratory decompensation.[58,59] Other studies have focused on the role of capnography with isolated etiologies for depressed level of consciousness. For example, Abramo documented the correlation between $EtCO_2$ monitoring and $PaCO_2$ from blood gas samples in nonintubated, actively seizing and postictal pediatric patients. In this study, sidestream capnography was found to correlate with hypoventilation and apnea better than oximetry, and had demonstrated value in the decision-making process for airway management.[60] A small case series reported a similar role for capnography in adult overdose patients, again providing adjunctive information supporting the decision to intubate.[61] Controlled, prospective studies looking at outcomes have not been completed; however, this early work supports a potential role for capnography as a means for continuous ventilatory monitoring in obtunded and unconscious patients.

Assessing Respiratory Illnesses

As an objective measurement of ventilation, capnography is suited well to assess respiratory illnesses in the ED, including: asthma, bronchiolitis, chronic obstructive pulmonary disease, croup, and cystic fibrosis. By measuring $EtCO_2$ and respiratory rate with each breath, capnography provides instantaneous feedback on the clinical status of the patient.

Using capnography, respiratory rate is measured directly from the airway, which provides a more reliable reading than conventional impedance monitoring. In upper airway obstruction and laryngospasm, impedance monitoring interprets chest wall movement as a valid breath, and consequently displays a respiratory rate even though the patient is not effectively ventilating. In contrast, capnography will detect the absence of ventilation in these patients, as demonstrated by a flatline capnogram (**Fig. 4D**).

End–tidal CO_2 has been shown to correlate with arterial CO_2 in adults and children who have normal lung function,[62–65] and in those who have underlying respiratory illness.[66,67] Therefore, capnography may be used as a noninvasive proxy measure for $PaCO_2$ when clinically indicated. The discriminating ability of absolute $EtCO_2$ values on clinical outcomes (eg, need for admission), however, has not been well shown.[68]

In contrast, the additional information that comes from continuous end–tidal CO_2 monitoring can be helpful in managing obstructive lung disease. Trends can provide a rapid assessment of the trajectory of the patient's ventilatory status (eg, worsening in spite of treatment [increasing $EtCO_2$], stabilizing [stable $EtCO_2$], or improving [decreasing $EtCO_2$]).

Recent attention has focused on waveform analysis as it relates to respiratory illness also. That is, characteristic changes in capnogram morphology correlate with underlying physiologic changes. For example, a wider Q angle and steeper plateau slope are indicative of slower CO_2 elimination and asynchronous alveolar ventilation, which correlate with increased airway obstruction and V/Q mismatch[69] (**Fig. 5**).

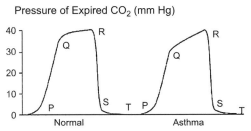

Pressure of Expired CO_2 (mm Hg)

Fig. 5. Capnogram of data from a normal subject and a subject with asthma. Note the wider Q angle and the steeper slope of the alveolar plateau (segment QR) in the asthma patient. P, onset of expiration; segment PQ, mixing of dead space and alveolar gases; segment QR, plateau phase representing alveolar gas delivery; R, end of expiration; segment RS, beginning of respiration; ST, low CO2 concentration in the air-way during the remainder of inspiration. (*From* Yaron M, Padyk P, Hutsinpiller M, et al. Utility of the expiratory capnogram in the assessment of bronchospasm. Ann Emerg Med 1996;28(4):403–7; with permission.)

Analyses of waveform changes can be translated into clinically useful information. The slope of the capnogram plateau has been shown to correlate with spirometric measures of obstructive airway pathology. Information regarding peak expiratory flow rate (PEFR) and forced expiratory volume in one second (FEV_1) can be inferred from capnographic analysis in patients who have asthma.[70,71] Therefore, capnography offers an effort-independent measure of the degree of bronchospasm, which may be particularly helpful in patients in whom young age or altered mental status precludes cooperation with pulmonary testing. In addition, assessing changes in the slope over time has been shown to be a reliable measure of response to therapy, with decreasing slope differences correlating with less severe respiratory impairment.[70,71] An alternative waveform analysis includes the $EtCO_2$ ratio (length of the alveolar plateau divided by the respiratory rate), which also correlates with the degree of airway resistance. In children who have asthma, the $EtCO_2$ ratio has been shown to have predictive ability in determining need for hospitalization.[72] Capnography can provide continuous, real-time objective information regarding a patient's ventilatory status. When used in conjunction with pulse oximetry and other clinical variables, it offers rapid assessment of severity of disease and may help guide therapeutic decisions in those who have acute and chronic obstructive lung disease.

FUTURE ADVANCED AIRWAY USES

Novel uses of capnography for airway management continue to emerge. Blind nasal intubation for EMS and in the ED has become rare since the advent of newer technologies; however, this remains a rescue option for the unanticipated difficult airway.[34] Capnography can be a useful adjunct for this technique, as passage of the tube toward the esophagus leads to declining $EtCO_2$ values and loss of the waveform, which suggests the need for tube redirection.[73] Similarly, small case series have described capnographic assistance during fiberoptic endotracheal intubation. Although the goal of fiberoptic bronchoscopy is to provide direct visualization of the airway before advancing the endotracheal tube over the scope, many factors may compromise visualization. In such circumstances, capnographic assessment through an open suction port has been shown to reliably demonstrate intratracheal scope positioning before advancing the endotracheal tube.[74] Use of a guiding stylet has become a well-recognized approach to difficult airway management also. Devises such as gum elastic bougies and stylets from laryngotracheal topical anesthesia (LTA) kits may be easier to position in the trachea when visualization is suboptimal, and they can serve as guides for subsequent endotracheal placement. $EtCO_2$ sampling by means of a modified stylet from an LTA kit has been shown to be an accurate way of determining endotracheal placement before tube placement.[75] Although there are no similar studies using elastic bougies which are more commonplace in the ED than LTAs, the recent introduction of ventilating bougie devices may make this feasible also. Finally, Coleman demonstrated the use of capnography in confirming intratracheal cannula placement before performing percutaneous dilutional tracheostomy.[76] Although this was not performed during emergent tracheostomy, the concept of using capnography to confirm intraluminal placement in this situation is intriguing and might be explored further.

Following successful intubation of a patient, capnography also has been shown to provide a means for optimizing endotracheal tube cuff filling. An appropriately inflated cuff allows for effective ventilation at the lowest possible positive pressure settings and may help ensure enough seal to prevent aspiration around the cuff. In a recent study, cuff filling was regulated to achieve the minimal pressure needed to prevent air leak, as determined by an $EtCO_2$ of less than 2 mm Hg proximal to the cuff (eg, at the nares). This method was found to be superior than determining the cuff pressure clinically.[77]

METABOLISM AND PERFUSION

This article has focused on the applications of capnography related to ventilation and airway management. It is worth noting, however, that as a reflection of CO_2 physiology, capnography can assess changes in perfusion and metabolism. Numerous studies in the emergency medicine literature have demonstrated the utility of capnography as a means of assessing perfusion during cardiac arrest. In particular, $EtCO_2$ monitoring can be used to evaluate the adequacy of cardiopulmonary resuscitation (CPR), and also serve as an early indicator of return of spontaneous circulation.[78–80] Likewise, capnography offers a quantitative, objective measure of the compensatory respiratory alkalosis in patients who have underlying metabolic acidosis. This has been applied in the management of patients who have diabetic ketoacidosis and gastroenteritis.[81–83] Such work demonstrates a trend toward expanded utility of capnography in the ED setting.

SUMMARY

Capnography provides a noninvasive means for measuring a patient's ventilatory status. It has been shown to be an effective clinical tool for:

Confirming and monitoring endotracheal intubations
Monitoring patients who have depressed mental status and during procedural sedation
Evaluating those who have obstructive airway diseases such as asthma

Many of these indications are endorsed by national position statements and guidelines. Additional novel uses for capnography as an adjunctive tool during airway management also have been published. In the future, as capnography becomes increasingly available and familiar, it can be expected that clinical indications for its use in emergency medicine will continue to grow.

REFERENCES

1. Aiken R, Clark-Kennedy A. On the fluctuation in the composition of the alveolar air during the respiratory cycle in muscular capacity. J Physiol 1928;65:389–411.
2. Smalhout B, Kalenda Z. An atlas of capnography. The Netherlands: Kerckebosche Zeist; 1975.
3. American Society of Anesthesiologists. Standards for basic anesthetic monitoring. 2005 Last amended October 25, 2005; Approved October 21, 1986: Cited December 2007. Available at: http://asahq.org/publicationsAndServices/standards/02.pdf. Accessed February 1, 2008.
4. Sanders AB, Atlas M, Ewy GA, et al. Expired PCO2 as an index of coronary perfusion pressure. Am J Emerg Med 1985;3(2):147–9.
5. Sanders AB. Capnometry in emergency medicine. Ann Emerg Med 1989;18(12): 1287–90.
6. Santos LJ, Varon J, Pic-Aluas L, et al. Practical uses of end–tidal carbon dioxide monitoring in the emergency department. J Emerg Med 1994;12(5):633–44.
7. Guidelines 2000 for cardiopulmonary resuscitation and emergency cardiovascular care. Part 6: advanced cardiovascular life support. Section 1: introduction to ACLS 2000. Overview of recommended changes in ACLS from the guidelines 2000 conference. The American heart association in collaboration with the international liaison committee on resuscitation. Circulation 2000;102(Suppl 8):I86–9.
8. O'Connor RE, Swor RA. Verification of endotracheal tube placement following intubation. National association of ems physicians standards and clinical practice committee. Prehosp Emerg Care 1999;3(3):248–50.
9. American College of Emergency Physicians. Verification of endotracheal intubation: policy statement. 2001. Cited December 2007. Available at: http://www.acep.org/practres.aspx?id=29846. Accessed February 1, 2008.
10. Swedlow DB. Capnometry and capnography: the anestherisa disaster early warning system. Semin Anesth 1986;V(3):194–205.
11. Thompson JE, Jaffe MB. Capnographic waveforms in the mechanically ventilated patient. Respir Care 2005;50(1):100–8.
12. Sullivan KJ, Kissoon N, Goodwin SR. End–tidal carbon dioxide monitoring in pediatric emergencies. Pediatr Emerg Care 2005;21(5):327–32.
13. Wang VJ, Krauss B. Carbon dioxide monitoring in emergency medicine training programs. Pediatr Emerg Care 2002;18(4):251–3.
14. Delorio NM. Continuous end–tidal carbon dioxide monitoring for confirmation of endotracheal tube placement is neither widely available nor consistently applied by emergency physicians. Emerg Med J 2005;22:490–3.
15. Guyton J, Hall J. Textbook of medical physiology. 10th edition. Philadelphia: W.B. Saunders Co.; 2000.
16. Hess D. Capnometry. In: Tobin MJ, editor. Principles and practice of intensive care monitoring. New York: McGraw-Hill; 1998. p. 377–400.
17. West J. Respiratory physiology: the essentials. 7th edition. Philadelphia: Lippincott Williams & Wilkins; 2005.
18. Weil MH, Rackow EC, Trevino R, et al. Difference in acid–base state between venous and arterial blood during cardiopulmonary resuscitation. N Engl J Med 1986;315(3):153–6.
19. Julian DG, Travis DM, Robin ED, et al. Effect of pulmonary artery occlusion upon end–tidal carbon dioxide tension. J Appl Phys 1960;15:87–91.
20. Krauss B, Hess DR. Capnography for procedural sedation and analgesia in the emergency department. Ann Emerg Med 2007;50(2):172–81.

21. Schwartz DE, Matthay MA, Cohen NH. Death and other complications of emergency airway management in critically ill adults. A prospective investigation of 297 tracheal intubations. Anesthesiology 1995;82(2):367–76.
22. Sakles JC, Laurin EG, Rantapaa AA, et al. Airway management in the emergency department: a one-year study of 610 tracheal intubations. Ann Emerg Med 1998; 31(3):325–32.
23. Timmermann A, Russo SG, Eich C, et al. The out-of-hospital esophageal and endobronchial intubations performed by emergency physicians. Anesth Analg 2007;104(3):619–23.
24. Katz SH, Falk JL. Misplaced endotracheal tubes by paramedics in an urban emergency medical services system. Ann Emerg Med 2001;37(1):32–7.
25. Roberts WA, Maniscalco WM, Cohen AR, et al. The use of capnography for recognition of esophageal intubation in the neonatal intensive care unit. Pediatr Pulmonol 1995;19(5):262–8.
26. Birmingham PK, Cheney FW, Ward RJ. Esophageal intubation: a review of detection techniques. Anesth Analg 1986;65(8):886–91.
27. Batra AK, Cohn MA. Uneventful prolonged misdiagnosis of esophageal intubation. Crit Care Med 1983;11(9):763–4.
28. Knapp S, Kofler J, Stoiser B, et al. The assessment of four different methods to verify tracheal tube placement in the critical care setting. Anesth Analg 1999; 88(4):766–70.
29. Vaghadia H, Jenkins LC, Ford RW. Comparison of end–tidal carbon dioxide, oxygen saturation, and clinical signs for the detection of oesophageal intubation. Can J Anaesth 1989;36(5):560–4.
30. Pollard BJ, Junius F. Accidental intubation of the oesophagus. Anaesth Intensive Care 1980;8(2):183–6.
31. Guggenberger H, Lenz G, Federle R. Early detection of inadvertent oesophageal intubation: pulse oximetry vs. capnography. Acta Anaesthesiol Scand 1989; 33(2):112–5.
32. Kelly JJ, Eynon CA, Kaplan JL, et al. Use of tube condensation as an indicator of endotracheal tube placement. Ann Emerg Med 1998;31(5):575–8.
33. Takeda T, Tanigawa K, Tanaka H, et al. The assessment of three methods to verify tracheal tube placement in the emergency setting. Resuscitation 2003;56(2): 153–7.
34. Practice guidelines for management of the difficult airway: an updated report by the American Society of Anesthesiologists task force on management of the difficult airway. Anesthesiology 2003;98(5):1269–77.
35. Clancy MJ. Position statement number 1. Emerg Med J 2001;18(5):329a.
36. Puntervoll SA, Soreide E, Jacewicz W, et al. Rapid detection of oesophageal intubation: take care when using colorimetric capnometry. Acta Anaesthesiol Scand 2002;46(4):455–7.
37. Qureshi S, Park K, Sturmann K, et al. The effect of carbonated beverages on colorimetric end–tidal CO(2) determination. Acad Emerg Med 2000;7(10):1169.
38. Conrardy PA, Goodman LR, Lainge F, et al. Alteration of endotracheal tube position. Flexion and extension of the neck. Crit Care Med 1976;4(1):7–12.
39. Gausche M, Lewis RJ, Stratton SJ, et al. Effect of out-of-hospital pediatric endotracheal intubation on survival and neurological outcome: a controlled clinical trial. JAMA 2000;283(6):783–90.
40. Jones JH, Murphy MP, Dickson RL, et al. Emergency physician-verified prehospital intubation, missed rates by ground paramedics. Acad Emerg Med 2003;10(5): 448b–9.

41. Jemmett ME, Kendall KM, Fourre MW, et al. Unrecognized misplaced endotracheal tubes in a mixed urban-to-rural EMS setting. Acad Emerg Med 2003; 10(5):481b–2.

42. Wayne MA, Friedland E. Prehospital use of succinylcholine: a 20-year review. Prehosp Emerg Care 1999;3(2):107–9.

43. Silvestri S, Ralls GA, Krauss B, et al. The effectiveness of out-of-hospital use of continuous end–tidal carbon dioxide monitoring on the rate of unrecognized misplaced intubation within a regional emergency medical services system. Ann Emerg Med 2005;45(5):497–503.

44. The Intensive Care Society. Guidelines for the transport of the critically ill adult. 2002. Cited 2007 December. Available at: http://www.ics.ac.uk/icmprof/downloads/ icstransport2002mem.pdf. Accessed February 1, 2008.

45. Wright SW. Conscious sedation in the emergency department: the value of capnography and pulse oximetry. Ann Emerg Med 1992;21(5):551–5.

46. Anderson JL, Junkins E, Pribble C, et al. Capnography and depth of sedation during propofol sedation in children. Ann Emerg Med 2007;49(1):9–13.

47. Deitch K, Chudnofsky CR, Dominici P. The utility of supplemental oxygen during emergency department procedural sedation and analgesia with midazolam and fentanyl: a randomized, controlled trial. Ann Emerg Med 2007;49(1):1–8.

48. Soto RG, Fu ES, Vila H Jr, et al. Capnography accurately detects apnea during monitored anesthesia care. Anesth Analg 2004;99(2):379–82, table of contents.

49. Fu ES, Downs JB, Schweiger JW, et al. Supplemental oxygen impairs detection of hypoventilation by pulse oximetry. Chest 2004;126(5):1552–8.

50. Yildizdas D, Yapicioglu H, Yilmaz HL, et al. Correlation of simultaneously obtained capillary, venous, and arterial blood gases of patients in a paediatric intensive care unit. Arch Dis Child 2004;89(2):176–80.

51. Hart LS, Berns SD, Houck CS, et al. The value of end–tidal CO2 monitoring when comparing three methods of conscious sedation for children undergoing painful procedures in the emergency department. Pediatr Emerg Care 1997;13(3):189–93.

52. Lightdale JR, Goldmann DA, Feldman HA, et al. Microstream capnography improves patient monitoring during moderate sedation: a randomized, controlled trial. Pediatrics 2006;117(6):e1170–8.

53. Miner JR, Heegaard W, Plummer D. End–tidal carbon dioxide monitoring during procedural sedation. Acad Emerg Med 2002;9(4):275–80.

54. Burton JH, Harrah JD, Germann CA, et al. Does end–tidal carbon dioxide monitoring detect respiratory events prior to current sedation monitoring practices? Acad Emerg Med 2006;13(5):500–4.

55. American Academy of Pediatrics, American Academy of Pediatric Dentistry, Cote CJ, et al. Guidelines for monitoring and management of pediatric patients during and after sedation for diagnostic and therapeutic procedures: an update. Pediatrics 2006;118(6):2587–602.

56. An Updated Report by the American Society of Anesthesiologists Task Force on Sedation and Analgesia by Non-Anethesiologists. Practice guidelines for sedation and analgesia by nonanesthesiologists. Anesthesiology 2002;96(4):1004–17.

57. Godwin SA, Caro DA, Wolf SJ, et al. Clinical policy: procedural sedation and analgesia in the emergency department. Ann Emerg Med 2005;45(2):177–96.

58. Kierzek G, Jactat T, Dumas F, et al. End–tidal carbon dioxide monitoring in the emergency department. Acad Emerg Med 2006;13(10):1086.

59. Wahlen BM, Bey T, Wolke BB. Measurement of end–tidal carbon dioxide in spontaneously breathing patients in the prehospital setting. A prospective evaluation of 350 patients. Resuscitation 2003;56(1):35–40.

60. Abramo TJ, Wiebe RA, Scott S, et al. Noninvasive capnometry monitoring for respiratory status during pediatric seizures. Crit Care Med 1997;25(7):1242–6.
61. Davis DP, Patel RJ. Noninvasive capnometry for continuous monitoring of mental status: a tale of 2 patients. Am J Emerg Med 2006;24(6):752–4.
62. Barton CW, Wang ES. Correlation of end–tidal CO2 measurements to arterial PaCO2 in nonintubated patients. Ann Emerg Med 1994;23(3):560–3.
63. Liu SY, Lee TS, Bongard F. Accuracy of capnography in nonintubated surgical patients. Chest 1992;102(5):1512–5.
64. McNulty SE, Roy J, Torjman M, et al. Relationship between arterial carbon dioxide and end–tidal carbon dioxide when a nasal sampling port is used. J Clin Monit 1990;6(2):93–8.
65. Friesen RH, Alswang M. End–tidal PCO2 monitoring via nasal cannulae in pediatric patients: accuracy and sources of error. J Clin Monit 1996;12(2):155–9.
66. Abramo TJ, Wiebe RA, Scott SM, et al. Noninvasive capnometry in a pediatric population with respiratory emergencies. Pediatr Emerg Care 1996;12(4):252–4.
67. Corbo J, Bijur P, Lahn M, et al. Concordance between capnography and arterial blood gas measurements of carbon dioxide in acute asthma. Ann Emerg Med 2005;46(4):323–7.
68. Guthrie BD, Adler MD, Powell EC. End–tidal carbon dioxide measurements in children with acute asthma. Acad Emerg Med 2007;14(12):1135–40.
69. You B, Peslin R, Duvivier C, et al. Expiratory capnography in asthma: evaluation of various shape indices. Eur Respir J 1994;7(2):318–23.
70. Yaron M, Padyk P, Hutsinpiller M, et al. Utility of the expiratory capnogram in the assessment of bronchospasm. Ann Emerg Med 1996;28(4):403–7.
71. Krauss B, Deykin A, Lam A, et al. Capnogram shape in obstructive lung disease. Anesth Analg 2005;100(3):884–8.
72. Kunkov S, Pinedo V, Silver EJ, et al. Predicting the need for hospitalization in acute childhood asthma using end–tidal capnography. Pediatr Emerg Care 2005;21(9):574–7.
73. Mentzelopoulos SD, Augustatou CG, Papageorgiou EP. Capnography-guided nasotracheal intubation of a patient with a difficult airway and unwanted respiratory depression. Anesth Analg 1998;87(3):734–6.
74. Wolf LH, Gravenstein D. Capnography during fiberoptic bronchoscopy to verify tracheal intubation. Anesth Analg 1997;85(3):701–3.
75. Bourke DL, Biehl J. The laryngotracheal topical anesthesia kit with capnography for difficult endotracheal intubation. Anesth Analg 1999;88(4):943–5.
76. Coleman NA, Power BM, van Heerden PV. The use of end–tidal carbon dioxide monitoring to confirm intratracheal cannula placement prior to percutaneous dilatational tracheostomy. Anaesth Intensive Care 2000;28(2):191–2.
77. Efrati S, Leonov Y, Oron A, et al. Optimization of endotracheal tube cuff filling by continuous upper airway carbon dioxide monitoring. Anesth Analg 2005;101(4):1081–8.
78. Garnett AR, Ornato JP, Gonzalez ER, et al. End–tidal carbon dioxide monitoring during cardiopulmonary resuscitation. JAMA 1987;257(4):512–5.
79. Falk JL, Rackow EC, Weil MH. End–tidal carbon dioxide concentration during cardiopulmonary resuscitation. N Engl J Med 1988;318(10):607–11.
80. Levine RL, Wayne MA, Miller CC. End–tidal carbon dioxide and outcome of out-of-hospital cardiac arrest. N Engl J Med 1997;337(5):301–6.
81. Fearon DM, Steele DW. End–tidal carbon dioxide predicts the presence and severity of acidosis in children with diabetes. Acad Emerg Med 2002;9(12):1373–8.

82. Garcia E, Abramo TJ, Okada P, et al. Capnometry for noninvasive continuous monitoring of metabolic status in pediatric diabetic ketoacidosis. Crit Care Med 2003;31(10):2539–43.
83. Nagler J, Wright RO, Krauss B. End–tidal carbon dioxide as a measure of acidosis among children with gastroenteritis. Pediatrics 2006;118(1):260–7.

Measurement of Exhaled Nitric Oxide in the Emergency Department in Patients with Asthma

Ani Aydin, MD[a], Breena Taira, MD[b], Adam J. Singer, MD, FACEP[b],*

KEYWORDS

• Asthma • Exhaled nitric oxide • Emergency department

Asthma is a chronic inflammatory respiratory disease characterized by acute exacerbations resulting in the narrowing of the smaller airways in response to certain triggers. According to the Centers for Disease Control and Prevention (CDC), 30.8 million Americans reported having been diagnosed with asthma in 2002. During that year, a higher prevalence was cited in children as compared with adults (122 of 1000 children versus 106 of 1000 adults).[1] Furthermore, 12 million Americans experienced an acute asthma attack in 2002.[1] Severe asthma exacerbations are potentially life-threatening events with a mortality rate of approximately 10%, and a 10% to 20% hospitalization rate.[2–5] Therefore, acute asthma exacerbations are common, life-threatening events that warrant prompt diagnosis and treatment in the emergency department.

Guidelines for the diagnosis and management of acute asthma attacks in the emergency department are outlined in the Expert Panel Report (ERP3), published by the National Asthma Education and Prevention Program (NAEPP) Coordinating Committee (CC), coordinated by the National Heart, Lung, and Blood Institute (NHLBI) of the National Institutes of Health.[6] In addition, new modalities and markers are on the horizon. For example, exhaled nitric oxide (NO) is a marker of airway inflammation, and its levels are reported to correlate to the level of airway obstruction both initially and in response to treatment.[7] In early 2008, a new hand-held device to measure exhaled

[a] Department of Emergency Medicine, New York University School of Medicine, First Avenue & 27th Street, New York, NY 10016, USA
[b] Department of Emergency Medicine, State University New York Stony Brook School of Medicine, HSC L3-058, Stony Brook, NY 11794-8350, USA
* Corresponding author.
E-mail address: adam.singer@stonybrook.edu (A.J. Singer).

Emerg Med Clin N Am 26 (2008) 899–904
doi:10.1016/j.emc.2008.08.003
0733-8627/08/$ – see front matter © 2008 Elsevier Inc. All rights reserved.

nitric oxide was approved by the US Food and Drug Administration (FDA), which makes such measurements in the emergency department more accessible for routine use.

A great deal of research has been conducted on the utility and usefulness of exhaled NO as a biomarker of airway inflammation and its role in the diagnosis of acute asthma exacerbations. This article reviews the pathophysiology of NO in asthma, evidence for the use of exhaled NO in acute asthma exacerbations, and the potential utility of devices available to emergency physicians for measuring exhaled NO.

PHYSIOLOGY AND PATHOPHYSIOLOGY OF NITRIC OXIDE IN THE AIRWAY OF ASTHMATICS

In the human body, NO is an unstable diffusible gas produced by the conversion of L-arginine to NO and L-citrulline by the enzyme NO synthase (NOS).[7,8] NO then is oxidized rapidly to nitrites (NO_2) and nitrates (NO_3), or inactivated when bound to hemoglobin.[7,8]

Several isoforms of NOS exist. NOS I, or nNOS, is a calcium-activated form of the enzyme present in neuronal cells, and it is involved in neurogenesis.[7,9] NOS III, or eNOS, another constitutive form of the enzyme, is expressed by endothelial cells throughout the body.[7,8] Finally, NOS II, or iNOS, is an inducible form of the enzyme. iNOS is involved in many aspects of asthma pathogenesis, including airway and smooth muscle tone, and inflammation.[7,8,10,11]

iNOS acts by means of the airway epithelium to produce NO. As the NO diffuses into the bronchial smooth muscle, it results in relaxation, or bronchodilation, by means of the activation of guanylyl cycle, which in turn produces guanosine 3′,5′-cyclic monophosphate (cGMP).[7,8] In the bronchial circulation, NO results in pulmonary vascular smooth muscle relaxation.[7,8] Although NO is a bronchodilator, it reportedly acts in asthma pathogenesis by modifying airway hyper-responsiveness and inflammation.[7,8] Alternatively, it simply may be a marker of inflammation in the asthmatic population.[7,8]

In the early 1990s the fractional exhaled NO (FE_{NO}) first was measured using chemiluminescence analyzers. The range of concentrations of NO in the exhaled breath of normal subjects is approximately 5 to 10 parts per billion.[7] Asthmatics have higher levels of FE_{NO}, and higher levels of iNOS expression in the airway epithelial cells.[7,12,13] This increase in FE_{NO} detected in asthmatics correlates with sputum eosinophils, bronchoalveolar lavage eosinophilia, the bronchial biopsy eosinophil score, blood eosinophilia, and bronchial hyperresponsiveness.[14–18] The rise in FE_{NO} in this population occurs before the symptoms of an asthma exacerbation, and therefore may be useful in early detection of an acute episode.[18,19]

FE_{NO} levels demonstrate a dose-dependent decrease after administration of anti-inflammatory medications, such as inhaled steroids in patients who have asthma, thereby demonstrating potential utility in the early detection of loss of control, and compliance with treatment.[7,8,18–21] With the recent approval of a hand-held device, serial measurement of FE_{NO} is possible in the emergency department setting.

EXHALED NITRIC OXIDE IN ASTHMATICS IN THE EMERGENCY DEPARTMENT

In 1999, the American Thoracic Society (ATS) issued guidelines for measuring of FE_{NO}, which were updated for the pediatric population in 2001 by the European Respiratory Society (ERS)/ATS Task Force.[22,23] As of 2003, the FDA approved the use of a stationary chemiluminescence analyzer (NIOX; Aerocrine AB, Solna, Sweden) to measure the FE_{NO} in patients who have asthma.[23] Limitations of this device include the machine's large size, the high cost, need for frequent calibration, necessity of precise atmospheric conditions, and the presence of trained laboratory personnel to run the examinations.[24] These restrictions thus far have limited its use in the emergency department.

Earlier this year, the FDA-approved a new portable hand-held device that uses electrochemical sensors, the NIOX-MINO (Aerocrine AB). The developers published the original validation study of the NIOX-MINO, comparing it with the gold standard, NIOX.[25] These results were recently corroborated by Menzies and colleagues,[26] who reported comparable results in 101 patients who had asthma and 50 controls. Finally, Maniscalco and colleagues[27] also found that results obtained from the NIOX-MINO were reproducible in a study consisting of 15 healthy subjects and 15 patients who had allergic rhinitis.

The portable device also has been studied in the pediatric population. McGill and colleagues[28] compared the NIOX with the hand-held NIOX-MINO in 55 children ranging from 4 to 15 years. A 6-second exhalation period was recorded, as opposed to the 10 seconds in the adults, as per the ERS/ATS guidelines, because of their smaller lung capacity.[21,28] The authors found that the FE_{NO} values obtained with the NIOX correlate with those from the hand-held NIOX-MINO, with a greater consistency at lower values.[28] They also found, however, that the FE_{NO} values were slightly lower using the NIOX-MINO.[28] They additionally argue that in younger children, the NIOX is preferable, as the auditory and visual incentives on the NIOX-MINO, versus the stationary device's sole visual cues, may confuse this population.[28] The ability to successfully use the NIOX-MINO improved from 40% at age 4 years to 100% at age 10 years, with good repeatability.[23,29]

In a larger study combining adults and children, Alving and colleagues[30] reported clinically acceptable agreement between the two devices and good repeatability with the hand-held version. Although there is a growing body of evidence for use of the NIOX-MINO, several studies cite the difference in values obtained between devices increases with increasing FE_{NO} levels.[25,26,28] To examine these discrepancies, Pizzimenti and colleagues[23] derived a correction equation to compare data obtained from both device types. The equation is as follows:

$$FE_{NO\ (NIOx)} = 1.656(SE = 0.61) + 0.808(SE = 0.009) \times FE_{NO\ (NIOx\text{-}MINO)}{}^{23}$$

This equation is very easy to use, but it is important to note that the authors derived the equation by using the same calibration gas in both FE_{NO} devices; the use of a different gas may change the derived relation.[23]

Given the ease of use, reproducibility, and validity of FE_{NO} using the new portable devices, one can foresee the use of FE_{NO} measurements in the emergency department. Baptist and colleagues recently conduced such a study[31] in 35 adults who had not received steroids for at least 1 week, and who presented to the emergency department with an acute exacerbation. The authors did not find any statistically significant correlation between the FE_{NO} levels and traditional asthma factors, such as the forced expiratory volume in 1 second (FEV_1), peak expiratory flow rate, spirometric measurements, asthma severity, asthma history, and demographic factors.[31] Therefore, these measures were not useful in determining which patients required hospitalization.[31] The authors, however, demonstrated good reproducibility with measures taken in the emergency department.[31] Given that FE_{NO} is a marker of inflammation, these authors argue that more research needs to be done in the emergency department setting to determine how best to incorporate this measure in the setting of an acute exacerbation.[31]

In a follow-up small pilot study, Baptist and colleagues[32] examined the FE_{NO} levels in 10 African American patients who were hospitalized for acute asthma exacerbations, using a hand-held device. Initial baseline FE_{NO} levels were taken upon presentation in the emergency department, followed by repeat measurements at 1, 4, 6, 8, 12, and 24 hours after admission, and 3 days after discharge from the hospital.[32] FEV_1 levels also were recorded at baseline in the emergency department, and 1, 6, 12, and 24 hours after admission to the hospital.[32] All patients received standard treatments for their exacerbations.[32] Interestingly, the authors noted a 52% increase in the FE_{NO} levels at 12 hours, and a 68% increase at 24 hours after treatment, which included steroids.[32] In addition, there was a positive correlation between the FE_{NO} and FEV_1 levels, although this correlation did not reach significance.[32] Of the eight patients who were reached after discharge, two being lost to follow-up, those who reported an improvement in their symptoms had higher increases in the FE_{NO} levels.[32] Although the authors postulated several theories concerning this increase in acute treatment and after discharge, larger-scale studies with more diverse populations need to be conducted to better understand their significance.

Although ongoing research must be conducted to find the best use for FE_{NO} measurements in the emergency department, the data collected thus far show that these devices can be used to predict exacerbations. For example, a patient who has an acute rise in his or her FE_{NO} level may require a course of steroids to prevent re-exacerbation of symptoms. Alternatively, for those who struggle with compliance with their medications, the FE_{NO} levels provide an educational opportunity as a quantifiable indicator of the importance of the prescribed medications. Serial FE_{NO} readings can be used to track response to treatment. Finally, in the pediatric population, these measures can help emergency medicine physicians quickly diagnose asthma in children who are unable to communicate their symptoms fully.

Current limitations of the NIOX -MINO devices, however, must be taken into consideration. For example, although one elevated FE_{NO} value can clue a physician into an acute asthma exacerbation, it would be best to know an individual patient's baseline level when prescribing medications. In addition, the smaller hand-held devices cannot be calibrated, as opposed to the larger, stationary devices. Variability between portable devices, therefore, might become a confounder. Although the FDA approved the NIOX -MINO for use early in 2008, and initial studies of its validity and reproducibility are promising, further studies are necessary to confirm its practicality in the emergency department. It is possible this device will be a useful tool in an emergency medicine physician's arsenal when diagnosing, treating, and referring patients who have asthma for follow-up evaluations.

REFERENCES

1. Available at: http://www.cdc.gov/nchs/products/pubs/pubd/hestats/asthma/asthma.htm. Accessed August 25, 2008.
2. McFadden ER Jr. Acute severe asthma. Am J Respir Crit Care Med 2003;168(7):740–59.
3. Restrepo RD, Peters J. Near-fatal asthma: recognition and management. Curr Opin Pulm Med 2008;14(1):13–23.
4. Pollack CV Jr, Pollack ES, Baren JM, et al. A prospective multicenter study of patient factors associated with hospital admission from the emergency department among children with acute asthma. Arch Pediatr Adolesc Med 2002;156(9):934–40.
5. Weber EJ, Silverman RA, Callaham ML, et al. A prospective multicenter study of factors associated with hospital admission among adults with acute asthma. Am J Med 2002;113(5):371–8.
6. Available at: http://www.nhlbi.nih.gov/guidelines/asthma/11_sec5_exacerb.pdf. Accessed August 25, 2008.

7. Dweik RA. The promise and reality of nitric oxide in the diagnosis and treatment of lung disease. Cleve Clin J Med 2001;68(6):486–93.
8. Kharitonov SA, Barnes PJ. Exhaled biomarkers. Chest 2006;130(5):1541–6.
9. Kennedy M. Signal-processing machines at the postsynaptic density. Science 2000;290(5492):750–4.
10. Batra J, Chatterjee R, Ghosh B. Inducible nitric oxide synthase (iNOS): role in asthma pathogenesis. Indian J Biochem Biophys 2007;44(5):303–9.
11. Redington AE, Meng QH, Springall DR, et al. Increased expression of inducible nitric oxide synthase and cyclo-oxygenase-2 in the airway epithelium of asthmatic subjects and regulation by corticosteroid treatment. Thorax 2001;56(5):335–6.
12. Kharitonov SA, Yates D, Robbins RA, et al. Increased nitric oxide in exhaled air of asthmatic patients. Lancet 1994;343(8890):133–5.
13. Alving K, Weitzberg E, Lundberg JM. Increased amount of nitric oxide in exhaled air of asthmatics. Eur Respir J 1993;6(9):1368–70.
14. Jatakanon A, Lim S, Kharitonov SA, et al. Correlation between exhaled nitric oxide, sputum eosinophils, and methacholine responsiveness in patients with mild asthma. Thorax 1998;53(2):91–5.
15. Warke TJ, Fitch PS, Brown V, et al. Exhaled nitric oxide correlates with airway eosinophils in childhood asthma. Thorax 2002;57(5):383–7.
16. Payne DN, Adcock IM, Wilson NM, et al. Relationship between exhaled nitric oxide and mucosal eosinophilic inflammation in children with difficult asthma, after treatment with oral prednisolone. Am J Respir Crit Care Med 2001;164 (8 Pt 1):1376–81.
17. Strunk RC, Szefler SJ, Phillips BR, et al. Relationship of exhaled nitric oxide to clinical and inflammatory markers of persistent asthma in children. J Allergy Clin Immunol 2003;112(5):883–92.
18. Jones SL, Kittelson J, Cowan JO, et al. The predictive value of exhaled nitric oxide measurements in assessing changes in asthma control. Am J Respir Crit Care Med 2001;164(5):738–43.
19. Kharitonov SA, Donnelly LE, Montuschi P, et al. Dose-dependent onset and cessation of action of inhaled budesonide on exhaled nitric oxide and symptoms in mild asthma. Thorax 2002;57(10):889–96.
20. van Rensen EL, Straathof KC, Veselic-Charvat MA, et al. Effect of inhaled steroids on airway hyper-responsiveness, sputum eosinophils, and exhaled nitric oxide levels in patients with asthma. Thorax 1999;54(5):403–8.
21. Recommendations for standardized procedures for the on-line and off-line measurement of exhaled lower respiratory nitric oxide and nasal nitric oxide in adults and children-1999. This official statement of the American Thoracic Society was adopted by the ATS Board of Directors, July 1999. Am J Respir Crit Care Med 1999;160(6):2104–17.
22. Baraldi E, de Jongste JC. European Respiratory Society; American Thoracic Society. Measurement of exhaled nitric oxide in children, 2001. Eur Respir J 2002;20(1):223–37.
23. Pizzimenti S, Bugiani M, Piccioni P, et al. Exhaled nitric oxide measurements: correction equation to compare hand-held device to stationary analyzer. Respir Med 2008;102:1272–5.
24. Khalili B, Boggs PB, Bahna SL. Reliability of a new hand-held device for the measurement of exhaled nitric oxide. Allergy 2007;62(10):1171–4.
25. Hemmingsson T, Linnarsson D, Gambert R. Novel hand-held device for exhaled nitric oxide—analysis in research and clinical applications. J Clin Monit Comput 2004;18(5–6):379–87.

26. Menzies D, Nair A, Lipworth BJ. Portable exhaled nitric oxide measurement: comparison with the gold standard technique. Chest 2007;131(2):410–4.
27. Maniscalco M, de Laurentiis G, Weitzberg E, et al. Validation study of nasal nitric oxide measurements using a hand-held electrochemical analyser. Eur J Clin Invest 2008;38(3):197–200.
28. McGill C, Malik G, Turner SW. Validation of a hand-held exhaled nitric oxide analyzer for use in children. Pediatr Pulmonol 2006;41(11):1053–7.
29. Buchvald F, Baraldi E, Carraro S, et al. Measurements of exhaled nitric oxide in healthy subjects age 4 to 17 years. J Allergy Clin Immunol 2005;115(6):1130–6.
30. Alving K, Janson C, Nordvall L. Performance of a new hand-held device for exhaled nitric oxide measurement in adults and children. Respir Res 2006; 7:67.
31. Baptist AP, Sengupta R, Pranathiageswaran S, et al. Evaluation of exhaled nitric oxide measurements in the emergency department for patients with acute asthma. Ann Allergy Asthma Immunol 2008;5:415–9.
32. Baptist AP, Shah B, Wang Y, et al. Exhaled nitric oxide levels during treatment in patients hospitalized with asthma. Allergy Asthma Proc 2008;29(2):171–6.

Heliox in Airway Management

Jane M. McGarvey, MD*, Charles V. Pollack, MA, MD, FACEP, FAAEM, FAHA

KEYWORDS

- Heliox • Airway management • Helium
- Helium-oxygen

Helium-oxygen ("heliox") mixtures have been used for decades in the treatment of various respiratory problems ranging from acute upper airway obstructions (UAOs) to lower airway derangements, such as asthma and exacerbations of chronic bronchitis. Studies from the 1930s to the present day have measured the impact of heliox use on a variety of outcomes, including peak flow, dyspnea scores, arterial blood gas values, peak airway pressures, exercise performance, and pulmonary function test variables. The data from these studies have often been conflicting and have confounded clinicians as to the specific and ultimate utility of heliox in airway management. Nevertheless, because of helium's unique physical properties, leading to its theoretic improvement of airflow in obstructed airways, interest and research have continued. This review presents a brief history of helium and helium-oxygen mixtures and their potential clinical uses, summarizes the results of past research into heliox in respiratory applications, explains the physiology of heliox, and presents more recent literature relating to heliox in the clinical setting.

HISTORY

The element helium was discovered in 1868 when the French astronomer Janssen observed a bright yellow line in the sun's atmosphere during a total solar eclipse in India. The gas was given its name later that year when the English astronomer Lockyer also observed it in the solar spectrum and, concluding that it was an element in the sun not found on Earth, named it after the Greek word for sun, *helios*. Once its physical properties were delineated, many useful applications for helium became apparent. Helium was found to exist naturally as a gas (except under extreme conditions) and to be lighter than air, making it ideal for filling balloons and airships. Its incombustibility became especially desirable in light of the Hindenburg disaster in 1936, after which helium quickly replaced hydrogen as the gas of choice for dirigibles. The Medical Department of the US Navy was the first organization to use helium in a clinical setting; its low solubility in

Department of Emergency Medicine, Pennsylvania Hospital, 800 Spruce Street, Philadelphia, PA 19107, USA
* Corresponding author.
E-mail address: jane.mcgarvey@uphs.upenn.edu (J.M. McGarvey).

Emerg Med Clin N Am 26 (2008) 905–920
doi:10.1016/j.emc.2008.07.007
0733-8627/08/$ – see front matter © 2008 Elsevier Inc. All rights reserved.

emed.theclinics.com

water made helium a good alternative to nitrogen in reducing the incidence of the nitrogen bubble formation responsible for "decompression sickness," and of "nitrogen narcosis" in underwater diving. The inert property of helium has made it useful in a wide range of applications, ranging from arc welding to gas chromatography and from preserving historical documents to pulmonary function testing and measuring lung volume.

PRIOR RESEARCH

In the 1930s, A.L. Barach tested various mixtures of helium and oxygen, finding benefit across a range of concentrations in asthmatic patients and infants with airway obstruction. He concluded that the low density of helium decreased the work of breathing and significantly improved ventilation. There was a paucity of systematic research on heliox until the 1970s; at that time, investigations into its potential benefit in UAO, postextubation stridor, croup, bronchiolitis, asthma, and chronic obstructive pulmonary disease (COPD) exacerbation showed mixed results.

CURRENT RESEARCH

Research in the past decade has focused on pediatric populations with UAOs and lower airway obstructions (LAOs), particularly asthma. In adults, many case reports and case series have been published on the benefit of heliox in UAO; the only randomized clinical trials have studied the use of heliox in asthma or COPD exacerbations. Other issues of concern include determination of the ideal gas mixture (at least 60% helium seems to be most effective; 80% helium means the gas mixture is hypoxic with respect to room air) and appropriate gas delivery vehicles.

PHYSIOLOGY OF HELIOX

In several studies, heliox has been found to decrease the work of breathing and improve gas delivery to the lungs. A review of the physical properties of helium and some of the laws of physics that apply to respiratory physiology can help to explain these results.

Helium is a colorless, odorless, tasteless, biologically inert, and therefore nontoxic gas. It is the second most abundant element in the universe (after hydrogen) but is relatively rare on Earth, requiring production by radioactive decay of heavier elements. It has the lowest boiling and melting points of all the elements, and therefore exists as a gas except under extreme conditions. Furthermore, helium diffuses rapidly because of its low atomic weight (4 g/mol) (**Table 1**).

The work of breathing is a function of respiratory system compliance and airway resistance. Respiratory system compliance is a static property determined by the elastic recoil of the lung and chest wall. Airway resistance, conversely, is a dynamic property

Table 1 Physical properties of selected respiratory gases				
	Helium	Oxygen	Nitrogen	Air
Density (g/L)	0.1785	1.429	1.2506	1.2929
Molecular weight (g/mol)	4.00	32.00	28.00	28.98
Boiling point (°C)	−268.78	−182.82	−195.65	−194.30
Melting point (°C)	−272.05	−192.65	−209.86	—

determined by several factors, including density and viscosity of the inspired gas, airway caliber and configuration, and flow rate.

The effect of a gas on flow through an airway is determined by several physical principles related to the viscosity and density of the gas. Viscosity is the property of a fluid or gas that affects the resistance of that substance to flow. As with any substance sliding along a surface, the interface of gas with an airway creates a certain amount of friction. These frictional forces cause resistance that produces energy losses, and thus a pressure drop along the airways. The more viscous a substance, the more friction is generated and the greater is the work of breathing for a given gas.

Viscosity also plays an important role in determining the type of airflow that occurs in a given airway: laminar, turbulent, or something in between (known as "transitional flow"). Most airflow through the respiratory tree is laminar. Steady laminar flow through a tube of uniform circular cross section is described by the Hagen-Poiseuille equation:

$$\dot{V} = \left(\pi r^4 \varDelta P\right)/(8\eta L)$$

where $\dot{V}$ indicates the laminar flow, r indicates the radius of the conducting tube, $\varDelta P$ indicates the pressure gradient, η indicates the viscosity of the gas, and L indicates the length of the conducting tube.

As shown in the equation, laminar flow increases with decreasing viscosity and is independent of density.

The lowest possible pressure drop attributable to friction occurs with laminar flow that does not transition to turbulent flow and does not experience "laminar separation." Under these conditions, in a straight tube, the gas particles travel in straight lines at constant velocity when under the influence of a steady-pressure gradient, such as inhalation and exhalation.

When partial airway obstruction occurs, however, airflow can become turbulent. Turbulent flow, as its name implies, is not as orderly as laminar flow. Instead, it is characterized by vortices, eddies, and other types of flow fluctuations. Although turbulent flow is much more complicated than laminar flow, the following equation offers some insight into its physical character:

$$\dot{V} = \left(4\pi r^5 \varDelta P\right)/(\rho L)$$

where ρ indicates density of gas.

As seen in this equation, turbulent flow (unlike laminar flow) is affected by the density (mass per unit volume) of a gas. Therefore, a less dense gas, such as a helium-oxygen mixture, flows better under turbulent conditions because, as seen in the equation, the flow increases or the pressure needed to generate the flow ($\varDelta P$) decreases.

As noted previously, resistance to airflow is attributable to frictional (viscous) forces that cause energy losses, and thus a pressure drop (and resulting decrease in efficiency of gas movement) along the airways. Resistance can be expressed as a pressure drop. The pressure drop along a single airway depends on the dimensions of the airway and the physical properties of the gas flowing through it. Airway dimensions and gas properties are reflected in the Reynolds number (Re). It is a dimensionless number used to predict whether a gas is going to develop a laminar or turbulent flow pattern. It is calculated as follows:

$$\mathrm{Re} = (\rho \mathrm{v} D)/\eta$$

where ρ indicates density, v indicates velocity, D indicates diameter (cm), and η indicates viscosity.

Re is the ratio of inertial forces (density-dependent, viscosity-independent) to viscous forces (viscosity-dependent, density-independent). The lower the Re for a given gas (<2000), the more likely that gas is to maintain laminar flow (because viscous forces, η, dominate over inertial or density-dependent forces). Conversely, the higher the Re, the more likely the gas is to become turbulent.

Bernoulli's principle can be used to describe flow along a streamline within a partially obstructed airway:

$$(P_1 - P_2) = (1/2)(\rho)(v_2^2 - v_1^2)$$

where $(P_1 - P_2)$ is the pressure required to produce flow, ρ is the density of the gas, and $(v_2^2 - v_1^2)$ is the velocity difference between P_1 and P_2.

Because the amount of pressure required to produce flow is directly proportional to the density of the gas, it follows from Bernoulli's principle that less pressure is needed to move the less dense gas, heliox, through a partially obstructed airway than air or oxygen.

In summary, in the lung periphery, gas velocities are low as a result of the large total cross-sectional area of numerous parallel pathways and the flow tends to be laminar with pressure losses proportional to $\dot{V}$ and the gas viscosity. In central airways, the total cross-sectional area is small. This leads to relatively high levels of gas velocity with turbulent flow, and pressure losses are proportional to the square of $\dot{V}$ and to gas density. Thus, there is a tremendous change in Re between the large number of small airways with low flow rate in the lung periphery and the small number of large-diameter airways with much higher flow rates in the central airways.

REVIEW OF CURRENT CLINICAL LITERATURE

In general, most heliox studies are limited by small sample sizes. Additionally, because UAO or severe LAO is generally an emergent condition, there has been a paucity of controlled studies done in these areas.

To assess objectively the value of each of the publications considered here, a classification system is used based on the study type (including case series) and the rigors of the study design (if any). This approach (**Box 1**) is modeled after the classification system used in the *Guidelines for the Acute Medical Management of Severe Traumatic Brain Injury in Infants, Children, and Adolescents*.[1] In each section, data are presented in the order of study classification, with the most reliable studies listed first.

Box 1
Classification of evidence

- Class I evidence represents randomized controlled trials—the "gold standard" of clinical trials. Some may be poorly designed, lack sufficient patient numbers, or have other methodologic inadequacies, however.

- Class II evidence represents nonrandomized clinical studies in which the data were collected prospectively and retrospective studies that were based on clearly reliable data. Types of studies so classified include observational studies, cohort studies, prevalence studies, and case-control studies.

- Class III evidence represents most retrospective studies. Evidence used in this class indicates clinical series, databases, registries, case reviews, case reports, and expert opinion.

RESEARCH ON THE USE OF HELIOX IN CHILDREN

The small anatomy and reactive physiology of infants and young children put them at greater risk for airway obstruction than older children and adults. Their upper and lower airways are small, predisposed to blockage by secretions, and vulnerable to edema and resultant airway narrowing. As noted previously, resistance to laminar airflow increases in inverse proportion to the fourth power of the airway radius (Hagen-Poiseuille's law); therefore, a small decrease in the radius of the airway results in a marked increase in resistance to airflow and the work of breathing. If heliox reduces resistance and improves the flow characteristics of breathing, it is then reasonable to expect heliox to benefit this age group especially.

UPPER AIRWAY OBSTRUCTION

There are many causes of UAO—acute, as in foreign body aspiration or acute epiglottitis, and more insidious in nature, such as a slow-growing mass. Regardless of the cause, UAO can precipitate acute ventilatory failure.[2] Obstruction increases airway resistance, causing increased work of breathing; this eventually leads to respiratory muscle fatigue and the life-threatening problems of hypercapnia and hypoxemia. The obvious goal of removing the obstruction may not always be accomplishable in an expedient manner; heliox may therefore be beneficial as a "therapeutic bridge" until more definitive treatment can be instituted.

Postextubation Stridor

With endotracheal intubation, the airway can become inflamed and swollen around the tube. Postextubation stridor (PES) may prolong length of stay in the recovery room or intensive care unit (ICU), particularly if airway obstruction is severe and reintubation proves necessary. Any therapy that decreases the work of breathing and decreases the need for reintubation is noteworthy.

Kemper and colleagues[3] studied 13 pediatric trauma or burn patients to investigate the benefit of heliox on PES. Heliox and oxygen-enriched room air were given in random order to each patient for 15 minutes after extubation. There were 15 extubations included in the analysis; 7 of those required additional treatment with racemic epinephrine or reintubation. The authors of this class I study reported significant improvement with heliox when compared with the control group, as measured by standard stridor scores (2.8 versus 3.7; $P < .005$), however, and concluded that it may be a useful adjunct in the treatment of pediatric PES.

Jaber and colleagues[4] conducted a prospective study of 18 patients recently extubated. The main end points were effort to breathe (assessed by the transdiaphragmatic pressure swings and the pressure-time index of the diaphragm), comfort, and gas exchange. This class II study showed improvement in the work of breathing and comfort levels with heliox but no significant difference in gas exchange.

Rodeberg and colleagues[5] studied eight pediatric burn patients in whom PES or retractions unresponsive to racemic epinephrine developed. These patients were given helium-oxygen mixtures with an initial helium concentration between 50% and 70%. Of the eight patients, only two experienced respiratory distress and required reintubation. Both of these patients had stridor for a longer time before the initiation of heliox therapy compared with those patients who did not require reintubation, which may have biased the results in this class III report. After initiation of heliox therapy, patients experienced a significant decrease in respiratory distress scores. These researchers concluded that heliox might have a role in relieving persistent stridor, and thereby aid in the prevention of respiratory distress and reintubation.

Polaner[6] presented a case report on the use of heliox and a laryngeal mask airway (LMA) device to avoid endotracheal intubation in an asthmatic child. The child presented with acute UAO attributable to a mediastinal mass, later diagnosed as lymphoma. In this class III report, the investigator argued that the use of heliox with the LMA prevented intubation with paralytics, both of which could exacerbate asthma symptoms.

Croup

Laryngotracheobronchitis, or croup, is the most common cause of UAO in young children.[2] Most life-threatening UAOs are glottic or supraglottic; rarely, however, viral croup (mostly parainfluenza), a subglottic infection, can cause severe respiratory compromise. Traditional advice of exposing the child to a steam-filled bathroom or to "cool night air" is not supported by evidence. Humidification of air may reduce edema of the airway and facilitate clearing of secretions, but the benefits of a vaporizer or mist tent are unproved.

In 1998, Terregino and colleagues[7] performed a randomized study of 15 patients with mild croup symptoms, comparing heliox (70:30 ratio) with oxygen-enriched air. This class I study showed a numeric benefit in croup score for the heliox group, but the difference did not reach statistical significance.

In 2001, Weber and colleagues[8] conducted a prospective, randomized, double-blind trial of 29 children with moderate to severe croup, all of whom first received treatment with humidified oxygen and corticosteroids. The children were then randomized to receive a 70:30 mixture of heliox or racemic epinephrine with supplemental oxygen alone. Clinical effect was evaluated through a modified croup score (skin color, air entry, retractions, level of consciousness, and degree of stridor). Both groups demonstrated improvement in croup score, and there was no significant difference between the two groups in terms of croup score, oxygen saturation, heart rate (HR), or respiratory rate (RR). This class I study demonstrated that heliox administration resulted in similar improvements in clinical measurements as compared with racemic epinephrine. No adverse effects were reported for either group.

In 1999, Smith and Biros[9] reported on five patients, all successfully treated for ventilatory insufficiency with heliox in the emergency department (ED). Three of the patients were children with croup. Measures assessed included stridor score, accessory muscle use, sternal retractions, and oxygen saturation by means of pulse oximetry. One child showed relief of stridor and retractions within 10 seconds of heliox administration. This class III study concluded that heliox may be a useful adjunct to standard therapies in the ED.

LOWER AIRWAY OBSTRUCTION

A study done in 2002 by Piva and colleagues[10] tested 20 children with chronic LAO, randomizing them to heliox or oxygen for ventilatory scintigraphy testing (ie, ventilation/perfusion [V/Q] scan). Results showed better gas distribution (lung deposition) with heliox in those with severe LAO; however, there was no difference between oxygen and heliox in milder obstruction, as designated by prior pulmonary function tests. These findings are supported by the previously reviewed respiratory physiology and the Re ($Re = (\rho v r)/\eta$). The narrower the airway (r), as in patients with the most severe obstruction, the higher was the flow rate (v) and, consequently, the higher was the Re number. This predicts more turbulent flow leading to increased particle deposition in the upper and central airways and, therefore, less penetration into the lungs. With milder obstructions, the airway diameter is not as markedly decreased and there is not a significant change in the flow rate. Therefore, changing the density of the gas (ρ) has less of an impact.

Based on this beneficial effect, Piva and colleagues[10] speculated that heliox may be beneficial in treating children with severe LAO. They cite two controversial issues concerning the use of heliox as being unresolved. One is the problem of using face masks to administer heliox. Because of the volatility of helium, it disperses easily; it is therefore recommended that administration should be through a "closed system." Face masks should be held firmly to minimize leakage, which could dilute the heliox mixture. This may prove difficult in small children, thereby reducing its effectiveness.

The second issue relates to the most efficacious ratio of helium to oxygen. Studies have found that heliox is most effective with an oxygen-to-helium ratio of between 80:20 and 60:40.[11,12] Therefore, the treatment given to patients who have severe LAO necessarily has a low fraction of inspired oxygen (FiO_2), and some amount of hypoxemia occurs. This disadvantage may be offset, however, by the benefit of improving ventilation with a lower density gas. The degree of hypoxemia to be considered safe in such situations is yet to be defined but clearly requires close monitoring in clinical practice.

Bronchiolitis

Respiratory syncytial virus (RSV) bronchiolitis is the most common severe lower respiratory tract infection in infants and young children.

In 2002, Martinon-Torres[13] studied 38 intubated infants in the pediatric intensive care unit (PICU) with moderate to severe RSV bronchiolitis. The first 19 patients admitted received supportive care and nebulized epinephrine. The subsequent 19 patients also received heliox by non-rebreather face mask. This nonrandomized class II study seemed to show that heliox therapy enhanced clinical respiratory status, according to the marked improvement in the patients' clinical scores and the reduction of the accompanying tachycardia and tachypnea. Another measure of improvement was reduced time in the PICU for heliox-treated patients.

In 1998, Hollman and colleagues[14] measured clinical asthma scores,[15] RRs and HRs, and oxygen saturation in 18 nonintubated PICU patients who had tested positive for RSV by rapid immunoassay. Thirteen of the patients were randomized; 5 children with severe bronchiolitis (clinical asthma score >5) were initially treated with heliox and scored after 20 minutes. There was a significant decrease in clinical asthma score in all patients treated with heliox for the duration of the treatment. In patients who had mild to moderate bronchiolitis (clinical asthma score <6), the beneficial effects of helium-oxygen were most pronounced in children with the greatest degree of respiratory compromise. RRs and HRs also improved but not statistically significantly so. The authors of this class I study concluded that heliox improves the overall respiratory status of children with acute RSV lower respiratory tract infection.

In 2000, Gross and colleagues[16] studied 10 mechanically ventilated children with bronchiolitis and found that heliox did not significantly improve gas exchange in these patients. The infants (aged 1–9 months) were mechanically ventilated in synchronized intermittent mandatory ventilation (SIMV) mode. These researchers used varying gas mixtures at 15-minute intervals: 50:50 nitrogen-oxygen, 50:50 heliox, 60:40 heliox, 70:30 heliox, and return to 50:50 nitrogen-oxygen. This class II study showed that neither ventilation nor oxygenation was noticeably improved using helium-oxygen mixtures over a nitrogen-oxygen mixture.

Status Asthmaticus

In 1997, Kudukis and colleagues[17] studied 18 pediatric patients with acute status asthmaticus. All patients received a continuously inhaled nebulized β-agonist and intravenous methylprednisolone. Patients were then randomized to receive inhaled heliox (80:20 ratio) or room air at 10 L/min by non-rebreather face mask for background breathing and in driving the nebulizer. In this class I study, heliox significantly lowered the pulsus paradoxus (PP), increased peak flow, and lessened the dyspnea score. Three of the patients had planned intubation cancelled because of their improvement. These data suggest that early intervention with heliox may relieve dyspnea and improve the work of breathing.

In 1996, Carter and colleagues[18] used a double-blind crossover design to study 11 pediatric inpatients who were admitted for acute asthma exacerbation. Patients were all pretreated with corticosteroids for at least 6 hours before randomized heliox (70:30 ratio) administration. This class I study showed only a small but significant improvement in peak expiratory flow rate (PEFR) and mean midexpiratory flow rate with heliox over oxygen; this result was found only in patients with less severe airway obstruction. The pretreatment with steroids may explain the minimal improvement. These investigators concluded that heliox was not beneficial for the population studied, however, because there was no difference with heliox in the dyspnea scores or the forced expiratory volume in 1 second (FEV_1) in patients with the more severe obstruction. These data are for late heliox administration as an inpatient, as opposed to other studies performed in the ED.

In 2003, Abd-Allah and colleagues[19] performed a retrospective review of 28 mechanically ventilated asthmatic patients, all of whom received helium-oxygen therapy as standard treatment at the study hospital. These investigators found that after patients received inhaled heliox, there was a significant decrease in mean peak inspiratory pressure (PIP; from 40.5 to 35.3 cm H_2O). Mean pH increased significantly (from 7.26 to 7.32), and mean partial pressure carbon dioxide (CO_2) decreased significantly (58.2 to 50.5 mm Hg). The authors of this class III report concluded that heliox is safe and may offer a clinical advantage in mechanically ventilated patients with status asthmaticus.

Adverse Effects

Most studies on the benefits of helium-oxygen mixtures have found no adverse side effects. In 1997, de Gamarra and colleagues[20] began a study of eight nonintubated neonates, four with bronchopulmonary dysplasia, but abandoned the study after immediate changes in behavior (eg, wakening, crying), decrease in skin temperature, and hypoxia with heliox administration. This has not been detected in other studies or reports.

RESEARCH ON THE USE OF HELIOX IN ADULTS
Upper Airway Obstruction

As with the pediatric population, much of the literature on the use of heliox in adults with UAO is limited to case descriptions.

In the previously mentioned 1999 case report by Smith and Biros,[9] two of the five patients were adults who had UAO: one with supraglottitis and one with laryngeal polyps and edema. This class III report examined two adults in severe respiratory distress who were treated in the ED and responded rapidly to heliox, avoiding mechanical ventilation. These investigators reported no adverse effects.

Thyroid masses

In 1997, Milner and colleagues[21] reported on the use of heliox with an LMA to allow for tracheostomy under conscious sedation in an extremely anxious patient. The patient was a 47-year-old woman with a history of Gardner's syndrome (inherited condition characterized by thyroid neoplasms, among other things) and subtotal thyroidectomy for papillary carcinoma 25 years earlier. The patient presented to the hospital with progressive UAO, tachypnea, and marked inspiratory stridor. Lateral soft tissue neck films showed a mass compressing the trachea. A CT scan confirmed a right-sided thyroid mass protruding into the trachea posteriorly. Excision of the mass was deemed to be impossible, and relief of the obstruction was clearly required before radiation. The patient's severe anxiety and the difficulty of surgical access obviated awake tracheostomy. The patient was given heliox (80:20 ratio) by means of a non-rebreathing face mask and reported subjective improvement in dyspnea. Anesthesia was induced with midazolam and small doses of propofol while maintaining spontaneous respirations. A size 3 LMA was inserted, and manual ventilation was started. Pulse oximetry ranged from the preheliox level of 94% to 97% throughout. When heliox was replaced by oxygen alone for insertion of the tracheostomy tube, a subjective increase in dyspnea was noted. These researchers noted that instrumentation of the trachea could have caused tumor hemorrhage and complete airway obstruction and concluded that heliox and the LMA allowed for the safe formation of a stable surgical airway in this patient.

Radiation injury
In 2001, Khanlou and Eiger[22] presented the case of a 69-year-old woman with UAO attributable to bilateral vocal cord paralysis subsequent to radiation therapy. Two days after therapy, she complained of vocal changes and episodic dyspnea. Her HR was noted to be 120 beats per minute, her RR was 26 breaths per minute, and oxygen saturation by pulse oximetry was 88% on room air. She was noted to be using accessory respiratory muscles and to have bilateral decreased breath sounds with audible inspiratory stridor. A chest radiograph showed small bilateral pleural effusions without infiltrates. An arterial blood gas on oxygen (5 L) by means of a non-rebreather face mask showed a pH of 7.35, P_{CO_2} of 45 mm Hg, and P_{O_2} of 64 mm Hg (calculated A-a gradient of 164.95 mm Hg). Bilateral vocal cord paralysis was suspected, and the patient was given heliox (80:20 ratio) with subjective and objective relief of dyspnea within minutes. A repeat arterial blood gas showed a pH of 7.37, P_{CO_2} of 42 mm Hg, and P_{O_2} of 82 mm Hg (calculated A-a gradient of 8.1 mm Hg). An emergency laryngoscopy confirmed the suspected diagnosis, and the patient underwent tracheostomy 4 hours later. In this class III report, these investigators concluded that heliox can be useful in UAO as a temporizing agent to allow time for definitive treatment.

Lymphoma or cancer
In 1988, Hessan and colleagues[23] studied eight adults with lymphoma involving the larynx or trachea. Involvement of the larynx and trachea by lymphoma is an uncommon problem that can cause life-threatening airway obstruction. High-grade obstruction, involvement of the soft tissue of the neck, and tracheal deviation can make intubation and tracheotomy hazardous, if not impossible. In addition, tracheotomy can be ineffective with obstruction of the distal trachea. Using a combination of radiotherapy, chemotherapy, corticosteroids, helium-oxygen mixtures, humidity, and ICU monitoring, these investigators reported a dramatic tumor response with relief of airway symptoms. This class II report showed that direct airway intervention, including tracheotomy, was usually successfully and safely avoided.

Angioedema
In 1989, Boorstein and colleagues[24] reported on the case of a 23-year-old woman with a history of asthma and recurrent tracheal angioedema unresponsive to bronchodilators and steroids and frequently requiring mechanical ventilation. During the episode

of respiratory distress reported on, the patient was given heliox by a non-rebreathing face mask. She improved clinically within minutes; oxygen saturation by means of pulse oximetry improved from 91% to 98%. The patient's condition stabilized, and intubation was not required during the subsequent hospitalization. In this class III report, the investigators concluded that heliox may be beneficial in certain patients as a non-invasive temporizing measure for ventilation around acute UAO.

Vocal cord dysfunction

Vocal cord dysfunction (VCD) is the nonphysiologic paradoxical closure of the true vocal folds on inspiration, with or without closure on expiration. It is a good example of a variable extrathoracic UAO, producing stridor and severe airway obstruction during inspiration but usually no significant obstruction during expiration. VCD has often been misdiagnosed as asthma with resultant mistreatment. Clinical presentation ranges from mild dyspnea to acute severe respiratory distress. The cause of VCD is poorly understood and is thought to be a combination of psychiatric, neurologic, and physiologic factors. Heliox has been found to be extremely effective in relieving some acute presentations of VCD.[25–27] As a therapeutic intervention, heliox does not directly relax the vocal cords but relaxes the patient by decreasing the work of breathing, which then leads to relaxation of the vocal cords.[28]

Lower Airway Obstruction

Asthma: acute exacerbation

In healthy patients, heliox has been shown to decrease airway resistance up to 40% and to increase maximum expiratory flow up to 50%. No such improvement has been observed in patients who have acute asthma, likely because flow limitation occurs in more distal airways, where flow is already laminar. In vitro studies have shown improvement in the PEFR as gas density decreases in airways where flow is turbulent, however.

In 1995, Kass and Castriotta[29] studied 12 adults with severe asthma in an unblinded class I study suggesting positive benefit to early treatment with heliox in adult asthmatics. The 12 patients all had acute respiratory acidosis (pH <7.35 and P_{CO_2} >44 mm Hg). All had been pretreated with 3-5 doses of nebulized albuterol before heliox administration. Five of the patients were mechanically ventilated, and the other 7 had heliox delivered by means of a face mask. All received a mixture of 60% to 70% helium and 30% to 40% oxygen. Results showed that this group had a significant decrease in P_{CO_2} (57.9 to 47.5 mm Hg) and a significant increase in pH (7.23 to 7.32) at a mean of 49.2 minutes after heliox administration. These researchers found that 4 of the patients were nonresponders and that these patients differed significantly from responders in that they had a longer duration of symptoms before treatment ($\geq$ 96 hours) and a higher pretreatment pH. These investigators concluded that heliox can benefit patients who have severe acute asthma with respiratory acidosis and a short duration of symptoms.

In 1999, Kass and Terregino[30] examined 23 adults who presented to a university hospital ED with acute severe asthma symptoms; values measured were PEFR, dyspnea score (a visual analog dyspnea scale from 0–10), HR, RR, and blood pressure (BP). Within 20 minutes of administration of heliox, there was a significant increase in percent of predicted PEFR (%PEFR) as compared with oxygen administration (58% versus 10%). There was also a significant decrease in the dyspnea scores and RR for the heliox group within the first 20 minutes. Additionally, there was a significant improvement in the dyspnea score between the baseline and 480-minute ratings. These researchers state that this is the first randomized controlled trial to demonstrate maintenance of improvement with heliox over 8 hours. One criticism of this class I study, however, is that the peak flow meters were not calibrated; therefore, patients were not known to have started from the same baseline.[31]

Another class I study was performed by Henderson and colleagues[32] in 1999; this study, however, showed no additional benefit from heliox. Over a period of 5 months, 205 patients were enrolled in a prospective single-blind study performed in an urban teaching hospital over a period of 5 months. All patients had mild to moderate asthma exacerbation. One group received three doses of albuterol aerosolized in oxygen 15 minutes apart, and the other group received three doses of albuterol aerosolized in a 70:30 helium-oxygen mixture 15 minutes apart. Although both groups showed significant improvement in PEFR and in FEV_1 from baseline after 45 minutes, the difference between the two groups was clinically and statistically insignificant ($P = .56$).

In 2000, Dorfman and colleagues[33] studied 39 adults, all of whom had experienced moderate to severe asthmatic symptoms for at least 40 hours before treatment in the ED with inhaled heliox versus oxygen. These researchers found no significant benefit in posttreatment %PEF between treatment groups. This was a class I study (unblinded) with all the subjects experiencing symptoms for at least 40 hours before study onset. Because many other studies have suggested better results with early intervention, the delay in treatment onset may have eliminated any potential benefit from heliox.

In 1995, Manthous and colleagues[34] evaluated heliox for its ability to produce a decrease in PP and increase in PEFR. In normal inspiration, the HR is elevated because of increased venous return. PP is an exaggeration of the normal variation in pulse during inspiration and is an important marker in asthmatics because it reflects the decrease in pleural pressure on inspiration attributable to decreased blood flow to the left heart from pulmonary vasodilatation or hyperinflation. The paradox is that clinically, on inspiration, an increase in HR can be detected yet not felt by way of the radial pulse because of this drop in BP. These researchers studied 27 adult asthmatics who presented to the ED with severe asthma exacerbation. This class II study demonstrated improvement in PEFR, decrease in hyperinflation as determined by a decrease in PP, and reduced work of breathing in the heliox group as opposed to controls (oxygen). These investigators concluded that heliox is likely useful for patients who are refractory to bronchodilator therapy or in whom intubation is expected.

In 1999, Schaeffer and colleagues[35] conducted a retrospective chart review of 22 ICU patients with status asthmaticus, all of whom required intubation. This class II study compared treatment with heliox versus treatment with placebo in mechanically ventilated patients. A significant drop in the A-a gradient of the heliox group allowed weaning of FIO_2 to decrease the risk for oxygen toxicity and allow a greater percentage of helium to be used. These researchers surmised that this allows for the full potential of heliox to be realized in even the most severe asthmatics.

In 1990, Gluck and colleagues[36] studied seven mechanically ventilated adults with status asthmaticus who developed a persistent respiratory acidosis associated with high PIP. A 60:40 heliox mixture was used, resulting in a dramatic resolution of the acidosis within 20 minutes. In six of the patients, there was a significant decrease in PIP, also within minutes of heliox administration. No adverse effects were reported.

In 2006, Rodrigo and colleagues[37] published a retrospective review of randomized controlled trials (single- or double-blind) on nonintubated adults and children with acute asthma exacerbations. Pulmonary function testing and clinical end points were used to assess the benefit between heliox and placebo (oxygen or air). These researchers analyzed 10 trials with 544 patients and found that heliox improved pulmonary function only in the subgroup of patients with the most severe baseline impairment. Because this finding is based on a small number of studies, these researchers concluded that the existing evidence does not support the routine use of heliox in all patients who have acute asthma.

Chronic obstructive pulmonary disease: acute exacerbation

Although the use of heliox in COPD has been investigated, few class I studies have been reported. Heliox has been shown to decrease arterial Pco_2 and CO_2 production, increase expiratory airflow, and decrease work of breathing in patients who have severe COPD.[38] These studies were performed using patients who had stable COPD rather than acute exacerbations.

In 2000, deBoisblanc and colleagues[39] studied 50 ED patients with acute exacerbations of COPD randomized to nebulizer treatments driven by heliox versus room air. Equivalency of aerosol delivery was ensured before the clinical trial using a method similar to that of Hess and colleagues.[40] This class I study did not demonstrate any significant physiologic benefits using FEV_1 as the primary end point. There was, however, a small statistically greater improvement in forced midexpiratory flow rate (FEF_{25-75}) between baseline and the 1-hour time point in the heliox group; this difference is of uncertain clinical significance.

In 2001, Gerbeaux and colleagues[41] performed a retrospective analysis over 18 months of 81 patients admitted with COPD exacerbation and respiratory acidosis. Heliox (78% helium, 22% oxygen) was used in 39 patients and not in 42 patients; the choice was not randomized. Standard therapeutic procedures were used equally in both groups (continuous inhaled terbutaline and ipratropium, prednisone [1 mg/kg], intravenous terbutaline, and supplemental oxygen). Mean time between the beginning of COPD exacerbation and ED arrival was 29 ± 19 hours. The authors of this class II study found a significant decrease in the number of intubations (50% versus 8%) and mortality rate (24% versus 3%) in the heliox group. For survivors in the heliox group, the length of ICU stay was also significantly lower (8 ± 6 days versus 18 ± 12 days), as was the total length of in-hospital stay (11 ± 7 days versus 17 ± 13 days).

Patients who have COPD often require positive-pressure mechanical ventilation to manage acute respiratory failure. The mechanical positive pressure, however, may cause hemodynamic changes, especially when incomplete emptying of the lung creates intrinsic positive end-expiratory pressure (PEEPi). PEEPi can lead to hypotension and decreased cardiac output and can also impede gas exchange. In 2005, Lee and colleagues[42] studied 25 consecutive mechanically ventilated patients who had COPD with systolic BP variations greater than 15 mm Hg to evaluate whether or not heliox would improve cardiac performance in these patients.

RR, airway pressure, flow, and inspiratory/expiratory ratio were measured directly from the ventilator. Arterial oxygen saturation was recorded using pulse oximetry. Ten patients had pulmonary artery catheters; right atrial pressure, pulmonary arterial pressure, and pulmonary arterial occlusion pressure were recorded throughout the respiratory cycle and measured at end-expiration in those subjects. HR, cardiac output, and cardiac index were also recorded. These researchers found in this class II study that mean pulmonary arterial pressure, right atrial pressure, and pulmonary arterial occlusion pressure all showed a statistically significant reduction when the subjects were breathing heliox. In addition, cardiac index increased by greater than 20% in the heliox group. There were no statistically significant changes in HR, mean arterial pressure, Pao_2, $Paco_2$, or pH between the control and heliox groups. Measurements of left ventricular performance improved: ΔPP (respiratory changes in systolic pressure variations) decreased by greater than 50% during heliox breathing and minimal pulse pressure (PP_{min}) occurring during expiration also increased significantly. Peak airway pressure, plateau pressure, PEEPi, and trapped lung volume at end-expiration ($V_{trapped}$), also known as functional residual capacity (FRC), all decreased significantly during heliox ventilation. Tassaux and colleagues[43] conducted a similar study but found no increase in cardiac performance; Lee and colleagues surmised that this may have been because their patients had less severe dynamic hyperinflation (75% of Lee and colleagues' subjects had PEEPi ≥ 10 cm H_2O compared with only 33% in the study by Tassaux and colleagues). These researchers concluded that heliox may be a useful addition to conventional therapies to improve cardiac performance in patients who have COPD with refractory PEEPi-associated hemodynamic changes.

Heliox with noninvasive pressure support ventilation (NIPSV) has been shown to reduce dyspnea, $Paco_2$, and the work of breathing more than NIPSV with air or oxygen in decompensated COPD. In 2003, Jolliet and colleagues[44] studied 123 ICU patients admitted with severe COPD exacerbation to evaluate whether it could also have beneficial consequences on outcome and hospitalization costs. Results of this class I study showed that there was no significant difference in intubation rate or length of stay in the ICU. The post-ICU hospital stay was shorter with helium-oxygen (air-oxygen for 19 $\pm$ 12 days versus helium-oxygen 13 $\pm$ 6 days; $P < .002$), and although cost of NIPSV gases was higher with heliox, the total hospitalization costs were lower by $3348 per patient with heliox. No complications were reported with heliox use. These researchers concluded that heliox NIPSV is safe and could prove to be cost-effective but cited as weaknesses of their study the fact that investigators were not blinded to treatment, that NIPSV/mechanical ventilation/weaning was not subject to a strict protocol, and that hospital (although not ICU) discharge did not follow practice guidelines.

Aerosol delivery
One complaint regarding heliox studies is that most allow room air entrainment (RAE) during aerosol delivery.[45] It is thought that RAE could significantly decrease the helium concentration to the point of diminishing its effect on reduction of turbulent gas flow and oxygen-drug delivery, thus raising questions as to the conclusions drawn in these studies. A few trials have used closed systems for gas delivery[18,46] and have demonstrated improvement in the study variables with heliox.

SUMMARY

Overall, the data continue to be inconclusive regarding the overall benefit of heliox in UAO and LAO; however, the following areas seem to be supported in the literature.

Heliox, because of its lower density than air or oxygen regardless of the concentration of helium in the mixture, increases gas particle deposition and improves air flow through constricted passageways by transforming turbulent flow into laminar flow; some studies have shown a concomitant decrease in the work of breathing. Benefits have been seen in intubated and nonintubated patients and in adults and children. Benefits are seen quickly, usually within an hour of initiation of treatment. All the studies on adults have shown no adverse effects from using heliox.

There have been disadvantages to the use of heliox cited in the literature. Heliox is more expensive than oxygen or room air. Also, special equipment may be required, such as premixed tanks, or training may be necessary on how to blend mixtures and avoid RAE. In intubated patients, tidal volumes recorded by the ventilator are not accurate, because flow meters are calibrated for oxygen-nitrogen rather than for oxygen-helium. Finally, heliox is an inert gas with no inherent therapeutic effects; therefore, it is not a definitive treatment. It is a temporizing measure to allow conventional treatments time to work.

REFERENCES

1. Adelson PD, Bratton SL, Carney NA, et al. Guidelines for the acute medical management of severe traumatic brain injury in infants, children, and adolescents. Introduction. Pediatr Crit Care Med 2003;4:S2–4.
2. Mason RJ. Murray and Nadel's textbook of respiratory medicine. 4th edition. Acute ventilatory failure.
3. Kemper KJ, Ritz RH, Benson MS, et al. Helium-oxygen mixture in the treatment of postextubation stridor in pediatric trauma patients. Crit Care Med 1991;19:356–9.
4. Jaber S, Carlucci A, Boussarsar M, et al. Helium-oxygen in the postextubation period decreases inspiratory effort. Am J Respir Crit Care Med 2001;164:633–7.
5. Rodeberg DA, Easter AJ, Washam MA, et al. Use of a helium-oxygen mixture in the treatment of postextubation stridor in pediatric patients with burns. J Burn Care Rehabil 1995;16:476–80.
6. Polaner DM. The use of heliox and the laryngeal mask airway in a child with an anterior mediastinal mass. Anesth Analg 1996;82:208–10.
7. Terregino CA, Nairn SJ, Chansky ME, et al. The effect of heliox on croup: a pilot study. Acad Emerg Med 1998;5:1130–3.
8. Weber JE, Chudnofsky CR, Younger JG, et al. A randomized comparison of helium-oxygen mixture (Heliox) and racemic epinephrine for the treatment of moderate to severe croup. Pediatrics 2001;107:E96.
9. Smith SW, Biros M. Relief of imminent respiratory failure from upper airway obstruction by use of helium-oxygen: a case series and brief review. Acad Emerg Med 1999;6:953–6.
10. Piva JP, Menna Barreto SS, Zelmanovitz F, et al. Heliox vs. oxygen for nebulized aerosol therapy in children with lower airway obstruction. Pediatr Crit Care Med 2002;3:6–10.
11. Tobias JD. Heliox in children with airway obstruction. Pediatr Emerg Care 1997;13:29–32.
12. Houck JR, Keamy MF III, McDonough JM. Effect of helium concentration on experimental upper airway obstruction. Ann Otol Rhinol Laryngol 1990;99:556–61.
13. Martinon-Torres F. Heliox therapy in infants with acute bronchiolitis. Pediatrics 2002;109:68–73.
14. Hollman G, Shen G, Zeng L, et al. Helium-oxygen improves clinical asthma scores in children with acute bronchiolitis. Crit Care Med 1998;26:1731–6.
15. Wood DW, Downes JJ, Lecks HI. A clinical scoring system for the diagnosis of respiratory failure. Am J Dis Child 1972;123:227–8.
16. Gross MF. Helium-oxygen mixture does not improve gas exchange in mechanically ventilated children with bronchiolitis. Crit Care Med 2000;4:3.
17. Kudukis TM, Manthous CA, Schmidt GA, et al. Inhaled helium-oxygen revisited: effect of inhaled helium-oxygen during the treatment of status asthmaticus in children. J Pediatr 1997;130:217–24.
18. Carter ER, Webb CR, Boffitt DR. Evaluation of heliox in children hospitalized with acute severe asthma. A randomized crossover trial. Chest 1996;109:1256–61.
19. Abd-Allah SA, Rogers MS, Terry M, et al. Helium-oxygen therapy for pediatric acute severe asthma requiring mechanical ventilation. Pediatr Crit Care Med 2003;4:353–7.
20. de Gamarra E, Moriette G, Farhat M, et al. Heliox® tolerance in spontaneously breathing neonates with bronchopulmonary dysplasia. Biol Neonate 1998;74:193–9.
21. Milner QJ, Abdy S, Allen JG. Management of severe tracheal obstruction with helium/oxygen and a laryngeal mask airway. Anaesthesia 1997;52:1087–9.
22. Khanlou H, Eiger G. Safety and efficacy of heliox as a treatment for upper airway obstruction due to radiation-induced laryngeal dysfunction. Heart Lung 2001;30:146–7.

23. Hessan H, Houck J, Harvey H. Airway obstruction due to lymphoma of the larynx and trachea. Laryngoscope 1988;98:176–80.
24. Boorstein JM, Boorstein SM, Humphries GN, et al. Using helium-oxygen mixtures in the emergency management of acute upper airway obstruction. Ann Emerg Med 1989;18:688–90.
25. Weir M. Vocal cord dysfunction mimics asthma and may respond to heliox. Clin Pediatr 2002;41:37–41.
26. Weir M, Ehl L. Vocal cord dysfunction mimicking exercise-induced broncho-spasm in adolescents. Pediatrics 1997;99:923–4.
27. Gose JE. Acute workup of vocal cord dysfunction. Ann Allergy Asthma Immunol 2003;91:318.
28. Hicks M, Brugman SM, Katial R. Vocal cord dysfunction/paradoxical vocal fold motion. Clinics in Office Practice. Prim Care 2008;35:81–103.
29. Kass JE, Castriotta RJ. Heliox therapy in acute severe asthma. Chest 1995;107:757–60.
30. Kass JE, Terregino CA. The effect of heliox in acute severe asthma: a randomized controlled trial. Chest 1999;116:296–300.
31. Carter ER. Heliox for Acute Severe Asthma. Chest 2000;117:1212–3.
32. Henderson SO, Acharya P, Kilaghbian T. Use of heliox-driven nebulizer therapy in the treatment of acute asthma. Ann Emerg Med 1999;33:141–6.
33. Dorfman TA, Shipley ER, Burton JH, et al. Inhaled heliox does not benefit ED pa-tients with moderate to severe asthma. Am J Emerg Med 2000;18:495–7.
34. Manthous CA, Hall JB, Caputo MA, et al. Heliox improves pulsus paradoxus and peak expiratory flow in nonintubated patients with severe asthma. Am J Respir Crit Care Med 1995;151:310–4.
35. Schaeffer EM, Pohlman A, Morgan S, et al. Oxygenation in status asthmaticus improves during ventilation with helium-oxygen. Crit Care Med 1999;27:2666–70.
36. Gluck EH, Onorato DJ, Castriotta R. Helium-oxygen mixtures in intubated patients with status asthmaticus and respiratory acidosis. Chest 1990;98:693–8.
37. Rodrigo G, Pollack CV, Rodrigo C, et al. Heliox for nonintubated acute asthma patients. Cochrane Database Syst Rev 2006;(4):CD002884.
38. Swidwa DM, Montenegro HD, Goldman MD, et al. Helium oxygen breathing in severe chronic obstructive pulmonary disease. Chest 1985;87:790–5.
39. deBoisblanc BP, DeBleiux P, Resweber S, et al. Randomized trial of the use of he-liox as a driving gas for updraft nebulization of bronchodilators in the emergent treatment of acute exacerbations of chronic obstructive pulmonary disease. Crit Care Med 2000;28:3177–80.
40. Hess DR, Acosta FL, Ritz RH, et al. The Effect of heliox on nebulizer function using a beta-agonist bronchodilator. Chest 1999;115:184–9.
41. Gerbeaux P, Gainnier M, Boussuges A, et al. Use of heliox in patients with severe exacerbation of chronic obstructive pulmonary disease. Crit Care Med 2001;29:2322–4.
42. Lee DL, Lee H, Chang H-W, et al. Heliox improves hemodynamics in mechani-cally ventilated patients with chronic obstructive pulmonary disease with systolic pressure variations. Crit Care Med 2005;33:968–73.
43. Tassaux D, Jolliet P, Roeseler J, et al. Effects of helium-oxygen on intrinsic positive end-expiratory pressure in intubated and mechanically ventilated patients with se-vere chronic obstructive pulmonary disease. Crit Care Med 2000;28:2721–8.
44. Jolliet P, Tassaux D, Roeseler J, et al. Helium-oxygen versus air-oxygen noninva-sive pressure support in decompensated chronic obstructive disease: a prospec-tive, multicenter study. Crit Care Med 2003;31:878–84.

45. Dhuper S, Choksi S, Selveraj S, et al. Room air entrainment during β-agonist delivery with heliox. Chest 2006;130:1063–71.
46. Kress JP, Noth I, Gehlbach BK, et al. The utility of albuterol nebulized with heliox during acute asthma exacerbations. Am J Respir Crit Care Med 2002;165:1317–21.

Advances with Surfactant

David C. Turell, MD, FAAP

KEYWORDS

- Surfactant • Respiratory distress syndrome
- Meconium aspiration syndrome
- Acute lung injury • Acute respiratory distress syndrome
- Surfactant-associated proteins
- Bronchopulmonary dysplasia
- Surfactant replacement therapy

Surfactant is a biologic agent found in the lungs that reduces surface tension, allowing for adequate respiration. This compound was discovered in the early twentieth century. Its use has had a dramatic impact in the field of neonatology, namely in the treatment of Respiratory Distress Syndrome (RDS) and Meconium Aspiration Syndrome (MAS). These pulmonary conditions are caused by a primary surfactant deficiency and surfactant inactivation, respectively. Recent research has focused on secondary surfactant deficiency as a result of lung injury from a variety of medical conditions.

In this article, the physiology of surfactant is reviewed along with the research that lead to its current clinical uses. Acute lung injury (ALI) and Acute Respiratory Distress Syndrome (ARDS) will also be reviewed because they represent a pulmonary disease process in which secondary deficiency and surfactant inactivation occur, and for which surfactant may prove to be an effective treatment. Finally, research using surfactant as a treatment for other pulmonary diseases, such as bronchiolitis and asthma, will be briefly highlighted. These studies may one day lead to new treatment opportunities in the realm of emergency medicine.

HISTORY

The physiologic concept of resistance to lung expansion as a result of surface tension was discovered by von Neergaard in 1929.[1,2] During the next few decades, research revealed the source of surfactant—the alveolar lining of the lungs—and its chemical characteristics.[3] Avery and Mead[4] reported in 1959 that saline extracts from the lungs of preterm infants with RDS lacked the low surface tension characteristic of pulmonary surfactant.

In the latter part of the twentieth century, especially as seen in the Vietnam War, soldiers with traumatic injuries resulting in significant blood loss reached medical care

Pediatric Urgent Care, Department of General Pediatrics, Children's Hospital, Cleveland Clinic, 9500 Euclid Avenue, Desk M73, Cleveland, OH 44195, USA
E-mail address: turelld@ccf.org

Emerg Med Clin N Am 26 (2008) 921–928
doi:10.1016/j.emc.2008.08.001
0733-8627/08/$ – see front matter © 2008 Elsevier Inc. All rights reserved.

with increasing speed because of the use of helicopters as air ambulances. In previous wars, many soldiers died either from direct injuries or indirectly from ones that resulted in massive blood loss before they could reach medical care. Many developed "shock lung"—a pulmonary deficiency seen in patients with significant injuries who develop hemorrhagic shock requiring blood transfusion even in the absence of direct thoracic trauma. Pathologic analysis of the lungs showed evidence of atelectasis. The lungs also contained fluid with high concentrations of protein. Expansion of the alveoli was achieved, but only at higher-than-expected pressures.[5]

PHYSIOLOGY

Surfactant is a chemical compound composed of phospholipids (90%) and proteins (10%). The main lipid component is saturated dipalmitoyl phosphatidylcholine (DPPC). The remaining lipids include free cholesterol and negatively charged phospholipids. Four surfactant-associated proteins (SP) have been identified and designated as SP-A, SP-B, SP-C, and SP-D. They are produced by and secreted from type II alveolar cells and Clara cells of the respiratory epithelium.[6,7] The hydrophilic character of SP-B and SP-C aids in the spread of surfactant within the terminal airway.[2] More recently, it has been discovered that the surface tension of conducting airways is about 15 mJ/m^2 in between the known extremes of 2 mJ/m^2 at the level of the alveoli and 32 mJ/m^2 at the trachea. This supports the concept that surface tension is regulated along the entire length of the airways of the respiratory tract and not just at the alveoli.[8]

The function of surfactant is twofold. First and most notably, it reduces surface tension in the alveoli, thereby stabilizing lung volume at low transpulmonary pressures. Laplace's law, $\Delta P = 2\gamma/r$, states that there is an inverse relationship between surface tension, γ, and the alveolar radius, r. The pressure gradient, ΔP, required to overcome the alveolar collapsing effect of surface tension would then rapidly become larger as the alveolar radius decreases during expiration.[9] In circumstances of surfactant deficiency or inactivation, larger alveoli overexpand to compensate for the collapse of the small alveoli, increasing the risk for pneumothorax. Surfactant replacement equalizes the pressures exerted on the different-sized alveoli and thus reduces the incidence of air leak and increases lung volumes. This, in turn, significantly increases the functional residual capacity of the lungs.[10]

In 2003, Prange[11] refuted the longstanding theory that Laplace's law fully explained the physics of the lungs at the level of alveoli, which were thought to be spherically shaped. In fact, each alveolus is polygonal rather than spherical in shape and is bound to another by connective tissue. They are grouped together in clusters that have an overall spherical appearance. Prange's research revealed that there must be additional physical forces to explain the mechanical workings of the alveoli.

Surfactant's secondary function, of equal importance, is to enhance macrophage activity as well as mucocilliary clearance, both of which enhance the lungs' defense against bacteria and viruses.[12] The apoproteins SP-A and SP-D have been shown to have effects on the inflammatory response of phagocytes and the regulation of pneumatocytes. These surfactant proteins are members of the collectin protein family. The most well-defined function of the collectins is to opsonize pathogens. They have carbon and nitrogen domains that are unique to carbohydrates found on nonhost bacteria and viruses.

Last, exogenous surfactant replacement does not inhibit the endogenous production and secretion of surfactant. The surfactant is absorbed slowly into lung tissues and then catabolized. Phospholipids are available as substrates in surfactant recycling pathways. This was first seen in studies on premature rabbits.[13]

PAST CLINICAL RESEARCH

Decades after surfactant was discovered to influence surface tension, clinical studies were performed to determine whether it could be used as a treatment for neonates with respiratory distress syndrome (RDS) since they have a primary deficiency of this substance. The American Academy of Pediatrics promoted such research to reduce mortality rates in prematurely born babies with respiratory insufficiency. In 1981, Notter and Shapiro[6] reviewed the current knowledge of surfactant to foster clinical studies on exogenous surfactant therapy and determine the best administration technique as well as the most effective form.

RDS is respiratory insufficiency seen in premature infants owing to an absolute surfactant deficiency. Oxygen support and mechanical ventilation are typically required. The major acute pulmonary complications of RDS are pneumothorax and pulmonary interstitial emphysema. The chronic lung disease that can result from prolonged oxygen exposure at high pressures is bronchopulmonary dysplasia (BPD).[14] The only consistently noted complication of surfactact use is pulmonary hemorrhage. The incidence of pulmonary hemorrhage in very low birth weight (VLBW) neonates with RDS is 5% to 7%, with an associated mortality rate of 50%.[15]

In 1990, Fujiwara and colleagues[16] administered surfactant to premature infants with RDS. The results showed that it reduced pulmonary morbidity, decreased the fraction of inspired oxygen (FIO_2) and mean arterial pressure (MAP) and significantly decreased the incidence of pulmonary interstitial emphysema and pneumothorax. Serial chest radiographs revealed consistent improvement in the surfactant replacement group. The author also noted that when the total duration of oxygen therapy was reduced, the number of infants who developed BPD decreased. With the introduction of Surfactant Replacement Therapy (SRT) in 1990, infant mortality rates significantly dropped. This was attributed primarily to fewer deaths from respiratory causes among preterm infants.

Pulmonary hemorrhage (PH) is a severe complication of RDS, but it is also a consistently noted complication of surfactant use. SRT results in a 47% increase in risk of PH, but this risk is considered small compared with the documented benefits of surfactant treatment for RDS. A study by Pandit and colleagues[17] in 1995 showed that despite the known risks of SRT on RDS, surfactant could still be used to overcome the surfactant insufficiency state, resulting in short-term improvements in oxygenation and ventilation. He postulated that there might be similar benefits in ARDS or other pulmonary injury/inflammation seen in children or adults.

MAS is also a significant cause of respiratory insufficiency in neonates. Meconium is a greenish-black viscous substance consisting of fetal waste products excreted from the ileum. Meconium aspiration is defined as the presence of meconium below the vocal cords. Meconium is released prematurely via the rectum, typically a result of some fetal insult or stress such as hypoxia or acidosis, acute or chronic. There are multiple mechanisms of respiratory insufficiency in MAS, but this article will focus only on surfactant. MAS is caused by surfactant inactivation and secondary surfactant deficiency. Surfactant is inactivated when it is exposed to the proteins and fatty acids found within the meconium. Synthesis of surfactant may decrease as well. This contributes to atelectasis, decreased lung compliance, intrapulmonary shunting, and hypoventilation.[18]

In 1990, Moses and colleagues[19] discovered that surfactant inactivation is related to both the consistency of the meconium and the concentration of the surfactant itself. This information suggested that preterm infants who aspirated thick meconium might benefit from treatment with exogenous surfactant. A small randomized trial showed that delivery of an intermittent bolus of high-dose surfactant improved oxygenation; resolved persistent pulmonary hypertension; and decreased the number of air leaks, need for extra-corporeal membrane oxygenation, and the duration of mechanical ventilation.[20]

Surfactant deficiency may also play a role in a potentially life-threatening syndrome seen in adults. Initially described as adult respiratory distress syndrome in the adult medical literature, ARDS is a diffuse inflammatory process that involves both lungs.[21] The American-European Consensus Conference on ARDS convened in 1994 and established diagnostic criteria for ALI and ARDS.[22] These five criteria include the following:

1. Acute onset of respiratory insufficiency.
2. Presence of a predisposing condition including intracranial hypertension, blood product transfusions, pneumonia, pulmonary contusion, cardiopulmonary bypass, sepsis, amniotic fluid embolus, and long-bone fracture.[22]
3. Bilateral infiltrates on frontal chest x-ray.
4. Severe hypoxemia evidenced by PaO_2/FiO_2 less than 200 mm Hg for ARDS, less than 300 mm Hg for ALI. ALI is a less severe form of ARDS, distinguished by the PaO_2/FiO_2 ratio.
5. Pulmonary artery occlusion (wedge) pressure less than 18 mm Hg or no clinical evidence of left atrial hypertension. Left-sided heart failure is not present.

These clinical criteria are not specific to ALI, and ARDS and can be seen with other causes of acute respiratory failure.

Surfactant production decreases during diffuse lung injury, presumably because the alveolar epithelium becomes damaged. This secondary surfactant deficiency may contribute to the disordered mechanical behavior of the lung in ARDS.[23] Systemic activation of circulating neutrophils subsequently results in damage to the epithelium of the capillaries at the alveoli-capillary interface. These leaky capillaries introduce exudate into the lung parenchyma, setting off an inflammatory cascade that leads to progressive respiratory insufficiency. The surfactant insufficiency seen in ALI/ARDS, similar to MAS, is caused by exposure to proteins. In ALI/ARDS, however, the source of proteins is the exudative exposure owing to capillary permeability. Fibrin deposition also occurs and is another characteristic of ARDS. This causes the pulmonary fibrosis that contributes to the decrease in lung compliance that is seen.[23]

CURRENT USES OF SURFACTANT

Surfactant is used routinely by neonatologists as a supportive adjunct for neonates with RDS and MAS. These patients can have severe hypoxemia and associated respiratory distress requiring respiratory support (eg, endotracheal intubation and mechanical ventilation). Intratracheal instillation of surfactant is performed to bathe the pulmonary tree and reduce surface tension, thereby decreasing the need for respiratory support. This is not a curative measure but rather a temporizing one.

There are two main types of surfactant that have been studied. Natural surfactant is the only type currently in use for patient care.[24,25] It is recovered from alveolar lavage or amniotic fluid. The other surfactant type is synthetic or recombinant surfactant. The first-generation synthetic surfactants were protein free. Because of the significant difference noted in efficacy between the two types, natural surfactants (eg, poractant alfa, calfactant, and beractant) are the only surfactants available for treatment. Investigations are under way to analyze newer synthetic surfactants whose components mimic the proteins and peptides found in natural surfactant.[26]

The doses and administration techniques were developed empirically from experience with animal models of RDS. The usual dose is 100 mg phospholipid per kilogram of body weight. The surfactant is suspended in 3 to 5 mL of saline per kilogram and delivered directly into the airway in divided aliquots through an endotracheal tube.[3] When newborn infants are in significant respiratory distress, they require mechanical ventilation at high pressures, which eases the administration of Surfactant Replacement Therapy (SRT). In contrast, when infants requiring low-pressure ventilation are treated with SRT, acute airway obstruction can occur. This complication is a result of the relatively large volume of fluid in the surfactant dose.

Surfactant is instilled through the endotracheal tube or by infusion through a side-hole adapter. Neither delivery mode is more advantageous than the other. Aerosolization of surfactant and continuous positive airway pressure assisted delivery of surfactant have been studied as a means to deliver surfactant to the lungs without the need for intubation. These techniques have not yet been proven to be effective.[26]

Two strategies have been used for treatment. Surfactant can be instilled prophylactically in premature babies at risk for developing RDS. Treatment is used to prevent the onset if respiratory insufficiency is caused by surfactant deficiency or surfactant inactivation. The other strategy is to wait to use surfactant until the diagnosis of RDS is established, which usually occurs before 24 hours of life. Subsequent human trials have established that the most beneficial timing for SRT is approximately 2 to 4 hours after birth. Delivery room SRT is reserved for the smallest infants at the highest risk of RDS because they are at a higher risk of complications.[26]

Multidose surfactant therapy can overcome surfactant inactivation. Exogenous surfactant is not lost when instilled into the lungs. Each additional treatment has been shown to further improve oxygenation and reduce the overall time of ventilatory support. The OSIRIS (open study of infants at high risk of or with respiratory insufficiency—the role of surfactant) study published in *The Lancet* in 1992 found that a two-dose treatment regimen was equivalent to multidose regimens of up to four doses.[27] The SRT is administered every 12 hours when given in multiple doses. Therapy is individualized based on the persistence of residual respiratory insufficiency risking pneumothorax or prolonged ventilatory support.[3]

RECENT CLINICAL RESEARCH

Animal studies were performed from 1995 to 1996 by Liu and colleagues[28,29] to determine the potential benefit of SRT in patients with asthma. Aeroallergens were introduced to the respiratory tract of guinea pigs after their lungs were sensitized with ovalbumin. This caused proteins to leak into the airways. The increase in airway resistance and decreased surfactant performance was consistent with surfactant dysfunction. Lung function declined less in the animals that received prophylactic treatment with surfactant.

It has also been shown that eosinophils produce lysophospholipase (LPLase), an enzyme that hydrolyzes pulmonary surfactant to an extent, which reduces its effectiveness.[30] In rat and rabbit fetus studies, treatment with B_2-adrenergic agonists released surfactant from alveoli, which then was extruded into the terminal-conducting airways.[31,32] Within the next few years, human trials had similar results in patients with asthma. Inflammatory proteins were proven to inactivate surfactant in asthmatic patients.[7]

In 1996, Novick and colleagues,[33] as part of the Transplantation-Immunobiology Group, reported that the lungs can become injured during lung transplant surgery when they are reperfused. This is the same mechanism of lung injury seen in extracorporeal mechanical oxygenation (ECMO) and the phenomenon previously described as "shock lung." Pulmonary ischemia results in direct injury to surfactant-producing cells. Upon reperfusion, within 10 to 18 hours after transfusion, pulmonary insufficiency typically develops. This correlates with a depletion of surfactant stores. Neutrophils release inflammatory mediators and produce superoxide anions, which can directly injure pulmonary endothelium, allowing proteins to enter into the pulmonary capillary beds.[33,34] Decreased production and inactivation of surfactant results in a surfactant deficiency and alteration of lung mechanics.

A pediatric study was performed in 1996 by Dargaville and colleagues[35] to determine whether there were any surfactant abnormalities in infants with acute viral bronchiolitis (AVB). Two groups of patients underwent alveolar lavage; one had been diagnosed with acute viral bronchiolitis and the other had no lung disease. The study measured SP-A and DPPC levels and documented overall surfactant functionality. All of the AVB infants were comparatively deficient in SP-A and DPPC. The AVB group also showed evidence of surfactant inactivation as a result of exudative protein exposure. In 2000, a randomized, controlled study in infants with RSV bronchiolitis showed definite improvements in oxygenation and ventilation after treatment with exogenous surfactant.[36]

Also in 2000, Mora and colleagues[37] conducted animal trials to induce injury to the lung endothelium similar to that seen in ALI/ARDS. Nebulized lipopolysaccharide (LPS) was administered to guinea pigs to reproduce lung injury caused by the neutrophil response to bacterial endotoxin. After 48 hours, lung mechanics were altered, and a surfactant deficiency was confirmed. The authors reported that instillation of surfactant was not as effective at maintaining lung function as had been hypothesized. They speculated that performing alveolar lavage before instilling surfactant might remove inflammatory mediators that are suspected to inhibit surfactant function.

Spragg and colleagues[38] performed a randomized, double-blinded, controlled prospective study in 2004 in which a protein C–based synthetic surfactant was administered to patients with ARDS. The treatment improved oxygenation within 24 hours; however, this did not reduce the number of days patients spent on mechanical ventilation or mortality rates. It was postulated that multidose treatment could lead to further improvements.[39]

A multicenter, randomized, blinded pediatric study by Wilson and colleagues[40,41] in 2005 used calfactant—a natural lung surfactant characterized by its high concentration of SP-B—in 153 children with ALI. SRT improved oxygenation and overall mortality, but failed to reduce the patients' ICU and hospital stays and time spent on a mechanical ventilator.

SUMMARY/SPECULATIVE USES IN EMERGENCY MEDICINE

The past century has yielded enormous medical advances. The discovery of surfactant has altered the field of neonatology, resulting in a significant reduction in neonatal mortality caused by respiratory insufficiency. Over the past 20 years, much attention has been given by the scientific and medical communities to exogenous surfactant and how it can be used as a therapy for pediatric and adult patients. So far, most clinical research in the fields of pediatrics, critical care, anesthesiology, and surgery has focused on using surfactant in the postoperative period or in cases of trauma or infection. Additionally, the use of SRT in patients with either surfactant deficiency or inactivation caused by inflammatory lung injury could turn out to be a significant area of clinical research in the field of emergency medicine. Can a patient presenting to an emergency department with an inflammatory lung condition, acute lung injury, or at a high risk to develop ARDS be treated with exogenous surfactant to avert significant pulmonary insufficiency and its subsequent medical and pharmacologic interventions, some of which have their own inherent risks? Further research and clinical trials will help us answer these questions.

REFERENCES

1. von Neergaard K. Neue auffassungen uber einen grundhegriff der atermmechanik: Retracktionskraft der lunge, abhangig von der berflachenspunning alveolen. Z Gestamte Exp Med 1929;66:373–94 [in German].
2. Warren WH. Is there a role for surfactant replacement therapy in adult pulmonary dysfunction? Crit Care Med 1998;26(10):1626–7.
3. Jobe AH. Natural surfactant and the surfactants in clinical use. N Engl J Med 1993;328(12):861–8.
4. Avery ME, Mead J. Surface properties in relation to atelectasis and hyaline membrane disease. Am J Dis Child 1959;97:517–23.
5. Bergofsky FH. Pulmonary insufficiency after nonthoracic trauma: shock lung. Am J Med Sci 1972;264(2):92–101.
6. Notter RH, Shapiro DL. Lung surfactant in an era of replacement therapy. Pediatrics 1981;68(6):781–9.
7. Hohlfeld JM. The role of surfactant in asthma. Respir Res 2002;3(1):1076–86.
8. Baritussio A. Lung surfactant, asthma, and allergens. Am J Respir Crit Care Med 2004;169:550–1.
9. Enhorning G, Chamberlain D, Contreras C, et al. Isoxsuprine-induced release of pulmonary surfactant in the rabbit fetus. Am J Obstet Gynecol 1977;129: 197–202.
10. Goldsmith LS, Greenspan JS, Rubenstein SD, et al. Immediate improvement in lung volume after exogenous surfactant: alveolar recruitment versus increased distension. J Pediatr 1991;119:424–8.
11. Prange H. LaPlace's law and the alveolus: a misconception of anatomy and a misunderstanding of physics. Adv Physiol Educ 2003;27:34–40.
12. Wright JR. Pulmonary surfactant: a front line of lung host defense. J Clin Invest 2003;111(10):1453–5.
13. Stewart-DeHaan PJ, Metcalfe IL, Harding PGR, et al. Effect of birth and surfactant treatment on phospholipid synthesis in the premature rabbit lungs. Biol Neonate 1980;38:238–47.
14. Northway WH Jr, Rosan RC, Porter DY. Pulmonary disease following respirator therapy of hyaline-membrane disease. bronchopulmonary dysplasia. N Engl J Med 1967;276(7):357–68.
15. Raju TN, Langenberg P. Pulmonary hemorrhage and exogenous surfactant therapy: a metaanalysis. J Pediatr 1993;123(4):603–10.
16. Fujiwara T, Konishi M, Chida S, et al. Surfactant replacement with a single postventilatory dose of reconstituted bovine surfactant in preterm neonates with respiratory distress syndrome: final analysis of a multicenter, double-blind, randomized trial and comparison with similar trials. Pediatrics 1990;86(5): 753–64.
17. Pandit PB, Dunn MS, Colucci EA. Surfactant therapy in neonates with respiratory deterioration due to pulmonary hemorrhage. Pediatrics 1995;95(1):32–6.
18. Klingner MC, Kruse J. Meconium aspiration syndrome: pathophysiology and prevention. J Am Board Fam Pract 1999;12(6):450–66.

19. Moses D, Holm BA, Spitale P, et al. Inhibition of pulmonary surfactant function by meconium. Am J Obstet Gynecol 1991;164:477–81.
20. Findlay RD, Taeush HW, Walther FJ. Surfactant replacement therapy for meconium aspiration syndrome. Pediatrics 1996;97:48–52.
21. Fulkerson WJ, MacIntyre N. Pathogenesis and treatment of the adult respiratory distress syndrome. Arch Intern Med 1996;156:29–38.
22. Bernard GR, Artigas A, Brigham KL, et al. The American-European consensus conference on ARDS: definitions, mechanisms, relevant outcomes, and clinical trial coordination. Am J Respir Crit Care Med 1994;149:818–24.
23. Marino P. Acute respiratory failure. In: Luppa PB, editor. The ICU book. 3rd edition. Philadelphia: Lipincott, Williams, and Williams; 2007. p. 421–36.
24. Holm B, Matalon S. Role of pulmonary surfactant in the development and treatment of adult respiratory distress syndrome. Anesth Analg 1989;140(2):805–18.
25. Kresch MJ, Lin WH, Thrall RS. Surfactant replacement therapy. Thorax 1996; 51(11):1137–54.
26. Engle W. Surfactant-replacement therapy for respiratory distress in the preterm and term neonate. Pediatrics 2008;121:419–32.
27. The OSIRIS Collaborative Group. Early versus delayed neonatal administration of synthetic surfactant—the judgement of OSIRIS. Lancet 1992;340:1363–9.
28. Liu M, Wang L, Enhorning G. Surfactant dysfunction develops when the immunized guinea-pig is challenged with ovalbumin aerosol. Clin Exp Allergy 1995; 25:1053–60.
29. Liu M, Wang L, Enhorning G. Pulmonary surfactant given prophylactically alleviates an asthma attack in guinea-pigs. Clin Exp Allergy 1996;26:270–5.
30. Enhorning G. Surfactant in airway disease. Chest 2008;133:975–80.
31. Dobbs LG, Mason RJ. Pulmonary alveolar type II cells isolated from rats: release of phosphatidylcholine in response to B-adrenergic stimulation. J Clin Invest 1979;63:378–87.
32. Cheng JB, Goldfein A, Bullard PL, et al. Glucocorticoids increase pulmonary beta-adrenergic receptors in fetal rabbit. Endocrinology 1989;107:1646–8.
33. Novick RJ, Gehman KE, Ali IS, et al. Lung preservation: the importance of endothelial and alveolar type II cell integrity. Ann Thorac Surg 1996;62(1):302–14.
34. Parajashingam R, Nicholson ML, Bell PR, et al. Non-cardiogenic pulmonary oedema in vascular surgery. Eur J Vasc Endovasc Surg 1999;17(2):93–105.
35. Dargaville PA, South M, McDougall PN. Surfactant abnormalities in infants with severe viral bronchiolitis. Arch Dis Child 1996;75(2):133–6.
36. Tibby SM, Hatherill M, Wright S, et al. Exogenous surfactant supplementation in infants with respiratory syncytial virus bronchiolitis. Am J Resp Crit Care Med 2000;162(4):1251–6.
37. Mora R, Arnold S, Marzan Y, et al. Determinants of surfactant function in acute lung injury and early recovery. Am J Physiol Lung Cell Mol Physiol 2000;279:342–9.
38. Spragg RG, Lewis JF, Walmrath HD, et al. Effect of recombinant protein C-based surfactant on the acute respiratory distress syndrome. N Engl J Med 2004;351(9):884–92.
39. Santacruz JF, Zavala ED, Arroliga A. Update in ARDS management: recent randomized controlled trials that changed our practice. Cleve Clin J Med 2006;73(3):217–35.
40. Wilson DF, Thomas NJ, Markowitz BP, et al. Effects of exogenous surfactant (calfactant) in pediatric acute lung injury: a randomized controlled trial. JAMA 2005; 293:470–6.
41. Hemmila M, Napolitano L. Severe respiratory failure: advanced treatment options. Crit Care Med 2006;34(9):278–90.

Use of Noninvasive Positive-Pressure Ventilation in the Emergency Department

Mark A. Hostetler, MD, MPH*

KEYWORDS

- Noninvasive • Positive pressure • Ventilation • BiPap • CPAP

Clinicians began using noninvasive positive-pressure ventilation (NPPV) techniques during the first half of the 20th century.[1] Although early methods were successful in supporting patients with severely comprised neuromusculature, it never gained wide acceptance because of bulky equipment and poor patient tolerance. During the early 1980s, however, NPPV saw a resurgence as nasal masks became more widely available.[2–6] Compared with invasive positive-pressure ventilation, NPPV was much easier to use, had fewer side effects, and was less costly to administer.[7] With time, NPPV progressively gained wide acceptance as the ventilator modality of first choice for patients with chronic respiratory failure, particularly in cases attributable to chronic restrictive thoracic disease.[8]

Ultimately, with improved equipment and experience, NPPV began being used for acute respiratory failure (ARF).[9] Noninvasive ventilation provides several advantages over invasive ventilation. NPPV maintains upper airway function and oronasal humidification; enhances patient comfort, reducing the need for sedation; and provides effective ventilation, avoiding many of the complications associated with invasive mechanical ventilation. Most importantly, NPPV has been shown to reduce patient morbidity and mortality and to reduce intensive care unit (ICU) length of stay and health care costs.[9,10]

To optimize the successful use of NPPV in the emergency department (ED), clinicians must acquire the necessary knowledge, experience, and skill in its proper application.[11] The purpose of this article is to provide a concise but thorough review of the current state of knowledge relating to the proper application of NPPV pertaining to its use in the ED.

Department of Pediatrics, The University of Chicago, Pritzker School of Medicine, Chicago, IL, 60637 USA
* The University of Chicago Medical Center, 5841 South Maryland Avenue, MC-0810, Chicago, IL 60637.
E-mail address: mhostetler@peds.bsd.uchicago.edu

Emerg Med Clin N Am 26 (2008) 929–939
doi:10.1016/j.emc.2008.07.008
0733-8627/08/$ – see front matter © 2008 Elsevier Inc. All rights reserved.

PATHOPHYSIOLOGY AND BIOPHYSICS OF NONINVASIVE POSITIVE-PRESSURE VENTILATION

Respiratory failure may be acute or chronic; however, the insult that precipitates the respiratory crisis is often a mild one superimposed on a severe underlying pathophysiologic defect or disease. It is for this reason that relatively small amounts of ventilatory assistance may restore equilibrium. In patients who have underlying obstructive or restrictive disease, inspiratory muscles fail, resulting in ventilatory failure. NPPV increases tidal volume while reducing respiratory rate, resulting in increased minute ventilation and improved gas exchange. In addition, supplemental positive end-expiratory pressure (PEEP) decreases muscle fatigue. Continuous positive airway pressure (CPAP) increases functional residual capacity and opens atelectatic alveoli, thus decreasing right-to-left intrapulmonary shunt and improving oxygenation. The opening of alveoli and increase in functional residual capacity improve lung compliance, further decreasing the work of breathing. In addition, by lowering ventricular transmural pressure, CPAP reduces afterload and increases cardiac output, which is something particularly helpful in patients who have pulmonary edema related to compromised left ventricular function.

EQUIPMENT AND SETUP

The equipment necessary for providing NPPV includes a positive-pressure ventilator and some type of patient interface, usually a mask.[12] There are a variety of masks commercially available. Masks used to provide noninvasive ventilation can be nasal masks or full-face oronasal masks that cover the nose and mouth.[13] Desirable features of a mask should include being transparent, lightweight, easy to secure, able to provide an adequate seal with low facial pressure, disposable or easy to clean, non-irritating to the skin, low dead space, and inexpensive. The choice of mask has a major impact on patient comfort and tolerance during noninvasive ventilation, because a poorly fitting mask decreases clinical effectiveness and patient compliance with this therapy. In addition to the mask itself, there is usually a means of attaching headgear or straps to act as a harness.

Newer commercially available masks have specially designed silicone or other soft rubber flanges to achieve a tighter air seal.[14] When correctly applied, these cushions help to minimize leak and improve comfort. The nasal portion of the mask should fit just above the junction of the nasal bone and cartilage. A common mistake is to choose a mask that is too large, resulting in air leaks and the tendency to excessively tighten the straps. To minimize air leak, it is advisable to pull out on the mask first and reseat the silicone flange. Maintaining a good seal between the chin and silicone seal may be difficult in edentulous patients.

A strap system is necessary to maintain correct position of most interfaces and is important for patient comfort. Most come preattached to the mask, and for ED use, simple disposable Velcro straps are most often used. A common mistake is to tighten the headgear excessively in an attempt to eliminate air leaks. As a rule of thumb, it should be possible to pass one or two fingers between the headgear and the face. Fitting the headgear too tightly may worsen an air leak and always decreases patient comfort and compliance.

Various ventilator types have been used to provide noninvasive ventilation, including standard critical care ventilators. Ventilators specifically designed to provide noninvasive ventilation are usually pressure limited and able to deliver so-called "bilevel" ventilation. These ventilators deliver a higher inspiratory pressure when triggered by the patient (inspiratory positive airway pressure [IPAP]), and then cycle into expiration after sensing a reduction in inspiratory flow or reaching an inspiratory time limit and deliver a lower expiratory pressure (expiratory positive air pressure [EPAP]). EPAP is synonymous with PEEP.

IMPLEMENTATION AND MANAGEMENT

Successful implementation and management of NPPV requires an initial series of clinical judgments and then close observation of the patient's response. First and foremost is the selection of appropriate patients.[15] In general, patients should be cooperative and capable of understanding the purpose of the therapy. Predictors of success include younger age, unimpaired consciousness, moderate rather than severe hypercarbia and acidemia, and prompt physiologic response (eg, improvement in heart and respiratory rates and gas exchange within 2 hours).[16] Second, intact swallowing and cough mechanisms are required, along with a modicum of airway secretions. Patients who have facial trauma or anatomic abnormalities that interfere with mask fitting or who have had upper airway surgery are poor candidates. Next, a mask and ventilator should be selected. Appropriate ventilator settings must be chosen based on the main goals of noninvasive ventilation.

Once a ventilator and mask are chosen, successful implementation of NPPV depends, in large part, on patient cooperation. The more comfortable the patient is and the better he or she understands the therapy, the more likely it is that the patient is going to be motivated and compliant with NPPV. Realize that a mask placed over the face may be frightening to a dyspneic patient. The patient should be allowed to acclimate to NPPV before strapping the mask on. It may be helpful to allow the patient to hold the mask in place initially before it is secured with the straps. Prompts like "let the machine breathe for you" may be helpful.

Begin with low settings (peak inspiratory pressure of 6–8 cm H_2O and expiratory pressure of 3–5 cm H_2O), and then slowly increase to the desired response (increments of 1–2 cm H_2O). The clinician should assess for the patient's level of distress, and observe for reduced work of breathing as evidenced by decreased respiratory rate, use of accessory muscles, and good patient-ventilator synchrony. Once the desired level has been achieved and the patient is comfortable and breathing in synchrony with the ventilator, the headgear straps may be fastened. Oxygen is titrated based on the patient's saturation by means of pulse oximetry (peripheral oxygen saturation [Spo_2]). Peak pressures greater than 20 cm H_2O are poorly tolerated and almost never needed.

The primary goal for most patients is to improve gas exchange abnormalities while optimizing patient safety and minimizing complications. In the acute setting, avoidance of intubation and its attendant complications is usually the highest priority. In general, the best indicators of success are reduced work of breathing as indicated by a reduction in respiratory rate and good synchrony between the patient and ventilator.[15] In general, arterial blood gases are the only clinically acceptable way of assessing $Paco_2$ levels as a measure of adequacy of ventilation. Arterial blood gases are recommended within the first 1 or 2 hours of initiation to demonstrate improvement or exclude deterioration and should be taken into consideration in conjunction with the patient's clinical status. An increase in $Paco_2$ in concert with poor synchrony or sustained respiratory distress would constitute an indication for prompt intubation.

Inhalational medications, such as albuterol, may be given simultaneously in-line with NPPV.[17–19] The best mode of delivery (nebulized versus metered dose inhaler [MDI]) remains controversial. Albuterol delivery with NPPV may be affected by the type of aerosol delivery device, by the location of the leak port, and by actuating the MDI at the proper time in the respiratory cycle.[14,20–22] According to at least one study, significantly more albuterol was delivered with the nebulizer than with the MDI ($P < .001$).[23]

Sedation is often considered to help decrease anxiety and facility delivery of NPPV. Practices vary widely within specialties and among geographic regions, however. In a survey of sedation practices during NPPV to treat ARF, physicians used sedation, analgesia, or physical restraint in only 15% to 30% of patients.[24] Overall, benzodiazepines alone (33%) or opioids alone (29%) were most frequently chosen as the sedation regimen of choice. The respondent's use of sedation seems to be inversely related to the frequency and experience in using NPPV to treat patients who have ARF. There is a lack of evidence to suggest that opioids or benzodiazepines actually exert respiratory depressant effects in patients receiving ventilatory assistance, however, particularly at the low doses commonly used for NPPV.

CONTRAINDICATIONS

Contraindications for NPPV include altered mental status, lack of protective airway reflexes, excessive secretions, or severe rather than moderate hypercarbia or acidemia. Based on 1033 consecutive patients who had chronic obstructive pulmonary disease (COPD), of whom 236 (22.8%) failed NPPV, the model showed that the highest risk for failure occurred in those with a Glasgow Coma Scale score less than 11, pH less than 7.25, and respiratory rate greater than 30 breaths per minute.[25]

COMPLICATIONS

Although generally safe and well tolerated, NPPV is not free of adverse side effects or complications. The most frequently encountered adverse effects are related to the mask and air pressure and flow. Pressure sores are most common and occur in up to 10% of patients when excessive pressure is applied for too long, leading to ulceration of the nasal bridge.[26] In the presence of skin breakdown, artificial skin may be applied to the area to afford greater protection, and efforts should be made to recheck mask fit and minimize strap tension. Children receiving prolonged periods of NPPV with obstructive sleep apnea (OSA), neuromuscular disorders, and cystic fibrosis (CF) may experience global facial flattening in as many as 68% of patients.[27–29] Discomfort related to air pressure is common, with complaints of pain or burning in the nose or ears. Gastric insufflation is another frequent problem related to air pressure. Although reported in up to 50% of patients using NPPV, this is rarely severe enough to interfere with therapy.

The most common significant complication related to NPPV is aspiration pneumonia, which is reported in 5% of patients.[30,31] Hypotension is an infrequent problem during NPPV. More serious complications of excessive inflation pressure, such as pulmonary barotraumas, occur rarely during NPPV, because inflation pressures are usually much lower than those used during invasive ventilation (<25 cm H_2O).

CLINICAL SCENARIOS AND USES

Randomized trials suggest that patients who have ARF are less likely to require endotracheal intubation and have better outcomes when NPPV is added to standard therapy.[32–34] In the acute setting, the addition of NPPV to standard care reduces the rate of endotracheal intubation (absolute risk reduction of 23%, 95% confidence interval: 10%–35%), ICU length of stay (absolute reduction of 2 days, 95% confidence interval: 1–3 days), and ICU mortality (absolute risk reduction of 17%, 95% confidence interval: 8%–26%).

Chronic Obstructive Pulmonary Disease

Multiple studies reveal that ARF related to COPD is highly amenable to NPPV.[8,16,31,32,35–44] Clinical success, defined as tolerance of NPPV by the patient with improvement in gas exchange and avoidance of endotracheal intubation, was reported in 51% to 93% of cases.[8,42,43] Studies show that clinicians can expect prompt improvements in respiratory rates, gas exchange, and sensation of respiratory distress when patients who have acute COPD exacerbations are treated with NPPV.[45] Success with NPPV can be predicted by less severely abnormal baseline clinical and gas exchange parameters in addition to less severe levels of acidosis.[25,46,47] Reduction in respiratory and heart rates, good synchrony with the ventilator, and improvement in $Paco_2$ within the first 2 hours are highly predictive of success. NPPV should now be considered the ventilation of choice for selected patients who have COPD exacerbations.

Asthma

Similar to COPD, NPPV is safe and effective for the treatment of ARF related to status asthmaticus.[48–51] NPPV has been used successfully in adults and children who have ARF.[48,50,52,53] NPPV seems to be highly effective in correcting gas exchange abnormalities and avoiding intubation in patients who have acute severe asthma.[48,50] Patients who have moderate to severe dyspnea and have not responded promptly to aerosolized bronchodilator treatments and seem to be at risk for developing respiratory muscle fatigue are the best candidates for NPPV therapy.

Pulmonary Edema

In patients who have pulmonary edema and compromised left ventricular function, CPAP may help to reduce afterload and increase cardiac output.[54] CPAP has been shown to be highly effective in reducing intubation rates (19% as compared with 47% among controls).[18,55–61] CPAP is also highly effective in reducing respiratory rates and dyspnea scores and in improving oxygenation, with most studies showing roughly 20% to 30% increases in Pao_2 or Pao_2 and fraction of inspired oxygen (Fio_2) within the first hour.[55,60,62] CPAP should be considered the modality of first choice for patients who have acute pulmonary edema. Caution is advised when patients have borderline low blood pressures (90–100 mm Hg), however, because they may become hemodynamically unstable.[63]

Pneumonia

The best available evidence indicates that NPPV can be successfully used to treat patients who have ARF attributable to acute pneumonia.[64] Overall success rates, however, can be confounded depending on the coexistence of COPD. Studies suggest that if a patient who has COPD also has pneumonia, the likelihood of success with NPPV is lower than for patients who have COPD who do not have pneumonia. The patient who has pneumonia and COPD seems to be more likely to succeed with NPPV than a patient who has ARF and no underlying lung disease, however.

Cystic Fibrosis

CF shares many pathophysiologic features similar to COPD and asthma, including severe expiratory airway obstruction and a tendency to develop hyperinflation and muscle fatigue. Similar to COPD and asthma, NPPV has been used as a means of partial ventilatory support.[65,66] Although formal studies are limited, case series reveal that patients with acute CF exacerbations had initial improvement or at least stabilization of gas exchange and were supported for periods ranging from 3 days to 36 days with NPPV.[66]

Acute Respiratory Distress Syndrome

NPPV is an effective technique for improving gas exchange and avoiding endotracheal intubation in selected patients who have ARF related to acute respiratory distress syndrome (ARDS).[67–69] In this setting, NPPV has been shown to decrease inspiratory muscle effort and work of breathing and to have a shorter duration of mechanical ventilation and ICU stay, and it has been associated with a lower risk for intubation and a lower 90-day mortality rate.[67] In ARDS, however, a transient loss of positive pressure during NPPV may seriously compromise lung recruitment and gas exchange; therefore, NPPV must be used with caution.

Obstructive Sleep Apnea

Severe OSA related to morbid obesity or anatomic issues can cause chronic carbon dioxide (CO_2) retention. Patients may present to the ED with an acute decompensation and ARF related to an intercurrent illness or poor adherence to a prescribed treatment regimen. Patients who have ARF related to OSA respond favorably to the institution of NPPV. Patients with moderate to severe CO_2 retention and acidemia ($Paco_2$ >50 mm Hg, pH <7.30) are the best candidates for NPPV.

Restrictive Disease

There are limited data supporting the use of NPPV in patients who have restrictive lung disease.[70] Theoretically, such patients would be difficult to manage noninvasively. This is attributable to the pathophysiologic changes associated with severe reductions in lung compliance and the need for high inflation pressures. It is conceivable, however, that NPPV could be helpful in instances of an acute reversible superimposed condition.

Neuromuscular Diseases

In patients who have progressive neuromuscular disease, NPPV has been shown to have a beneficial effect on nocturnal hypoventilation, hospitalization rates, and quality of life.[4–7,71–73] Although NPPV is not a cure for these diseases, it seems to have a substantial positive impact on patients who have neuromuscular disease, particularly during acute decompensations.[73]

Pulmonary Embolus, Trauma, Transplant

Successful application of CPAP and NPPV has been reported in cases of other forms of ARF, such as acute pulmonary embolism.[1,8] In addition, CPAP and NPPV have been successfully applied to patients with trauma, including flail chest, and patients recovering from organ transplantation.[74–76] In one study using CPAP (5–10 mm H_2O), oxygenation was consistently improved and only 2 of 33 patients (1 of 6 with flail chest) required intubation.[76]

Pediatric Uses

NPPV has been shown to be effective in pediatric-aged patients who have acute or chronic respiratory disease.[48,52,53,72,73,77] NPPV may be particularly attractive, at least in part because of the high morbidity and morality rates associated with endotracheal intubation and mechanical ventilation in children. In addition, the recent availability of soft nasal masks in a range of pediatric sizes and the introduction of portable pressure-targeted ventilators have encouraged greater use of NPPV. Important differences exist between children and adults in the anatomy and mechanical function of the respiratory system, however.

During infancy, resistance of the nasal airway is relatively high and the nasopharyngeal airway is particularly prone to obstruction. Adenotonsillar hypertrophy is the most important cause of OSA in the pediatric population, and the adenoids and tonsils often enlarge in response to recurrent infections and allergies. In addition, thick copious secretions are common in children with respiratory tract infections and can obstruct the nasopharyngeal airway.

Several respiratory conditions are amenable to a trial of NPPV in pediatric-aged patients: restrictive disorders, such as muscular dystrophies, spinal muscular atrophy, and thoracic kyphoscoliosis; obstructive disorders, such as CF, status asthmaticus, bronchiolitis obliterans, OSA, and obesity hypoventilation syndrome; impaired central respiratory drive, such as central hypoventilation syndrome and infectious and metabolic encephalopathies; and acute hypoxemic respiratory failure attributable to pneumonia or acute chest syndrome in sickle cell anemia. In such cases, NPPV has been associated with a decrease in the respiratory rate, heart rate, and oxygen requirement. Nevertheless, clinicians should be aware of a relatively high rate of failure related to intolerance from agitation. Children 8 years of age and older are the best candidates because they are most likely to cooperate and understand the process.

SUMMARY

NPPV has been used to assist ventilation and avoid intubation in many forms of ARF. There is abundant level I evidence supporting the use of NPPV in ARF related to chronic COPD, asthma, and acute cardiogenic pulmonary edema.[37]

The exact role of NPPV in acute and chronic settings continues to evolve. Advances in technology have led to masks and ventilators specifically designed for the administration of NPPV that are more comfortable and enhance patient acceptance and success rates. Even in the best of hands, however, NPPV fails in as many as 40% of cases. In appropriate patients, a trial of NPPV is often recommended, with attention to the patient populations as described most or least likely to benefit. The prudent clinician should always be prepared to intubate the patient after 1 or 2 hours without improvement.

REFERENCES

1. Barach AL, Martin J, Eckman M. Positive pressure respiration and its application to the treatment of acute pulmonary edema. Ann Intern Med 1938;12:754–95.
2. Alba A, Khan A, Lee M. Mouth IPPV for sleep. Rehabilitation Gazette 1984;24: 47–9.
3. Bach JR, Alba AS, Bohatiuk G, et al. Mouth intermittent positive pressure ventilation in the management of post-polio respiratory insufficiency. Chest 1987;91: 859–64.
4. Ellis ER, Bye PT, Bruderer JW, et al. Treatment of respiratory failure during sleep in patients with neuromuscular disease: positive-pressure ventilation through a nose mask. Am Rev Respir Dis 1987;135:148–52.
5. Kerby GR, Mayer LS, Pingleton SK. Nocturnal positive pressure ventilation via nasal mask. Am Rev Respir Dis 1987;135:738–40.
6. Rideau Y, Gatin G, Bach J, et al. Prolongation of life in Duchenne's muscular dystrophy. Acta Neurol 1983;5:118–24.

7. Bach JR, Intintola P, Alba AS, et al. The ventilator-assisted individual cost analysis of institutionalization versus rehabilitation and in-home management. Chest 1992; 101:26–30.
8. Kramer N, Meyer TJ, Meharg J, et al. Randomized, prospective trial of noninvasive positive pressure ventilation in acute respiratory failure. Am J Respir Crit Care Med 1995;151:1799–806.
9. Plant PK, Owen JL, Elliott MW. Early use of noninvasive ventilation for acute exacerbations of chronic obstructive pulmonary disease on general respiratory wards: a multicentre randomized controlled trial. Lancet 2000;355:1931–5.
10. Plant PK, Owen JL, Parrott S, et al. Cost effectiveness of ward based non-invasive ventilation for acute exacerbations of chronic obstructive pulmonary disease: economic analysis of randomized controlled trial. BMJ 2003;326:956–9.
11. Wood KA, Lewis L, Von Harz B, et al. The use of noninvasive positive pressure ventilation in the emergency department. Chest 1998;113:1339–46.
12. Wysocki M, Richard JC, Meshaka P. Noninvasive proportional assist ventilation compared with noninvasive pressure support ventilation in hypercapneic acute respiratory failure. Crit Care Med 2002;30:323–9.
13. Kwok H, McCormack J, Cece R, et al. Controlled trial of oronasal versus nasal mask ventilation in the treatment of acute respiratory failure. Crit Care Med 2003;31:468–73.
14. Smaldone GC. Assessing new technologies: patient-device interactions and deposition. Respir Care 2005;50(9):1151–60.
15. Plant PK, Owen JL, Elliott MW. Non-invasive ventilation in acute exacerbations of chronic obstructive pulmonary disease: long term survival and predictors of in-hospital outcome. Thorax 2001;56:708–12.
16. Mehta S, Hill NS. Noninvasive ventilation. Am J Respir Crit Care Med 2001;163(2): 540–77.
17. Dhand R, Tobin MJ. Inhaled bronchodilator therapy in mechanically ventilated patients. Am J Respir Crit Care Med 1997;156(1):3–10.
18. Nava S, Karakurt S, Rampulla C, et al. Salbutamol delivery during non-invasive mechanical ventilation in patients with chronic obstructive pulmonary disease: a randomized controlled study. Intensive Care Med 2001;27(10):1627–35.
19. Pollack CV Jr, Fleisch KB, Dowsey K. Treatment of acute bronchospasm with beta-adrenergic agonist aerosols delivered by a nasal bilevel positive airway pressure circuit. Ann Emerg Med 1995;26(5):552–7.
20. Chatmongkolchart S, Schettino GP, Dillman C, et al. In vitro evaluation of aerosol bronchodilator delivery during noninvasive positive pressure ventilation: effect of ventilator settings and nebulizer position. Crit Care Med 2003;30(11):2215–9.
21. Dolovich M. Influence of inspiratory flow rate, particle size, and airway caliber on aerosolized drug delivery to the lung. Respir Care 2000;56(6):597–608.
22. Parkes SN, Bersten AD. Aerosol kinetics and bronchodilator efficacy during continuous positive airway pressure delivered by face mask. Thorax 1997;52(2): 171–5.
23. Branconnier MP, Hess DR. Albuterol delivery during noninvasive ventilation. Respir Care 2005;50(12):1649–53.
24. Devlin JW, Nava S, Fong JJ, et al. Survey of sedation practices during noninvasive positive-pressure ventilation to treat acute respiratory failure. Crit Care Med 2007;35(10):1–9.
25. Confalonieri M, Garuti G, Cattaruzza MS, et al. A chart of failure risk for noninvasive ventilation in patients with COPD exacerbations. Eur Respir J 2005;25: 348–55.

26. Gregoretti C, Confalonieri M, Navalesi P, et al. Evaluation of patient skin break-down and comfort with a new face mask for noninvasive ventilation: a multi-center study. Intensive Care Med 2002;28:278–84.
27. Faroux B, Lavis JF, Nicot F, et al. Facial side effects during noninvasive positive pressure ventilation in children. Intensive Care Med 2005;31:965–9.
28. Li KK, Riley RW, Guilleminault C. An unreported risk in the use of home nasal continuous positive airway pressure and home nasal ventilation in children: mid-face hypoplasia. Chest 2000;117:916–8.
29. Villa MP, Pagani J, Ambrosio R, et al. Mid-face hypoplasia after long-term nasal ventilation. Am J Respir Crit Care Med 2002;166:1142–3.
30. Girou E, Schortgen F, Declaux C. Association of noninvasive ventilation with nos-ocomial infections and survival in critically ill patients. JAMA 2000;284:2361–7.
31. Meduri GU, Abou-Shala N, Fox RC, et al. Noninvasive face mask mechanical ventilation in patients with acute hypercapnic respiratory failure. Chest 1991;103: 174–82.
32. Keenan SP, Sinuff T, Cook DJ, et al. Does noninvasive positive pressure ventilation improve outcome in acute hypoxemic respiratory failure? A systematic review. Crit Care Med 2004;22(12):2516–23.
33. Peter JV, Moran JL, Phillips-Hughes J, et al. Noninvasive ventilation in acute respiratory failure—a meta-analysis update. Crit Care Med 2002;30:555–62.
34. Ram FS, Picot J, Lightowler J, et al. Noninvasive positive pressure ventilation for treatment of respiratory failure due to exacerbations of chronic obstructive pulmonary disease [update of Cochrane Database Syst Rev 2003;1:CD004104]. Cochrane Database Syst Rev 2004;(1):CD004101.
35. Bott J, Carroll MP, Conway JH, et al. Randomised controlled trial of nasal ventilation in acute ventilatory failure due to chronic obstructive airways disease. Lancet 1993;341:1555–7.
36. Brochard L, Mancebo J, Wysocki M, et al. Noninvasive ventilation for acute exacerbations of chronic obstructive pulmonary disease. N Engl J Med 1995;333: 817–22.
37. Caples SM, Gay PC. Noninvasive positive pressure ventilation in the intensive care unit: a concise review. Crit Care Med 2005;33:2651–8.
38. Celikel T, Sungur M, Ceyhan B, et al. Comparison of noninvasive positive pressure ventilation with standard medical therapy in hypercapnic acute respiratory failure. Chest 1998;114:1636–42.
39. Delclaux C, L'Her E, Alberti, et al. Treatment of acute hypoxemic nonhypercapnic respiratory insufficiency with continuous positive airway pressure delivered by a face mask: a randomized controlled trial. JAMA 2000;284:2352–60.
40. Ferrer M, Dsquinas A, Leon M, et al. Noninvasive ventilation in severe hypoxemic respiratory failure. A randomized clinical trial. Am J Respir Crit Care Med 2003; 168:1438–44.
41. Hess DR. The evidence for noninvasive positive-pressure ventilation in the care of patients in acute respiratory failure: a systematic review of the literature. Respir Care 2004;49:810–29.
42. Keenan SP, Kernerman PD, Cook DJ, et al. The effect of noninvasive positive pressure ventilation on mortality in patients admitted with acute respiratory failure: a meta-analysis. Crit Care Med 1997;25:1685–92.
43. Lightowler JV, Wedzicha JA, Elliott MW, et al. Non-invasive positive pressure ventilation to treat respiratory failure resulting from exacerbations of chronic obstructive pulmonary disease: Cochrane systematic review and meta-analysis. BMJ 2003;326(7382):185–9.

44. Martin TJ, Hovis JD, Costantino JP, et al. A randomized, prospective evaluation of noninvasive ventilation for acute respiratory failure. Am J Respir Crit Care 2000; 161:807–13.

45. Antonelli M, Conti G, Rocco M, et al. A comparison of noninvasive positive-pressure ventilation and conventional mechanical ventilation in patients with respiratory failure. N Engl J Med 1998;l339:429–35.

46. Antonelli M, Conti G, Moro ML, et al. Predictors of failure of noninvasive positive pressure ventilation in patients with acute hypoxemic respiratory failure. A multicenter study. Intensive Care Med 2001;27:1718–28.

47. Keenan SP, Sinuff T, Cook DJ, et al. Which patients with acute exacerbation of chronic obstructive pulmonary disease benefit from noninvasive positive-pressure ventilation? A systematic review of the literature. Ann Intern Med 2003; 138:861–70.

48. Akingbola OA, Simakajornboon N, Hadley EF, et al. Noninvasive positive-pressure ventilation in pediatric status asthmaticus. Pediatr Crit Care Med 2002; 3(2):181–4.

49. Meduri GU, Cook TR, Turner RE, et al. Noninvasive positive pressure ventilation in status asthmaticus. Chest 1996;110:767–74.

50. Needleman JP, Sykes JA, Schroeder SA, et al. Noninvasive positive pressure ventilation in the treatment of pediatric status asthmaticus. Pediatric Asthma, Allergy, & Immunology 2004;17(4):272–7.

51. Soroksky A, Stav D, Shpirer I. A pilot prospective, randomized, placebo-controlled trial of bilevel positive airway pressure in acute asthmatic attack. Chest 2003;123:1018–25.

52. Fortenberry JD, Torro JD, Jefferson LS, et al. Management of pediatric acute hypoxemic respiratory insufficiency with bilevel positive pressure (BiPAP) nasal mask ventilation. Chest 1995;108:1059–61.

53. Padman R, Lawless ST, Kettrick RG. Noninvasive ventilation via bilevel positive airway pressure support in pediatric practice. Crit Care Med 1998;26:169–73.

54. L'Her E, Duquesne F, Girou E. Noninvasive continuous positive airway pressure in elderly cardiogenic pulmonary edema patients. Intensive Care Med 2004;30: 882–8.

55. Bersten AD, Holt AW, Vedig AE, et al. Treatment of severe cardiogenic pulmonary edema with continuous positive airway pressure delivered by face mask. N Engl J Med 1991;325:1825–30.

56. Crane SD, Elliott MW, Gilligan P, et al. Randomised controlled comparison of continuous positive airways pressure, bilevel noninvasive ventilation, and standard treatment in emergency department patients with acute cardiogenic pulmonary oedema. Emerg Med J 2004;21:155–61.

57. Hoffmann B, Welte T. The use of noninvasive pressure support ventilation for severe respiratory insufficiency due to pulmonary oedema. Intensive Care Med 1999;25:15–20.

58. Levitt MA. A prospective, randomized trial of BiPAP in severe acute congestive heart failure. J Emerg Med 2001;21:363–9.

59. Masip J, Betbese AJ, Paez J, et al. Noninvasive pressure support ventilation versus conventional oxygen therapy in acute cardiogenic pulmonary oedema: a randomized trial. Lancet 2000;356:2126–32.

60. Mehta S, Jay GD, Woolard RH, et al. Randomized, prospective trial of bilevel versus continuous positive airway pressure in acute pulmonary edema. Crit Care Med 1997;25:620–8.

61. Nava S, Carbone G, DiBattista N, et al. Noninvasive ventilation in cardiogenic pulmonary edema: a multicenter, randomized trial. Am J Respir Crit Care Med 2003; 168:1432–7.
62. Rusterholtz T, Kempf J, Berton C, et al. Noninvasive pressure support ventilation (NIPSV) with face mask in patients with acute cardiogenic pulmonary edema (ACPE). Intensive Care Med 1999;25:21–8.
63. Lin M, Yang Y, Chiang H, et al. Reappraisal of continuous positive airway pressure therapy in acute cardiogenic pulmonary edema: short-term results and long-term follow-up. Chest 1995;107:1379–86.
64. Confalonieri M, Potena A, Carbone G, et al. Acute respiratory failure in patients with severe community-acquired pneumonia: a prospective randomized evaluation of noninvasive ventilation. Am J Respir Crit Care Med 1999;160:1585–91.
65. Fauroux B, Itti E, Pigeot J, et al. Optimization of aerosol deposition by pressure support in children with cystic fibrosis. Am J Respir Crit Care Med 2000; 162(6):2265–71.
66. Hodson ME, Madden BP, Steven MH, et al. Noninvasive mechanical ventilation for cystic fibrosis patients: a potential bridge to transplantation. Eur Respir J 1991;4:524–7.
67. Antonelli M, Conti G, Esquinas A, et al. A multiple-center survey on the use in clinical practice of noninvasive ventilation as a first-line intervention for acute respiratory distress syndrome. Crit Care Med 2007;35(1):18–25.
68. Cheung TM, Yam LY, So LK, et al. Effectiveness of noninvasive positive pressure ventilation in the treatment of acute respiratory failure in severe acute respiratory syndrome. Chest 2004;126:845–50.
69. Rocker GM, MacKenzie MG, Williams B, et al. Noninvasive positive pressure ventilation: successful outcome in patients with acute lung injury/ARDS. Chest 1999; 115:173–7.
70. Baydur A, Layne E, Aral H, et al. Long term non-invasive ventilation in the community for patients with musculoskeletal disorders: 46 year experience and review. Thorax 2000;55:4–11.
71. Bach JR, O'Brien R, Krotenberg, et al. Management of end stage respiratory failure in Duchenne muscular dystrophy. Muscle Nerve 1987;10:177–82.
72. Niranjan V, Bach JR. Noninvasive management of pediatric neuromuscular ventilatory failure. Crit Care Med 1998;26:2061–5.
73. Katz S, Selvadurai H, Keilty K, et al. Outcome of non-invasive positive pressure ventilation in paediatric neuromuscular disease. Arch Dis Child 2004;89:121–4.
74. Antonelli M, Conti G, Bufi M, et al. Noninvasive ventilation for treatment of acute respiratory failure in patients undergoing solid organ transplantation: a randomized trial. JAMA 2000;283:235–41.
75. Auriant I, Jallot A, Herve P, et al. Noninvasive ventilation reduces mortality in acute respiratory failure following lung resection. Am J Respir Crit Care Med 2001;164:1231–5.
76. Hurst JM, DeHaven CB, Branson RD. Use of CPAP mask as the sole mode of ventilatory support in trauma patients with mild to moderate respiratory insufficiency. J Trauma 1985;25:1065–8.
77. Conti G, Antonelli M, Navalesi P, et al. Noninvasive vs. conventional mechanical ventilation in patients with chronic obstructive pulmonary disease after failure of medical treatment in the ward: a randomized trial. Intensive Care Med 2002;28: 1701–7.

Permissive Hypercapnia

Alex Rogovik, MD, PhD[a], Ran Goldman, MD[a,b,c,*]

KEYWORDS

• Permissive hypercapnia • Mechanical ventilation • Lung

Mechanical ventilation using high tidal volume (VT) and transpulmonary pressure can damage the lung, causing ventilator-induced lung injury. Several mechanisms have been offered to explain this damage. Repetitive overstretching and damage to lung tissue and cyclic alveolar recruitment may result in mechanical stress and mechano-trauma.[1] Increased mechanical stress may activate immune response in the lung,[2] with the potential for intrapulmonary inflammatory mediators and bacteria to cross an impaired alveolar-capillary barrier.[3,4] Therefore the use of low-lung-stretch ventilatory strategies that reduce mechanical trauma and the associated inflammatory effects is increasing.[5,6] Permissive hypercapnia, a ventilatory strategy for acute respiratory failure in which the lungs are ventilated with a low inspiratory volume and pressure, has been accepted progressively in critical care for adult, pediatric, and neonatal patients requiring mechanical ventilation, and it is one of the central components of current protective ventilatory strategies. Permissive hypercapnia is used to minimize lung damage during mechanical ventilation; its limitations are the resulting hypoventilation, CO_2 retention, and acidosis. Hypoxemia is caused by decreasing the alveolar oxygen tension and alveolar collapse during hypoventilation. The alveolar collapse can be offset in part, however, by increasing the end-expiratory volume.

PHYSIOLOGIC EFFECTS OF HYPERCAPNIA
Systemic Physiologic Effects

In healthy subjects, hypercapnia is associated with air hunger and distress. Because of decreased CO_2 elimination and consequent hypercapnia, respiratory acidosis occurs during hypoventilation. Laboratory studies have shown that acute hypercapnia,

[a] Pediatric Research in Emergency Therapeutics (PRETx) Program, Division of Pediatric Emergency Medicine, Room K4-226, Ambulatory Care Building, BC Children's Hospital, 4480 Oak Street, Vancouver, BC V6H 3V4, Canada
[b] Department of Pediatrics, University of British Columbia, 4480 Oak Street, BC Children's Hospital, Vancouver, BC V6H 3V4, Canada
[c] Child & Family Research Institute (CFRI), Vancouver, BC, Canada
* Corresponding author.
E-mail address: rgoldman@cw.bc.ca (R. Goldman).

Emerg Med Clin N Am 26 (2008) 941–952
doi:10.1016/j.emc.2008.08.002
0733-8627/08/$ – see front matter © 2008 Elsevier Inc. All rights reserved.

emed.theclinics.com

induced within 1 hour, is associated with significant increases in cardiac output, organ blood flow, and intracranial pressure.[7]

Systemic physiologic effects of hypercapnia in humans are respiratory (increased minute ventilation, subjective discomfort, air hunger, anxiety, fatigue), cardiovascular (increased cardiac output, tachycardia, systemic and pulmonary hypertension), neurologic (increased cerebral blood flow, headache, cerebral edema), and metabolic (endogenous catecholamines and corticosteroids release, increased tissue O_2 unloading, decreased effect of exogenous vasopressors). In extreme hypercapnia and in high-risk patients hypercapnia can cause myocardial depression and dysrhythmias, cerebral hemorrhage and herniation, stupor, and coma.[8]

The role of hypercapnia in protective lung ventilation per se, apart from the reduced lung stretch, remains unclear because of a lack of clinical data comparing the efficacy of protective lung ventilatory strategies in the presence and absence of hypercapnia. Experimental studies suggest that tissue oxygenation can be unchanged or improved during permissive hypercapnia with increased cardiac output, reduced differences in arterial and venous O_2 content, and reduced blood lactate concentration.[9,10] In dogs, permissive hypercapnia produced by inhaled CO_2 produced gradual and significant increases in the hemoglobin concentration and arterial oxygen content, increasing oxygen-carrying capacity.[11]

Animal studies of peripheral microcirculation showed that when Pa_{CO_2} increases up to 80 mm Hg, vessel diameter, blood-flow velocity, and blood-flow rate increase markedly, with slight increase in cardiac output;[12] however, when Pa_{CO_2} exceeded 100 mm Hg, all these variables decreased. In addition, hypercapnic acidosis may reduce cellular oxygen demand.[13]

Hypercapnic acidosis attenuated acute experimental endotoxin-induced lung injury, improving the decrement in oxygenation and lung compliance and reducing alveolar neutrophil infiltration and histologic indices of lung injury.[14]

One small clinical study, however, showed that acute moderate changes in Pa_{CO_2} have no major effect on splanchnic perfusion and metabolism.[15] In another study in patients who had severe acute respiratory distress syndrome (ARDS),[16] the Pa_{CO_2} increase from 38 to 57 mm Hg, and the pH decrease from 7.41 to 7.31 at 24 hours did not induce significant changes in arterial oxygenation, pulmonary vascular resistance, systemic vascular resistance, cardiac index, or systemic oxygen delivery and consumption.

Anti-Inflammatory Action

Hypercapnic acidosis may interfere with the coordination of the immune response. In one in vitro study,[17] CO_2 produced profound reversible inhibition of lipopolysaccharide-stimulated cytokine release by peritoneal macrophages, possibly explaining the lack of systemic inflammation after laparoscopic surgery with CO_2. Macrophages incubated in CO_2 produced significantly less tumor necrosis factor and interleukin (IL)-1 in response to lipopolysaccharide compared with those incubated in air or helium;[18] the authors attributed this finding to cellular acidification.

According to other authors, neutrophils respond to hypercarbia by decreasing intracellular oxidant production and the release of IL-8 from lipopolysaccharide-stimulated cells.[19] This hypothesis suggests that CO_2 can modify neutrophil activity significantly by altering pH. Extracellular acidosis may intensify acute inflammatory responses by inducing neutrophil activation, delaying spontaneous apoptosis, and extending neutrophil functional lifespan.[20] Hypercapnic acidosis may increase neutrophil CD18 expression and enhance neutrophil adhesion.[21] There is a direct positive correlation between the intracellular pH value and the locomotor response of neutrophils to a chemotactic gradient.[22]

Spreading and several functions of neutrophils were inhibited at an acidic pH.[23] This observation indicates that neutrophils release superoxide upon spreading, generating a burst of intracellular acid production, and the coordinated activation of intracellular pH regulatory mechanisms along with the oxidase is essential for sustained microbicidal activity.

Hypercapnic acidosis can have anti-inflammatory effects through a mechanism that inhibits activation of nuclear factor-κB,[24] leading to down-regulation of intercellular adhesion molecule-1 and IL-8, which in turn inhibit neutrophil adherence to pulmonary endothelial cells.[25]

Hypercapnic acidosis seems to attenuate free radical production and may attenuate tissue injury following pulmonary ischemia and reperfusion.[26] The production of superoxide radicals by chemotactic factor-stimulated human neutrophils in vitro was decreased at acidic pH.[27] There are, however, concerns regarding the formation of nitration products from peroxynitrite, a potent free radical.[28,29]

In general, the available experimental data are inconclusive as to whether hypercapnic acidosis interferes with the coordination of the immune response.

IMPLEMENTATION OF PERMISSIVE HYPERCAPNIA

Implementation of permissive hypercapnia requires ventilation with decreased VT and low alveolar pressure.[8] The VT should be reduced gradually to 7 mL/kg or less[30] to allow a progressive rise in the $Paco_2$, not to exceed 10 mm Hg/h, to a maximum of 80 to 100 mm Hg, to maintain the static peak airway pressure at less than 40 cm H_2O and arterial oxygen saturation (SaO_2) greater than 90%.[31]

The strategies of permissive hypercapnia are continuing to develop. The initial approach aimed at avoiding end-inspiratory lung trauma by using small VTs, limiting the plateau airway pressure to 30 to 35 cm H_2O, and allowing a slow rise of $Paco_2$.[32-36] It has been suggested that the use of small VTs that avoid tissue overdistention and the acceptance of the consequent elevation of $Paco_2$ minimize the risk of barotrauma in patients who have asthma and ARDS.[36] Adoption of the ARDS Network low-VT protocol for routine ventilator management was associated with lower mortality in 292 patients who had acute lung injury (ALI)/ARDS than seen in recent historical controls.[37]

Further development of this strategy emphasized the importance of alveolar recruitment to avoid the end-expiratory lung trauma by applying positive end-expiratory pressure (PEEP) and optimizing gas exchange.[38,39,40]

Although in most patients PEEP induces alveolar hyperinflation during mechanical ventilation with conventional VT, at low VT a significant alveolar collapse is present, and PEEP is able to expand these units, improving gas exchange and hemodynamics.[38] In patients who have ALI, a PEEP of at least 15 cm H_2O is needed to prevent the decay of respiratory system compliance because of low VT ventilation.[40]

In a study of the hemodynamic effects of hypercapnia in adult patients who have ARDS,[41] the acute combined use of permissive hypercapnia, VT less than 6 mL/kg, distending pressures above PEEP of less than 20 cm H_2O, and PEEP 2 cm H_2O above the lower inflection point resulted in an immediate increase in heart rate, cardiac output, oxygen delivery, and mixed venous partial pressure of oxygen. The mean pulmonary arterial pressure increased markedly (by 8.8 mm Hg), but the pulmonary vascular resistance did not change. A multivariate analysis suggested that these acute hyperdynamic effects were related to respiratory acidosis, with no depressant effects ascribed to high PEEP levels,[41] and transitory pulmonary hypertension and high cardiac output were attenuated significantly within 36 hours.

In patients who had ARDS, adding increased PEEP to low VT resulted in improved survival at 28 days, a higher rate of weaning from mechanical ventilation, and a lower rate of barotrauma than seen with conventional ventilation.[42] In another study in patients who had ARDS, a high PEEP/low VT ventilatory strategy also improved ICU mortality, hospital mortality, and ventilator-free days at day 28 as compared with patients receiving conventional ventilation.[43]

Higher levels of sedation may be required to manage patients with permissive hypercapnia. In a study by Vinayak and colleagues,[44] higher doses of propofol but not midazolam were required to sedate patients managed with permissive hypercapnia. Hypercapnia should be avoided in trauma patients who have evidence of brain injury, because it can worsen intracranial pressure.[31]

Clinical Studies

A growing body of evidence supports the use of permissive hypercapnia in ALI and ARDS, status asthmaticus, and neonatal respiratory failure.

Acute lung injury and acute respiratory distress syndrome

Patients who have ALI and ARDS require ventilatory support, and ALI/ARDS are complicated further by ventilator-induced lung injury. The causes of the ALI and ARDS include pneumonia, sepsis or generalized infection, aspiration, shock, trauma/multiple fractures, acute pancreatitis, multiple transfusions, inhalation injury, burns, pulmonary contusion, and drug overdose.[32,34,42,45]

Protective ventilation involving end-expiratory pressures above the lower inflection point on the static pressure-volume curve, a VT of less than 6 mL/kg, driving pressures of less than 20 cm H_2O above the PEEP value, permissive hypercapnia, and preferential use of pressure-limited ventilatory modes resulted in improved survival at 28 days, a higher rate of weaning from mechanical ventilation, and a lower rate of barotrauma in 29 patients who had ARDS;[42] however, this treatment was not associated with a higher rate of survival to hospital discharge.

A further large, multicenter, randomized trial in 861 patients who had ALI and ARDS[32] demonstrated that ventilation with a lower VT, which involved an initial VT of 6 mL/kg predicted body weight and a plateau pressure of 30 cm H_2O or less, significantly decreased mortality (31% vs. 40%) and increased the number of days without ventilator use during the first 28 days (12 $\pm$ 11 days vs. 10 $\pm$ 11 days). A high-PEEP/low-VT ventilatory strategy improved outcome in 53 patients who had persistent ARDS compared with 50 control patients receiving conventional ventilation:[43] ICU mortality (53% vs. 32%), hospital mortality (56% vs. 34%), and ventilator-free days at day 28 (6 vs. 11) all favored the low-VT strategy, and the number of organ failures was higher in the control group.

One hundred and twenty patients at high risk for ARDS were assigned randomly to pressure- and volume-limited ventilation, with the peak inspiratory pressure maintained at 30 cm H_2O or less and the VT at 8 mL/kg body weight or less, or to conventional ventilation (control group).[34] In the limited-ventilation group, permissive hypercapnia (defined as $Paco_2$ > 50 mm Hg) was more common (52% vs. 28%), more marked (54 $\pm$ 19 mm Hg vs. 46 $\pm$ 10 mm Hg), and more prolonged (146 $\pm$ 265 hours vs. 25 $\pm$ 22 hours) than in the control group. Permissive hypercapnia did not seem to reduce mortality and might increase morbidity, however, the incidence of barotrauma, the multiple-organ dysfunction score, and the number of episodes of organ failure were similar in the two groups, and more patients in the limited-ventilation group than in the control group required paralytic agents and dialysis for renal failure.[34] A study comparing traditional versus reduced VT ventilation conducted in 52 patients who had ARDS in eight ICUs demonstrated the safety of the reduced-VT strategy.[45] There were, however, no significant differences in requirements for PEEP, fluid intakes/outputs, requirements for vasopressors, sedatives, or neuromuscular-blocking agents, percentage of patients who achieved unassisted breathing, ventilator days, or mortality.[45] Another multicenter trial compared 116 patients who had ARDS and no organ failure (other than the lung) ventilated with different VTs (7.1 ± 1.3 vs. 10.3 ± 1.7 mL/kg at day 1) and plateau pressure resulting in different $Paco_2$ (60 ± 15 vs. 41 ± 8 mm Hg) and pH (7.28 ± 0.09 vs. 7.4 ± 0.09) but with a similar level of oxygenation.[33] In this trial, mortality at day 60, the duration of mechanical ventilation, the incidence of pneumothorax, and the secondary occurrence of multiple organ failure were not reduced.[33]

A meta-analysis of six trials involving 1297 adult patients who had ALI or ARDS, comparing ventilation using either lower VT or low airway driving pressure versus ventilation with VT in the range of 10 to 15 mL/kg, found that mortality at day 28 and at the end of hospital stay was reduced significantly by lung-protective ventilation allowing hypercapnia.[30]

Kregenow and colleagues[46] tested the hypothesis that hypercapnic acidosis is associated with reduced mortality in patients who have ALI, independent of changes in mechanical ventilation in a previously conducted randomized, multicenter trial (n = 861) comparing 12 mL/kg with 6 mL/kg.[32] After controlling for comorbidities and severity of lung injury, they found that hypercapnic acidosis was associated with reduced 28-day mortality in the group treated with VTs of 12 mL/kg predicted body weight.

Despite data supporting the use of protective ventilatory strategies and permissive hypercapnia in patients who have ALI and ARDS, many clinicians do not use these strategies. A survey of experienced ICU nurses and respiratory therapists has shown that clinicians had used lung-protective ventilation in a median of 20% (interquartile range, 10%–50%) patients who had ALI or ARDS.[47] Barriers to using lung-protective ventilation were physician unwillingness to relinquish control of ventilator, physician recognition of ALI or ARDS, and physician perceptions of patient contraindications to low VTs. Barriers to continuing patients on lung-protective ventilation were concerns about patient discomfort and tachypnea and concerns about hypercapnia, acidosis, and hypoxemia.[47]

Status asthmaticus

Controlled hypoventilation with permissive hypercapnia is a relatively safe strategy in the ventilatory management of asthma,[48] and it may reduce morbidity and mortality compared with conventional normocapnic ventilation in the management of status asthmaticus.[49] The aim of controlled hypoventilation with permissive hypercapnia in status asthmaticus is to reduce potentially life-threatening side effects such as lung barotrauma and cardiovascular collapse by using low minute ventilation (≤ 10 L/min), low VT (6–10 mL/kg), and low respiratory rate (10–14 cycles/min), taking care that expiratory time be sufficient (≥ 4 seconds).[49] A low incidence of barotrauma and no mortality were reported with a ventilation strategy involving permissive hypercapnia in patients who had near-fatal asthma in an inner-city hospital.[50] Hypercapnia and associated acidosis are well tolerated in the absence of contraindications such as pre-existing intracranial hypertension;[48] however, inhalation anesthesia may be necessary. Pressure-controlled ventilation is an effective ventilatory strategy in severe status asthmaticus in children and represents a therapeutic option in their management.[51]

Neonatal respiratory failure

Permissive hypercapnia seems to be an effective and safe approach to decrease morbidity from bronchopulmonary dysplasia in premature infants.[52] Retrospective studies reported a lower incidence of bronchopulmonary dysplasia in infants whose $Paco_2$ values were higher during the first 4 days after birth.[53,54] Kamper and colleagues[55] have shown that ventilatory treatment in 407 extremely premature and extremely low-birth-weight infants based on the principle of permissive hypercapnia and early nasal continuous positive airway pressure supplemented with surfactant resulted in a lower incidence of chronic lung disease than reported with conventional treatment, with comparable survival rates and sensorineural outcomes. Application of a treatment protocol using gentle ventilation and permissive hypercapnia for congenital diaphragmatic hernia produced a significant increase in survival and a concomitant decrease in morbidity; the rate of pneumothorax also was decreased significantly.[56]

Two trials[57,58] involving 269 newborn infants were included in a Cochrane meta-analysis of permissive hypercapnia for the prevention of morbidity and mortality in mechanically ventilated newborn infants.[59] There was no evidence that permissive hypercapnia reduced the incidence of death or chronic lung disease at 36 weeks, grade 3 or 4 intraventricular hemorrhage, or periventricular leukomalacia. There were no differences in any other reported outcomes when permissive hypercapnia was compared with routine ventilation in newborn infants. One trial, however, reported that permissive hypercapnia reduced the incidence of chronic lung disease in the subgroup of newborns weighing 501 to 750 g.[58] A recent randomized, controlled trial in 86 extremely preterm infants under 28 weeks' gestational age with optimized ventilation including continuous tracheal gas insufflation, prophylactic surfactant administration, low oxygen saturation target, and moderate permissive hypercapnia resulted in a very gentle ventilation; the rate of survival without bronchopulmonary dysplasia was remarkably high for the whole population (78%) and for the subgroup of infants weighing less than 1000 g at birth (75%).[60]

There are, however, concerns regarding the use of permissive hypercapnia in ventilated very-low-birth-weight infants during the first week of life, because impaired autoregulation during this period may be associated with increased vulnerability to brain injury.[61] A retrospective cohort study of 574 very-low-birth-weight infants has shown that, in addition to traditional risk factors, the maximum $Paco_2$ during the first 3 days of life seems to be a dose-dependent predictor of severe intraventricular hemorrhage.[62] According to Fabres and colleagues,[63] both the extremes of arterial CO_2 pressure and the magnitude of fluctuations in arterial CO_2 pressure are associated with severe intraventricular hemorrhage in preterm infants, and it may be prudent to avoid extreme hypocapnia and hypercapnia during the period of risk for intraventricular hemorrhage. Although managing ventilatory support to keep $Paco_2$ values above 40 mm Hg in preterm infants seems to be beneficial and safe,[52] ventilatory strategies targeting high levels of $Paco_2$ (> 55 mm Hg) should be undertaken only in the context of well-designed, controlled clinical trials to establish the safe range for CO_2 in ventilated newborns and to examine the role of protective ventilatory techniques in achieving this target.[59]

A study of physical outcome and school performance in a cohort of very-low-birth-weight infants treated with early nasal continuous positive airway pressure and a minimal handling regimen with permissive hypercapnia[64] found a relatively low incidence of handicaps and impairments, with near-average school performances that were not different from their siblings', indicating that these infants fare at least as well as survivors after conventional treatment.

PERMISSIVE HYPERCAPNIA IN SEPSIS

Sevransky and colleagues,[65] in their review of mechanical ventilation in sepsis-induced ALI/ARDS, recommend using permissive hypercapnia. A large prospective study (n = 861)[32] of ventilation with lower VTs as compared with traditional VTs for ALI and ARDS, which included patients who had sepsis (27%) and pneumonia (34%), showed that mechanical ventilation with a lower VT results in decreased mortality and increases the number of days without ventilator use. O'Croinin and colleagues,[66] however, argue that the potential for hypercapnia to exert deleterious effects in the context of sepsis and to result in significant adverse consequences is clear. Although hypercapnic acidosis has been shown to be protective against experimental endotoxin-induced lung injury,[14] and the potential for CO_2 to inhibit bacterial growth and metabolism has been demonstrated,[67] several concerns regarding the safety of hypercapnia in sepsis exist, based on experimental studies. Hypercapnic acidosis may inhibit the chemotactic and bactericidal activity of neutrophils and macrophages,[22,23,66,68] render some antibiotics less effective,[69] and potentially increase tissue destruction through neutrophil necrosis.[19] In addition, a study by Stewart and colleagues,[34] which included 42% patients who had pneumonia and 39% who had sepsis, suggested that permissive hypercapnia did not seem to reduce mortality and might increase morbidity. The multiple-organ dysfunction scores and the number of episodes of organ failure were similar in the two groups; the number of patients who required dialysis for renal failure was greater in the limited-ventilation group.[34]

In contrast, another study of protective ventilation involving permissive hypercapnia conducted in 53 patients who had ARDS (with sepsis in 86% of the group receiving protective ventilation and 79% of the group receiving conventional ventilation)[42] resulted in improved survival at 28 days, a higher rate of weaning from mechanical ventilation, and a lower rate of barotrauma in patients receiving protective ventilation.

In general, caution is advised in using permissive hypercapnia in patients who have sepsis, although most clinical data support its use.

ADVERSE EVENTS

Although moderate hypercapnia has beneficial effects, these benefits may be counterbalanced by a potential for adverse effects of hypercapnic acidosis at high levels. Permissive hypercapnia, via the combined effects of increased cardiac output and decreased alveolar ventilation, can increase pulmonary shunt and impair pulmonary gas exchange in ARDS.[70] An experimental study demonstrated that severe hypercapnia produced by 15% CO_2 worsened neurologic injury compared with normocapnia (3% CO_2) or 12% CO_2,[71] presumably because of more severe cardiovascular depression that leads to greater cerebral ischemia and ultimate brain damage. Two other laboratory studies reported that intestinal lesions[72] and lung inflammation and injuries[73] were induced in rats by experimentally created severe acidosis, which is unlikely in the clinical setting.

Therefore correction of acidosis is important, and most authors prefer to correct it by increasing the mechanical respiratory rate.[8] It has been shown that in patients who have severe ARDS treated with permissive hypercapnia increasing the respiratory rate and reducing instrumental dead space during conventional mechanical ventilation is as efficient as expiratory washout in reducing Pa_{CO_2}.[74] pH as low as 7.15 can be tolerated before the administration of intravenous buffering agents (bicarbonate or tromethamine) is initiated.[31]

PHARMACOLOGIC BUFFERING OF HYPERCAPNIC ACIDOSIS

In critically ill patients, subjective discomfort caused by hypercapnic acidosis can be mitigated with the appropriate buffering and sedation. A slowly established hypercapnia, in which acidosis is buffered, would have minimal adverse effects.[8] There are concerns, however, that the protective effects of hypercapnic acidosis in ALI result from the acidosis rather than CO_2, and that buffering hypercapnic acidosis may worsen ALI, causing pulmonary vasodilation.[26]

Hypercapnia at normal pH also may enhance cell injury, as evidenced by the impairment of monolayer barrier function and increased induction of apoptosis[28] via modifying nitric oxide–dependent pathways. In addition, CO_2 can enhance nitration of surfactant protein A by activated alveolar macrophages and decrease its function.[29]

Buffering with bicarbonate raises systemic CO_2 levels and may worsen an intracellular acidosis.[66,75] Although intracellular acidification occurs after the addition of sodium bicarbonate to a suspension of human leucocytes in vitro, the effect is minimal when the conditions approximate those seen in clinical practice.[75] Another option is the use of tromethamine acetate,[76,77] which does not increase CO_2 production. Tromethamine buffer may attenuate the reversible depression of myocardial contractility and hemodynamic alterations during rapid permissive hypercapnia[78] and allow the benefit of decreased airway pressures to be realized while minimizing the adverse hemodynamic effects of hypercapnic acidosis. The initial loading dose of tromethamine acetate is 0.3 mol/L, and the maximum daily dose is 15 mmol/kg for an adult;[76] in large doses, it may induce respiratory depression and hypoglycemia, which will require ventilatory assistance and glucose administration.

SUMMARY

Permissive hypercapnia is one of the central components of current protective ventilatory strategies in critical care for adult, pediatric, and neonatal patients requiring mechanical ventilation. Moderate permissive hypercapnia seems to be effective and safe in ALI and ARDS, status asthmaticus, and neonatal respiratory failure. Patients at risk include those who have head trauma, high intracranial pressure, hemodynamic instability, and myocardial dysfunction. The optimal ventilatory strategy for hypercapnia remains to be established.

REFERENCES

1. Boussarsar M, Thierry G, Jaber S, et al. Relationship between ventilatory settings and barotrauma in the acute respiratory distress syndrome. Intensive Care Med 2002;28:406–13.
2. Dreyfuss D, Ricard JD, Saumon G. On the physiologic and clinical relevance of lung-borne cytokines during ventilator induced lung injury. Am J Respir Crit Care Med 2003;167:1467–71.
3. Tremblay L, Valenza F, Ribeiro SP, et al. Injurious ventilatory strategies increase cytokines and c-fos mRNA expression in an isolated rat lung model. J Clin Invest 1997;99:944–52.
4. Nahum A, Hoyt J, Schmitz L, et al. Effect of mechanical ventilation strategy on dissemination of intratracheally instilled Escherichia coli in dogs. Crit Care Med 1997;25:1733–43.
5. Moloney ED, Griffiths MJ. Protective ventilation of patients with acute respiratory distress syndrome. Br J Anaesth 2004;92:261–70.
6. Ricard JD, Dreyfuss D, Saumon G. Ventilator-induced lung injury. Eur Respir J 2003;42:2s–9s.
7. Cardenas VJ Jr, Zwischenberger JB, Tao W, et al. Correction of blood pH attenuates changes in hemodynamics and organ blood flow during permissive hypercapnia. Crit Care Med 1996;24:827–34.

8. Bigatello LM, Patroniti N, Sangalli F. Permissive hypercapnia. Curr Opin Crit Care 2001;7:34–40.

9. Hickling KG, Joyce C. Permissive hypercapnia in ARDS and its effect on tissue oxygenation. Acta Anaesthesiol Scand Suppl 1995;107:201–8.

10. Ratnaraj J, Kabon B, Talcott MR, et al. Supplemental oxygen and carbon dioxide each increase subcutaneous and intestinal intramural oxygenation. Anesth Analg 2004;99:207–11.

11. Torbati D, Mangino MJ, Garcia E, et al. Acute hypercapnia increases the oxygen-carrying capacity of the blood in ventilated dogs. Crit Care Med 1998;26:1863–7.

12. Komori M, Takada K, Tomizawa Y, et al. Permissive range of hypercapnia for improved peripheral microcirculation and cardiac output in rabbits. Crit Care Med 2007;35:2171–5.

13. Hassett P, Laffey JG. Permissive hypercapnia: balancing risks and benefits in the peripheral microcirculation. Crit Care Med 2007;35:2229–31.

14. Laffey JG, Honan D, Hopkins N, et al. Hypercapnic acidosis attenuates endotoxin-induced acute lung injury. Am J Respir Crit Care Med 2004;169:46–56.

15. Kiefer P, Nunes S, Kosonen P, et al. Effect of an acute increase in PCO2 on splanchnic perfusion and metabolism. Intensive Care Med 2001;27:775–8.

16. McIntyre RC Jr, Haenel JB, Moore FA, et al. Cardiopulmonary effects of permissive hypercapnia in the management of adult respiratory distress syndrome. J Trauma 1994;37:433–8.

17. West MA, Baker J, Bellingham J. Kinetics of decreased LPS-stimulated cytokine release by macrophages exposed to CO2. J Surg Res 1996;63:269–74.

18. West MA, Hackam DJ, Baker J, et al. Mechanism of decreased in vitro murine macrophage cytokine release after exposure to carbon dioxide: relevance to laparoscopic surgery. Ann Surg 1997;226:179–90.

19. Coakley RJ, Taggart C, Greene C, et al. Ambient pCO2 modulates intracellular pH, intracellular oxidant generation, and interleukin-8 secretion in human neutrophils. J Leukoc Biol 2002;71:603–10.

20. Trevani AS, Andonegui G, Giordano M, et al. Extracellular acidification induces human neutrophil activation. J Immunol 1999;162:4849–57.

21. Serrano CV Jr, Fraticelli A, Paniccia R, et al. pH dependence of neutrophil-endothelial cell adhesion and adhesion molecule expression. Am J Physiol 1996;271:C962–70.

22. Simchowitz L, Cragoe EJ Jr. Regulation of human neutrophil chemotaxis by intracellular pH. J Biol Chem 1986;261:6492–500.

23. Demaurex N, Downey GP, Waddell TK, et al. Intracellular pH regulation during spreading of human neutrophils. J Cell Biol 1996;133:1391–402.

24. Tak PP, Firestein GS. NF-kappaB: a key role in inflammatory diseases. J Clin Invest 2001;107:7–11.

25. Takeshita K, Suzuki Y, Nishio K, et al. Hypercapnic acidosis attenuates endotoxin-induced nuclear factor-[kappa]B activation. Am J Respir Cell Mol Biol 2003;29:124–32.

26. Laffey JG, Engelberts D, Kavanagh BP. Buffering hypercapnic acidosis worsens acute lung injury. Am J Respir Crit Care Med 2000;161:141–6.

27. Simchowitz L. Intracellular pH modulates the generation of superoxide radicals by human neutrophils. J Clin Invest 1985;76:1079–89.

28. Lang JD Jr, Chumley P, Eiserich JP, et al. Hypercapnia induces injury to alveolar epithelial cells via a nitric oxide-dependent pathway. Am J Physiol Lung Cell Mol Physiol 2000;279:L994–1002.

29. Zhu S, Basiouny KF, Crow JP, et al. Carbon dioxide enhances nitration of surfactant protein A by activated alveolar macrophages. Am J Physiol Lung Cell Mol Physiol 2000;278:L1025–31.

30. Petrucci N, Iacovelli W. Lung protective ventilation strategy for the acute respiratory distress syndrome. Cochrane Database Syst Rev 2007;(3):CD003844.
31. Hemmila MR, Napolitano LM. Severe respiratory failure: advanced treatment options. Crit Care Med 2006;34:S278–90.
32. The Acute Respiratory Distress Syndrome Network. Ventilation with lower tidal volumes as compared with traditional tidal volumes for acute lung injury and the acute respiratory distress syndrome. N Engl J Med 2000;342:1301–8.
33. Brochard L, Roudot-Thoraval F, Roupie E, et al. Tidal volume reduction for prevention of ventilator-induced lung injury in acute respiratory distress syndrome. The Multicenter Trial Group on Tidal Volume reduction in ARDS. Am J Respir Crit Care Med 1998;158:1831–8.
34. Stewart TE, Meade MO, Cook DJ, et al. Evaluation of a ventilation strategy to prevent barotrauma in patients at high risk for acute respiratory distress syndrome. Pressure- and Volume-Limited Ventilation Strategy Group. N Engl J Med 1998; 338:355–61.
35. Hickling KG, Henderson SJ, Jackson R. Low mortality associated with low volume pressure limited ventilation with permissive hypercapnia in severe adult respiratory distress syndrome. Intensive Care Med 1990;16:372–7.
36. Slutsky AS. Mechanical ventilation. American College of Chest Physicians' Consensus Conference. Chest 1993;104:1833–59.
37. Kallet RH, Jasmer RM, Pittet JF, et al. Clinical implementation of the ARDS Network protocol is associated with reduced hospital mortality compared with historical controls. Crit Care Med 2005;33:925–9.
38. Ranieri VM, Mascia L, Fiore T, et al. Cardiorespiratory effects of positive end-expiratory pressure during progressive tidal volume reduction (permissive hypercapnia) in patients with acute respiratory distress syndrome. Anesthesiology 1995;83:710–20.
39. Webb HH, Tierney DF. Experimental pulmonary edema due to intermittent positive pressure ventilation with high inflation pressures. Protection by positive end-expiratory pressure. Am Rev Respir Dis 1974;110:556–65.
40. Cereda M, Foti G, Musch G, et al. Positive end-expiratory pressure prevents the loss of respiratory compliance during low tidal volume ventilation in acute lung injury patients. Chest 1996;109:480–5.
41. Carvalho CR, Barbas CS, Medeiros DM, et al. Temporal hemodynamic effects of permissive hypercapnia associated with ideal PEEP in ARDS. Am J Respir Crit Care Med 1997;156:1458–66.
42. Amato MB, Barbas CS, Medeiros DM, et al. Effect of a protective-ventilation strategy on mortality in the acute respiratory distress syndrome. N Engl J Med 1998;338:347–54.
43. Villar J, Kacmarek RM, Pérez-Méndez L, et al. A high positive end-expiratory pressure, low tidal volume ventilatory strategy improves outcome in persistent acute respiratory distress syndrome: a randomized, controlled trial. Crit Care Med 2006;34:1311–8.
44. Vinayak AG, Gehlbach B, Pohlman AS, et al. The relationship between sedative infusion requirements and permissive hypercapnia in critically ill, mechanically ventilated patients. Crit Care Med 2006;34:1668–73.
45. Brower RG, Shanholtz CB, Fessler HE, et al. Prospective, randomized, controlled clinical trial comparing traditional versus reduced tidal volume ventilation in acute respiratory distress syndrome patients. Crit Care Med 1999;27: 1492–8.
46. Kregenow DA, Rubenfeld GD, Hudson LD, et al. Hypercapnic acidosis and mortality in acute lung injury. Crit Care Med 2006;34:1–7.

47. Rubenfeld GD, Cooper C, Carter G, et al. Barriers to providing lung-protective ventilation to patients with acute lung injury. Crit Care Med 2004;32:1289–93.
48. Mutlu GM, Factor P, Schwartz DE, et al. Severe status asthmaticus: management with permissive hypercapnia and inhalation anesthesia. Crit Care Med 2002;30: 477–80.
49. Oddo M, Feihl F, Schaller MD, et al. Management of mechanical ventilation in acute severe asthma: practical aspects. Intensive Care Med 2006;32:501–10.
50. Dhuper S, Maggiore D, Chung V, et al. Profile of near-fatal asthma in an inner-city hospital. Chest 2003;124:1880–4.
51. Sarnaik AP, Daphtary KM, Meert KL, et al. Pressure-controlled ventilation in children with severe status asthmaticus. Pediatr Crit Care Med 2004;5:133–8.
52. Miller JD, Carlo WA. Safety and effectiveness of permissive hypercapnia in the preterm infant. Curr Opin Pediatr 2007;19:142–4.
53. Kraybill EN, Runyun DK, Bose CL, et al. Risk factors for chronic lung disease in infants with birth weights of 751 to 1000 grams. J Pediatr 1989;115:115–20.
54. Garland JS, Buck RK, Allred EN, et al. Hypocarbia before surfactant therapy appears to increase bronchopulmonary dysplasia risk in infants with respiratory distress syndrome. Arch Pediatr Adolesc Med 1995;149:617–22.
55. Kamper J, Feilberg Jørgensen N, Jonsbo F, et al. Danish ETFOL Study Group. The Danish national study in infants with extremely low gestational age and birthweight (the ETFOL study): respiratory morbidity and outcome. Acta Paediatr 2004;93:225–32.
56. Bagolan P, Casaccia G, Crescenzi F, et al. Impact of a current treatment protocol on outcome of high-risk congenital diaphragmatic hernia. J Pediatr Surg 2004;39: 313–8.
57. Mariani G, Cifuentes J, Carlo WA. Randomized trial of permissive hypercapnia in preterm infants. Pediatrics 1999;104:1082–8.
58. Carlo WA, Stark AR, Bauer C, et al. Effects of minimal ventilation in a multicenter randomized controlled trial of ventilator support and early corticosteroid therapy in extremely low birthweight infants. Pediatrics 1999;104(3 Suppl):738–9.
59. Woodgate PG, Davies MW. Permissive hypercapnia for the prevention of morbidity and mortality in mechanically ventilated newborn infants. Cochrane Database Syst Rev 2001;(2):CD002061.
60. Danan C, Durrmeyer X, Brochard L, et al. A randomized trial of delayed extubation for the reduction of reintubation in extremely preterm infants. Pediatr Pulmonol 2008;43:117–24.
61. Kaiser JR, Gauss CH, Williams DK. The effects of hypercapnia on cerebral autoregulation in ventilated very low birth weight infants. Pediatr Res 2005;58:931–5.
62. Kaiser JR, Gauss CH, Pont MM, et al. Hypercapnia during the first 3 days of life is associated with severe intraventricular hemorrhage in very low birth weight infants. J Perinatol 2006;26:279–85.
63. Fabres J, Carlo WA, Phillips V, et al. Both extremes of arterial carbon dioxide pressure and the magnitude of fluctuations in arterial carbon dioxide pressure are associated with severe intraventricular hemorrhage in preterm infants. Pediatrics 2007;119:299–305.
64. Dahl M, Kamper J. Physical outcome and school performance of very-low-birthweight infants treated with minimal handling and early nasal CPAP. Acta Paediatr 2006;95:1099–103.
65. Sevransky JE, Levy MM, Marini JJ. Mechanical ventilation in sepsis-induced acute lung injury/acute respiratory distress syndrome: an evidence-based review. Crit Care Med 2004;32(11 Suppl):S548–53.

66. O'Croinin D, Ni Chonghaile M, Higgins B, et al. Bench-to-bedside review: permissive hypercapnia. Crit Care 2005;9:51–9.
67. Dixon NM, Kell DB. The inhibition by CO_2 of the growth and metabolism of microorganisms. J Appl Bacteriol 1989;67:109–36.
68. Rotstein OD, Fiegel VD, Simmons RL, et al. The deleterious effect of reduced pH and hypoxia on neutrophil migration in vitro. J Surg Res 1988;45:298–303.
69. Simmen HP, Battaglia H, Kossmann T, et al. Effect of peritoneal fluid pH on outcome of aminoglycoside treatment of intraabdominal infections. World J Surg 1993;17:393–7.
70. Feihl F, Eckert P, Brimioulle S, et al. Permissive hypercapnia impairs pulmonary gas exchange in the acute respiratory distress syndrome. Am J Respir Crit Care Med 2000;162:209–15.
71. Vannucci RC, Towfighi J, Brucklacher RM, et al. Effect of extreme hypercapnia on hypoxic-ischemic brain damage in the immature rat. Pediatr Res 2001;49:799–803.
72. Pedoto A, Nandi J, Oler A, et al. Role of nitric oxide in acidosis-induced intestinal injury in anesthetized rats. J Lab Clin Med 2001;138:270–6.
73. Pedoto A, Caruso JE, Nandi J, et al. Acidosis stimulates nitric oxide production and lung damage in rats. Am J Respir Crit Care Med 1999;159:397–402.
74. Richecoeur J, Lu Q, Vieira SR, et al. Expiratory washout versus optimization of mechanical ventilation during permissive hypercapnia in patients with severe acute respiratory distress syndrome. Am J Respir Crit Care Med 1999;160:77–85.
75. Goldsmith DJ, Forni LG, Hilton PJ. Bicarbonate therapy and intracellular acidosis. Clin Sci (Lond) 1997;93:593–8.
76. Nahas GG, Sutin KM, Fermon C, et al. Guidelines for the treatment of acidaemia with THAM. Drugs 1998;55:191–224.
77. Kallet RH, Jasmer RM, Luce JM, et al. The treatment of acidosis in acute lung injury with tris-hydroxymethyl aminomethane (THAM). Am J Respir Crit Care Med 2000;161:1149–53.
78. Weber T, Tschernich H, Sitzwohl C, et al. Tromethamine buffer modifies the depressant effect of permissive hypercapnia on myocardial contractility in patients with acute respiratory distress syndrome. Am J Respir Crit Care Med 2000;162:1361–5.

Extracorporeal Membrane Oxygenation

Onsy Ayad, MD[a,b], Ann Dietrich, MD, FAAP, FACEP[b,c,*],
Leslie Mihalov, MD[b,c]

KEYWORDS

- ECMO • Respiratory failure • Circulatory failure

Extracorporeal membrane oxygenation (ECMO) is an advanced technology that is available at a limited number of facilities. It is a supportive modality that is used in acute severe reversible cardiac or respiratory failure in patients of all ages when there is a high risk for dying from the primary disease despite maximal conventional intensive care supportive measures (**Fig. 1**). ECMO has been used successfully since the 1970s for neonates with persistent pulmonary hypertension refractory to conventional therapy. Hypothermic cardiopulmonary arrest, failed traditional therapies for respiratory diseases, and protracted resuscitation have also been situations in which ECMO has been effective. Similar to cardiac bypass, ECMO is a means by which venous blood is removed from the patient, oxygenated and ventilated, and returned to the arterial or venous circulation of the patient (**Fig. 2**).

ECMO is labor-intensive and expensive, however, with an estimated total hospital cost of $20,000 to $90,000 per patient, and it should be targeted to patients likely to benefit from the therapy. In 2006, the Extracorporeal Life Support Organization (ELSO) reported a survival rate to intensive care unit (ICU) discharge of 65% in a cohort of 32,905 patients. The current reported survival rates are 77% for neonatal respiratory failure, 56% for pediatric respiratory failure, 53% for adult respiratory failure, 43% for pediatric cardiac failure, and 32% for adult cardiac failure.

Early initiation of this technology may be life saving for critically ill patients with specific respiratory or cardiac diseases. Early identification of patients who may benefit from this technology and timely transfer to facilities prepared to use this

[a] Nationwide Children's Hospital, 700 Children's Drive, Columbus, OH, USA
[b] The Ohio State University College of Medicine, 370 West 9th Avenue, Columbus, OH 43210, USA
[c] Section of Pediatric Emergency Medicine, Nationwide Children's Hospital, 700 Children's Drive, Columbus, OH, USA
* Corresponding author. Section of Emergency Medicine, Nationwide Children's Hospital, 700 Children's Drive, Columbus, OH.
E-mail address: adietric@columbus.rr.com (A. Dietrich).

Emerg Med Clin N Am 26 (2008) 953–959
doi:10.1016/j.emc.2008.07.010
0733-8627/08/$ – see front matter © 2008 Elsevier Inc. All rights reserved.
emed.theclinics.com

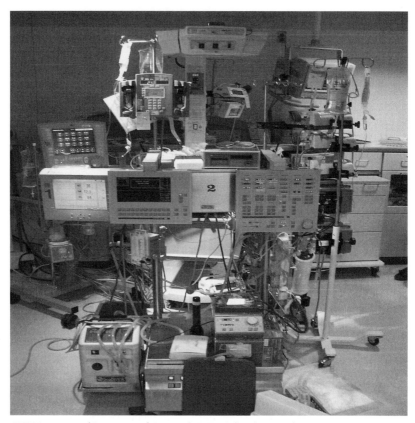

Fig. 1. ECMO system. (*Courtesy of* O. Ayad, MD, Columbus, OH).

technology if conventional therapies are not effective may improve outcomes for a select subset of patients.

RESPIRATORY DISEASES

ECMO has been used for patients with primary acute hypoxic respiratory failure (AHRF) of various causes. Causes of AHRF include viral pneumonia (most common), bacterial pneumonia, aspiration, acute respiratory distress syndrome (ARDS), postoperative or posttraumatic ARDS, pulmonary hemorrhage, and burn injuries. Cochran and colleagues[1] reviewed 10 years of experience with pediatric ECMO used for 27 children and adolescents with life-threatening pulmonary conditions unresponsive to conventional intensive care therapy. Most patients were male, and the mean age of the patients was 28 months. Venoarterial access was ultimately used in all but 1 patient. The most frequent diagnoses were presumed viral pneumonia, respiratory syncytial virus (RSV), bronchiolitis, and pertussis pneumonia. The overall survival rate was 67%. Although the number of patients in any category was limited, patients who had pertussis and documented bacterial pneumonia had higher mortality rates than patients with other diagnoses. The mean duration of ECMO was 12.2 days. Reasons for early termination included unrelenting pulmonary hypertension, multiple organ dysfunction, and intracerebral bleeding.

VENOARTERIAL ECMO CIRCUIT

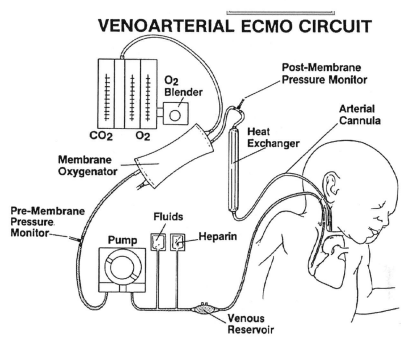

Fig. 2. Venoarterial ECMO circuit. (*From* Walker G, Liddell M, Davis C. Extracorporeal life support—state of the art. Paediatr Respir Rev 2003;4(2):147–52; with permission.)

Other studies have tried to predict which patients would not benefit from ECMO. An A-a gradient of greater than 450 mm Hg for more than 16 hours and a mean airway pressure of greater than 23 cm H_2O were highly predictive of mortality.[2,3] This differs from the results noted by Cochran and colleagues,[1] who found a survival rate of 67% in a pediatric population with a mean A-a gradient of 580 mm Hg and a mean airway pressure of 29.9 cm H_2O.

It has been demonstrated that the earlier the referral, especially before significant barotrauma or volutrauma, the better is the outcome.[1]

ECMO survival also varies, depending on the etiology of the respiratory failure. Survival is highest in cases of aspiration pneumonia (65%) and lowest in *Pneumocystis* pneumonia (41%) and pertussis (30%). In one series, when all patients were stratified into mortality risk quartiles (based on oxygenation index and pediatric risk of mortality [PRISM] score), the proportion of deaths among ECMO-treated patients in the 50% to 75% mortality risk quartile was less than half of the proportion in non–ECMO-treated patients (28.6% vs. 71.4%; $P < .05$; **Fig. 3**).[3]

REFRACTORY CIRCULATORY FAILURE

Initially, the use of ECMO was contraindicated for patients who had septicemia because of concerns that contamination of the circuit would result in certain death. Several studies have not supported these concerns.[4–6] The American College of Critical Care Medicine has published guidelines regarding the management of septic shock in children.[7] The recommendation is to consider ECMO for children who are unresponsive to all conventional treatment. Septic shock frequently has a different hemodynamic manifestation in neonates, infants and children, and adults. In

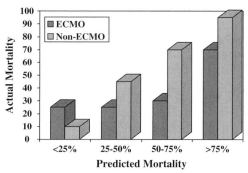

Fig. 3. ARDS: Pediatric ECMO. (*From* Green TP, Timmons OD, Fackler JC, et al. The impact of extracorporeal membrane oxygenation on survival in pediatric patients with acute respiratory failure. Crit Care Med 1996;24:323–9; with permission.)

neonates, most have persistent pulmonary hypertension. In infants and young children, decreased left ventricular function and low cardiac output are more common, and in adults, the pattern is usually distributive shock. ECMO may be particularly advantageous in children with impaired ventricular function. Studies used to establish these recommendations had fewer than 13 patients in each series, however.[5,6] A more recent review of 45 children who received venoarterial ECMO for hemodynamic support has added more credibility to the recommendations, with a 47% survival rate to hospital discharge. The use of ECMO in children with septic shock and multiple organ failure is controversial, with some institutions not placing these patients on ECMO because of dismal survival rates.

Potential indications for ECMO support in refractory circulatory failure include failure to wean from cardiopulmonary bypass, cardiopulmonary failure after surgical repair, severe ventricular failure (eg, in myocarditis and cardiomyopathy), severe hypoxemia in cyanotic congenital heart disease if surgery is temporarily contraindicated, a bridge for cardiac transplantation, and refractory septic shock.

CARDIAC ARREST

The use of ECMO for patients who have cardiac arrest is increasing in frequency. The survival rate after pediatric cardiopulmonary arrest is dismal. Young and Seidel reported a 13% survival to hospital discharge.[8] Out-of-hospital arrests had the worst survival rates at 8.4%, whereas in-ICU or in-hospital arrests had slightly better survival rates (20% and 24%, respectively). In a 5.5-year study examining factors predictive of survival to hospital discharge for pediatric ICU arrests, de Mos and colleagues[9] found high in-hospital mortality and morbidity rates and that the use of postarrest ECMO within 24 hours was associated with reduced mortality; the overall survival rate increased to 25%. Factors associated with mortality included the presence of renal dysfunction and an epinephrine infusion at the time of the arrest.

Alsoufi and colleagues[10] reported on pediatric patients who had refractory cardiac arrest (N = 80, age range: 1 day to 17.6 years). Most patients had cardiac disease (71 [88.8%] of 80). Criteria for initiation of ECMO included a witnessed arrest in a pediatric patient, (including infants and children), lack of recovery of cardiac function within 5 to 10 minutes of institution of cardiopulmonary resuscitation (CPR), absence of coexisting conditions that would preclude survival, and ability to institute ECMO within a short period (25–40 minutes). The median duration of CPR for patients with a favorable versus unfavorable outcome was 46 minutes versus 41 minutes. Favorable outcomes occurred in 67% of patients who had myocarditis, 50% of those who had cardiomyopathy, 36% following cardiotomy, and 6% of those who had unoperated congenital heart disease. Unfortunately, only 1 (11.1%) of 9 patients who had a noncardiac etiology survived.

Several other series have reported favorable outcomes with the use of ECMO for cardiac arrest. In the study by Duncan,[11] of 11 children with congenital heart disease and cardiac arrest, 7 (63.6%) survived to hospital discharge and 4 (36.4%) were neurologically intact. A retrospective review of 57 adults receiving ECMO after a cardiac arrest showed improved survival rates (>15 minutes, 32% hospital survival; 15–60 minutes, 48% hospital survival; and >60 minutes, 12% survival).[12] Hamrick and colleagues[13] failed to find the same results in pediatric patients with a survival rate of only 6%.

The duration of arrest before institution of ECMO is controversial, with wide variations in the reported data. A review found no difference between survivors and nonsurvivors regarding length of CPR before cannulation.[14] In the adult literature, Chen and colleagues[12] reported that more patients survived if the initial CPR duration was less than 60 minutes.

Laboratory testing has been postulated to be predictive of survival. In adults, the Pao_2 was a predictor of positive neurologic outcome; patients with a Pao_2 between 12 and 442 mm Hg predicted a return of consciousness, whereas those who did not regain consciousness had a Pao_2 between 34 and 58 mm Hg. Doski and colleagues[15] did not find arterial blood gas values to be predictors for survival of pediatric patients. Horisberger and colleagues[16] found that the initial base deficit was related to survival in pediatric patients. In this series, 10% of CPR recipients with a base deficit greater than 20 survived 1 year compared with a survival rate of 86% in CPR recipients with a base deficit less than or equal to 15.

Ideally, a permanent on-site team is available to allow for early efficient transition to ECMO. Ghez and colleagues[17] explored the use of an on-call ECMO response team for patients who had cardiac disease and were undergoing CPR in the pediatric intensive care unit (PICU) or pediatric cardiac catheterization laboratory. Although the study was retrospective and only consisted of 15 episodes in 14 patients, mean CPR time before ECMO was 44 ± 27 minutes, with a 57% survival to discharge. The survival rate improved to 64% in a pediatric study from Boston Children's Hospital comparing a historical control with patients treated by a rapid-response ECMO team that initiated ECMO within 15 minutes of notification. Rapid-deployment ECMO requires an in-house dedicated team using a modified ECMO circuit and the capability to initiate cannulation within 10 to 15 minutes of beginning CPR.

HYPOTHERMIC CARDIOPULMONARY ARREST

Initially, extracorporeal circulation was considered the ideal method for resuscitation of hypothermic cardiac arrest. Ruttman and colleagues[18,19] studied a consecutive series of 59 patients who had hypothermia and cardiopulmonary arrest. Thirty-four patients were resuscitated by standard extracorporeal circulation, and 25 patients were resuscitated by ECMO. Spontaneous circulation was restored in 32 patients (32 [54.2%] of 59), and 12 (12 [20.3%] of 59) survived. ECMO-assisted resuscitation showed a sixfold higher chance for survival.[18] Asphyxia-related hypothermia (avalanche or drowning) was the most predictive adverse factor for survival (relative risk [RR] = 0.09, 95% confidence interval [CI]: 0.01–0.60). In a subgroup analysis of avalanche victims, ECMO-assisted resuscitation was found to be superior to ECC-assisted rewarming with respect to survival (RR = 7.6, 95% CI: 1.4–50.8).[18]

COMPLICATIONS OF EXTRACORPOREAL MEMBRANE OXYGENATION

Complications during ECMO are the rule rather than the exception. As of 2005, there was an average of 2.7 complications per case as reported by the ELSO registry. Complications encountered during ECMO can be classified as mechanical or patient related. Mechanical complications include thrombosis in any ECMO circuit component, cannula problems (malposition, kinking, perforation of a vessel, and dislodgement), oxygenator failure, tubing rupture, or pump malfunction. Patient-related complications include surgical or cannula site bleeding, intracranial infarct or bleed, hemolysis, renal insufficiency requiring dialysis or hemofiltration, hypertension, seizures, electrolyte abnormalities, pneumothorax, cardiac dysfunction or arrhythmias, gastrointestinal hemorrhage, and infection.

SUMMARY

In summary, ECMO is an important tool to provide oxygen delivery and carbon dioxide removal in addition to cardiac support for patients with intractable reversible respiratory or cardiovascular collapse unresponsive to conventional treatment. Even though ECMO can be a life-saving modality, it is expensive and labor-intensive and carries a significant complication risk. Early recognition and prompt referral of patients who may benefit from ECMO in addition to careful patient selection, continuous communication between ECMO centers and their referral base, and meticulous care can improve the outcome of these critically ill patients who previously had no chance of survival.

REFERENCES

1. Cochran JB, Habib DM, Webb S, et al. Pediatric extracorporeal membrane oxygenation (ECMO): a review of the first ten years of experience at the Medical University of South Carolina. J S C Med Assoc 2005;101(4):104–7.
2. Tamburro RF, Bugnitz MC, Stidham GL. Alveolar-arterial oxygen gradient as a predictor of outcome in patients with nonneonatal pediatric respiratory failure. J Pediatr 1991;119(6):935–8.
3. Green TP, Timmons OD, Fackler JC, et al. The impact of extracorporeal membrane oxygenation on survival in pediatric patients with acute respiratory failure. Pediatric Critical Care Study Group. Crit Care Med 1996;24(2):323–9.
4. MacLaren G, Butt W, Best D, et al. Extracorporeal membrane oxygenation for refractory septic shock in children: one institution's experience. Pediatr Crit Care Med 2007;8(5):1–5.
5. Beca J, Butt W. Extracorporeal membrane oxygenation for refractory septic shock in children. Pediatrics 1994;93(5):726–9.
6. Goldman AP, Kerr SJ, Butt W, et al. Extracorporeal support for intractable cardiorespiratory failure due to meningococcal disease. Lancet 1997;349(9050):466–9.
7. Carcillo JA, Fields AI, American College of Critical Care Medicine Task Force Committee Members. Clinical practice parameters for hemodynamic support of pediatric and neonatal patients in septic shock. Crit Care Med 2002;30(6):1365–78.
8. Young KD, Seidel JS. Pediatric cardiopulmonary resuscitation: a collective review. Ann Emerg Med 1999;33(2):195–205.

9. de Mos N, van Litsenburg RR, McCrindle B, et al. Pediatric in-intensive-care-unit cardiac arrest: incidence, survival, and predictive factors. Crit Care Med 2006; 34(4):1209–15.

10. Alsoufi B, Al-Radi OO, Nazer RI, et al. Survival outcomes after rescue extracorporeal cardiopulmonary resuscitation in pediatric patients with refractory cardiac arrest. J Thorac Cardiovasc Surg 2007;134(4):952–9.

11. Duncan BW. Mechanical circulatory support in children: extracorporeal membrane oxygenation and ventricular assist devices. Expert Rev Med Devices 2005;2(3):239–41.

12. Chen YS, Chao A, Yu HY, et al. Analysis and results of prolonged resuscitation in cardiac arrest patients rescued by extracorporeal membrane oxygenation. J Am Coll Cardiol 2003;41(2):197–203.

13. Hamrick SE, Gremmels DB, Keet CA, et al. Neurodevelopmental outcome of infants supported with extracorporeal membrane oxygenation after cardiac surgery. Pediatrics 2003;111(6 Pt 1):e671–5.

14. Morris MC, Wernovsky G, Nadkarni VM. Survival outcomes after extracorporeal cardiopulmonary resuscitation instituted during active chest compressions following refractory in-hospital pediatric cardiac arrest. Pediatr Crit Care Med 2004;5(5):440–6.

15. Doski JJ, Butler TJ, Louder DS, et al. Outcome of infants requiring cardiopulmonary resuscitation before extracorporeal membrane oxygenation. J Pediatr Surg 1997;32(9):1318–21.

16. Horisberger T, Fischer E, Fanconi S. One-year survival and neurological outcome after pediatric cardiopulmonary resuscitation. Intensive Care Med 2002;28(3): 365–8 [Epub 2002 Feb 13].

17. Ghez O, Fouilloux V, Charpentier A, et al. Absence of rapid deployment extracorporeal membrane oxygenation (ECMO) team does not preclude resuscitation ECMO in pediatric cardiac patients with good results. ASAIO J 2007;53(6):692–5.

18. Ruttmann E, Weissenbacher A, Ulmer H, et al. Prolonged extracorporeal membrane oxygenation-assisted support provides improved survival in hypothermic patients with cardiocirculatory arrest. J Thorac Cardiovasc Surg 2007;134(3): 594–600.

19. Available at: http://www.elso.med.umich.edu/Registry.htm. Accessed April 15, 2008.

Pediatric Airway Management

Genevieve Santillanes, MD[a], Marianne Gausche-Hill, MD, FACEP, FAAP[b],*

KEYWORDS

- Pediatric assessment triangle • Position • Suction
- Oxygen • Delivery • Airway management

Pediatric airway problems are seen commonly in pediatric and general emergency departments; in fact, several studies have shown respiratory distress to be the fourth most common chief complaint in children presenting to the emergency department.[1,2] Furthermore, airway management often is required in children who have other presenting complaints such as trauma and seizures. The peak age of respiratory distress in children is under 2 years of age, an age at which the airway is significantly different from an adult airway.[1,2]

Management of the pediatric airway is often stressful to providers. One reason is that while management of an adult airway is familiar to emergency medicine physicians, management of the pediatric airway is a less frequent but more complex process. The wide variation in equipment sizes and medication doses adds additional steps in airway management. Dose and equipment size calculations are nonautomatic activities that require mental effort.[3] This cognitive activity takes away from the time spent on patient assessment and management decisions.

This article reviews the pediatric airway, highlighting the anatomic and physiologic differences between infant, pediatric and adult airways, and how these differences impact assessment and management of the pediatric airway.

ANATOMIC AND PHYSIOLOGIC DIFFERENCES

Significant differences exist between neonatal and adult airways. As children grow, their airways adopt a form more similar to adults. In general, by the age of 8, the airway is very similar to an adult airway.

[a] Departments of Emergency Medicine and Pediatrics, Harbor-University of California Los Angeles Medical Center, Torrance, CA, USA
[b] Department of Emergency Medicine, Harbor-University of California Los Angeles Medical Center, David Geffen School of Medicine at University of California Los Angeles, 1000 West Carson Street, Torrance, CA 90509, USA
* Corresponding author. Department of Emergency Medicine, Harbor-University of California Los Angeles Medical Center, 1000 West Carson Street, Box 21, Torrance, CA 90509.
E-mail address: mgausche@emedharbor.edu (M. Gausche-Hill).

Emerg Med Clin N Am 26 (2008) 961–975
doi:10.1016/j.emc.2008.08.004
0733-8627/08/$ – see front matter © 2008 Elsevier Inc. All rights reserved.

emed.theclinics.com

Several of these airway differences make infants and young children susceptible to upper airway obstruction. Infants and young children have a relatively large occiput. When lying supine on a flat surface, this results in neck flexion and potential airway obstruction. The increased soft tissue and the flexible trachea can result in pressure on the tracheal rings and airway obstruction. External pressure such as cricoid pressure can cause tracheal collapse and airway obstruction. Infants and young children also have a proportionally larger tongue within the oral cavity, which is a common cause of airway obstruction.

Other airway differences make infants and young children more susceptible to respiratory failure. Infants have a lower percentage of type 1 or slow-twitch skeletal muscle fibers in their intercostal muscles and diaphragm.[4] Type 1 muscle fibers are less prone to fatigue. Infants also have lower stores of glycogen and fat in their respiratory muscles.[5] These differences predispose infants to respiratory muscle fatigue. Furthermore, young infants preferentially breathe through their noses,[6,7] and during oral breathing, must use soft palate muscles to maintain an open oral airway.[8]

Infants have more horizontal ribs and a flatter diaphragm than adults. They also air trap because of their high respiratory rate. Although this increases their functional residual capacity, it also means that they are less able to increase their tidal volume to compensate for changes in respiratory rate or increased oxygen demand. Because minute ventilation equals respiratory rate multiplied by tidal volume, infants must increase minute ventilation by increasing their respiratory rate. There is a limit, however, to the increase in respiratory rate before tidal volume is compromised. These factors are further reasons infants have less reserve and are more susceptible to respiratory failure.

Awake infants have 40% of the functional residual capacity of adults.[9] This functional residual capacity is achieved, however, because they hold their respiratory muscles in a slightly inspiratory position.[10] Because infants have a compliant chest wall, decreased muscle tone in deep sleep and sedated states lead to a significantly decreased functional residual capacity. During an apneic state, an infant has only 10% of the functional residual capacity of an adult.[9] This decreased functional residual capacity means that infants have less oxygen available in their lungs for gas exchange during exhalation or apnea. Infants have a higher metabolic rate than adults and metabolize at least 6 mL of oxygen per minute, while adults metabolize only 3 mL of oxygen per minute.[9] In addition, term newborn infants have only half of the alveoli seen in an adult.[11] All of these factors cause infants to desaturate much more quickly than adults during periods of apnea.

The child's relatively smaller airway results in increased airway resistance, making infants and children more prone to respiratory failure. Poiseuille's law of resistance demonstrates this. Resistance is inversely proportional to the radius to the power of four ($R \propto 1/r^4$). Therefore, small changes in airway diameter have a large impact on overall airway resistance.

Some pediatric airway differences are especially important to understand to increase likelihood of successful endotracheal intubation. These differences include the relatively large tongue within the oral cavity, the high and anterior airway, and the more acute angle between the tracheal opening and the epiglottis. These differences can make visualization of the airway and manipulation of the endotracheal tube (ETT) tube more difficult in children.

Another difference is that in adults, the narrowest diameter of the airway is at the vocal cords, while in children, the narrowest diameter is at the cricoid ring. This means that an ETT may fit through the vocal cords but be too large to pass through the cricoid ring in a child. In addition, a foreign body can be lodged below the level of the vocal cords in a child, necessitating either basic life support maneuvers to dislodge it into the oropharynx, or a surgical airway to bypass the obstruction.

ASSESSMENT

Assessing the child for signs respiratory distress or failure can be challenging. One initial approach to assessment is the Pediatric Assessment Triangle (PAT).[12] The PAT is a brief visual and auditory assessment that is performed without touching the child. This initial brief assessment can be extremely helpful, because children often become frightened and agitated when approached by a medical provider and may be difficult to assess. The PAT is an assessment of appearance, work of breathing, and circulation to the skin. The TICLS mnemonic summarizes a brief assessment of overall appearance: tone, interactiveness, consolability, look/gaze and speech/cry. After an assessment of general appearance, the work of breathing should be assessed, focusing on audible airway sounds and visual clues to increased work of breathing. The last component of the PAT is the circulation to the skin, looking for pallor, mottling, and cyanosis. The PAT can be completed in less than 30 seconds and determines if immediate resuscitation is necessary. **Table 1** outlines how abnormalities in the triangle may be used to create a general impression of the physiologic abnormality. This impression then drives immediate management priorities (**Box 1**). Once the PAT is completed, if immediate resuscitation is not required, a more complete assessment can be done (**Fig. 1**).

The complete assessment of the pediatric airway includes visual inspection of the child and assessment of respiratory rate, oxygen saturation and auscultation. The resting posture can provide important clues to level and cause of respiratory distress. A sniffing position is indicative of upper airway obstruction; the child leans forward in an attempt to open the upper airway and improve airflow. Another concerning posture is the tripod position. The child leans forward on outstretched arms to maximize use of accessory muscles of respiration. A child who refuses to lie down may be attempting to maintain a compromised airway. An obviously agitated child may be hypoxic.

Particular attention should be paid to use of accessory muscles of respiration. Retractions are a commonly seen sign of respiratory distress, in which skin and soft tissue are drawn inward during respiration. Retractions can occur in the substernal, intercostal, supraclavicular, and suprasternal areas. Because retractions can occur in any of these areas, it is important to undress the child for a complete assessment. Nasal flaring is another form of accessory muscle use and represents exaggerated

Table 1
Components of the Pediatric Assessment Triangle and the general impression

Stable	Respiratory Distress	Respiratory Failure	Shock	Central Nervous System/Metabolic	Cardio-Pulmonary Failure
Appearance					
Normal	Normal	Abnormal	Normal/ abnormal	Abnormal	Abnormal
Breathing					
Normal	Abnormal	Abnormal	Normal	Normal	Abnormal
Circulation					
Normal	Normal	Normal/ abnormal	Abnormal	Normal	Abnormal

Box 1
Management priorities by general impression

Stable

　Continue assessment

　Specific therapy based on possible etiologies

Respiratory distress

　Position of comfort

　Supplemental oxygen/suction as needed

　Specific therapy based on possible etiologies: (albuterol, diphenhydramine, epinephrine)

Respiratory failure

　Position the head and open the airway

　Provide 100% oxygen

　Initiate bag–mask ventilation as needed

　Initiate foreign body removal as needed

　Advanced airway as needed

Shock

　Provide oxygen as needed

　Obtain vascular access

　Begin fluid resuscitation

　Specific therapy based on possible etiologies

Central nervous system/metabolic

　Provide oxygen as needed

　Obtain rapid glucose as needed

　Specific therapy based on possible etiologies

Cardiopulmonary failure/arrest

　Position the head and open the airway

　Initiate bag–mask ventilation with 100% oxygen

　Begin chest compressions as needed

　Specific therapy as based on possible etiologies (defibrillation, epinephrine, amiodarone)

---

nostril opening during respiratory distress. Nasal flaring is an attempt to decrease airway resistance. Another form of accessory muscle use seen in infants who have severe respiratory distress is head bobbing. In head bobbing, the neck muscles are used to increase inspiratory pressure. The neck is extended during inhalation and relaxed during exhalation.

Abdominal breathing can be normal in young infants but may become exaggerated during respiratory distress. Paradoxical breathing or chest collapse during inspiration can be seen in infants. This occurs because, as high negative intrathoracic pressure is generated, the compliant chest wall is pulled inward. An ominous sign of impending respiratory failure is seesaw breathing. Seesaw breathing is a combination of

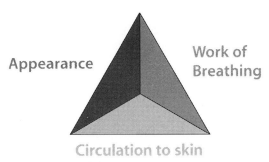

Fig. 1. The Pediatric Assessment Triangle components: appearance, work of breathing, and circulation to skin. (*From* Dieckmann RA. Pediatric assessment. In: Gausche-Hill M, Fuchs S, Yamamoto L, editors. APLS: the pediatric emergency medicine resource. 4th edition. Sudbury (MA): Jones and Bartlett; 2004. p. 25; with permission.)

paradoxical respiration and abdominal breathing. The chest retracts during inspiration and the abdomen bulges out; the converse happens during exhalation. Seesaw breathing is an ineffective form of breathing, and the infant is likely to fatigue quickly.

Resting respiratory rate should be assessed before disturbing the child (**Box 2**). Infants frequently have periodic breathing, so it is important to count respirations over a full minute and frequently reassess respiratory rate.[13] Oxygen saturation also should be measured.

Both audible and auscultated respiratory sounds can provide clues as to cause of respiratory distress. Expiratory wheezing is a very common sign of respiratory distress. This high-pitched sound is made during attempts at exhalation against an intrathoracic airway obstruction. The obstruction can be intrinsic such as airway constriction caused by asthma, extrinsic such as a mass or vascular structure compressing the airway, or caused by a foreign object within the airway. Wheezing can occur in both inspiratory and expiratory phases with severe obstruction. Wheezing generally is heard only with a stethoscope, but in severe cases, it may audible without a stethoscope.

Inspiratory stridor is a high-pitched sound that is caused by turbulent air flow across an extrathoracic airway obstruction. Causes of stridor include laryngotracheobronchitis (croup), retropharyngeal abscesses, and upper airway foreign bodies. Changes in the quality of voice or cry can be another clue to the cause of respiratory distress.

Box 2
Normal respiratory rates in infants and children

Neonates—24 to 50 breaths per minute

1 month to 1 year—24 to 38 breaths per minute

1 to 3 years—22 to 30 breaths per minute

4 to 6 years—20 to 24 breaths per minute

7 to 9 years—18 to 24 breaths per minute

10 to 14 years—16 to 22 breaths per minute

14 to 18 years—14 to 20 breaths per minute

Data from Loughlin CE. Pulmonology. In: Robertson J, Silkofski N, editors. The Harriet Lane handbook. 17th edition. Philadelphia: Elsevier; 2005. p. 613–30.

A muffled or hot potato voice might indicate a retropharyngeal or peritonsillar abscess. Laryngotracheobronchitis usually causes a hoarse voice and cry. Snoring noises may be a clue to partial airway obstruction from the tongue falling back into the posterior oropharynx as may be seen in seizing patients. Gurgling sounds can be an indication of blood or secretions in the airway.

Another sign of respiratory distress is grunting. Grunting is the sound produced when an infant exhales against a partially closed glottis and serves to increase end–expiratory pressure. It is seen frequently in alveolar diseases such as pneumonia and pulmonary edema and in diseases of the small airways such as bronchiolitis.[10]

Once a child in severe respiratory distress fatigues, many of these signs of respiratory distress diminish. Disappearance of retractions or slowing of respiratory rate in a child previously noted to be in severe respiratory distress can be an ominous sign of fatigue and impending respiratory arrest.

MANAGEMENT OF THE PEDIATRIC AIRWAY

Airway management should proceed in an orderly, stepwise fashion. Timely basic airway maneuvers may prevent the need for intubation and mechanical ventilation. Even when intubation is required, the early steps of airway management remain important. Successful intubation is difficult or impossible if the early steps of proper positioning and suctioning are omitted.

Airway Positioning

The first step in airway positioning is to place the head in a midline sniffing position with the neck extended and chin lifted. This can be accomplished with a head lift and chin tilt in medical patients. If there is any concern about cervical spine injury, a jaw thrust is preferred. The prominent occiput of young children impacts ideal head positioning. To counteract the natural neck flexion seen in children, a towel roll should be placed under the shoulders of the child (**Figs. 2** and **3**). Proper positioning opens the airway and improves ventilation. In some patients, proper positioning is all that is needed to correct respiratory distress. If intubation is required, proper positioning can improve visualization of the vocal cords.

Supplemental Oxygen

Supplemental oxygen should be provided to children in respiratory distress. Choice of oxygen delivery device depends on the situation and degree of respiratory distress. In a child who has mild hypoxia, a simple nasal cannula may be sufficient. A child who is fighting the oxygen delivery device vigorously can increase his or her oxygen demand. In an awake, agitated child, blow-by oxygen sometimes is tolerated better and might be a better choice. In cases of moderate hypoxia, a simple facemask might be more appropriate. In moderate-to-severe hypoxia, or if preoxygenation for intubation is desired, a nonrebreather mask is preferred.

Suction

Because infants preferentially breathe through their noses, obstruction of the nares with secretions can lead to severe respiratory distress. Suctioning the nose can improve the respiratory status of a young infant with bronchiolitis or an upper respiratory infection dramatically.

Excessive secretions can pool in the posterior oropharynx and cause airway obstruction. This is especially true in cases of oral or nasal bleeding, bronchiolitis,

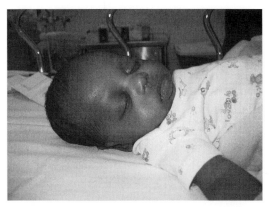

Fig. 2. Infant with neck in flexed position and partial airway obstruction.

or seizures. Suctioning is important to decrease obstruction and to improve visualization during laryngoscopy.

Airway Adjuncts

As discussed previously, infants and young children have a proportionally larger tongue than adults. This large tongue is a common cause of airway obstruction, especially in children who are seizing, postictal, or obtunded. Placement of a nasal or oral airway can reverse this obstruction. Oral airways should be used only in comatose patients without a gag reflex. The appropriate size of oral airway can be determined by holding the airway along the side of the child's face. The flange should be placed at the corner of the mouth, and the tip should reach the angle of the mandible (**Fig. 4**). Nasal airways can be placed in awake or semiconscious patients, but they cannot be used if there is possible basilar skull fracture, cerebrospinal fluid (CSF) leak, or coagulopathy. Nasal airways should be placed cautiously in young infants, because the large

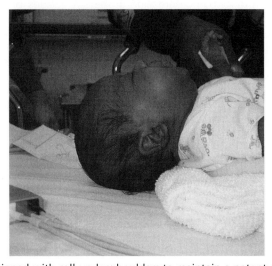

Fig. 3. Infant positioned with roll under shoulders to maintain a patent airway.

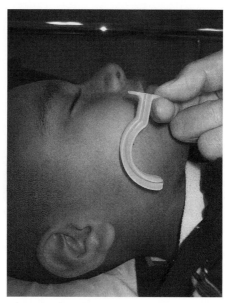

Fig. 4. Measuring correct length of oral airway.

adenoids and tonsils can be traumatized during insertion, resulting in bleeding. The nasal airway should be inserted with the bevel pointed away from the nasal septum to minimize risk of bleeding. Correct length can be determined by placing the airway along the side of the face extending from the nostril to the tragus of the ear, and the width of the nasopharyngeal airway should be less than that of the nostril (**Figs. 5** and **6**).

Bag–Mask Ventilation

Care must be taken to avoid compression of the soft tissues of the neck in young children during bag–mask ventilation (BMV). The provider should hold the jaw and avoid compressing the submental soft tissues. In young children, the airway can be compressed easily, or the tongue can be pushed up into the airway, causing an obstruction. One technique of BMV taught is the E-C clamp[14] (**Fig. 7**). In this technique the thumb and index fingers of the left hand form a C that holds the mask on the child's face. The other three fingers form an E and are placed on the angle of the jaw to lift the jaw into the mask. The right hand is free to squeeze the ventilation bag to deliver respirations.

Care must also be taken not to overventilate young children. The bag should be squeezed only until chest rise is seen. Normal tidal volume is 6 to 8 mL/kg, but with dead space of the device, one can estimate the volume needed to initiate chest rise as 10 mL/kg. Using this estimate, a 10 kg 1- year-old child requires only 80 to 100 mL per breath. This is equivalent to 6 tablespoons of air. Overventilation can lead to gastric distention and emesis or difficulty ventilating because of an elevated hemi-diaphragm. Time allowed for passive exhalation should be longer than inspiratory time. One method that is taught to prevent the likelihood of overexpansion of the chest and allow adequate exhalation time during BMV ventilation is to say "squeeze-release-release" while bagging. The ventilation bag is squeezed only until chest rise is initiated, while the provider

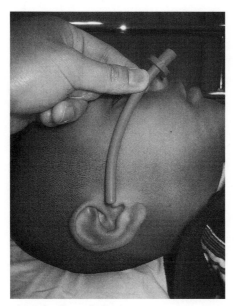

Fig. 5. Measuring correct length of nasal airway.

says "squeeze," and then the provider's hand relaxes to allow for the bag to re-expand during exhalation as the provider says "release, release."[14]

During rapid sequence intubation, gentle cricoid pressure should be maintained from the time of chemical paralysis until endotracheal intubation is confirmed. Children have flexible tracheal rings that can be collapsed if excessive pressure is applied

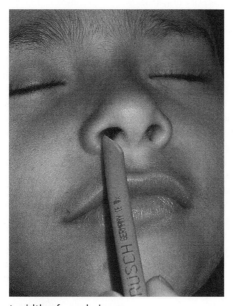

Fig. 6. Measuring correct width of nasal airway.

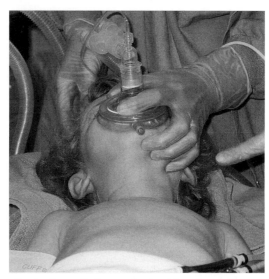

Fig. 7. E-C clamp method of ventilating patient with a bag-valve mask. Notice that the physician is lifting jaw into mask.

during the Sellick maneuver. Care must be taken to avoid obstructing the tracheal lumen or distorting airway landmarks with excessive pressure; if the intubator cannot visualize the airway (only pink mucosa is seen), it may be that excessive cricoid pressure is being used.

Endotracheal Intubation

One challenge in intubating children is determining the appropriate size of equipment. Equipment sizes are listed on length-based resuscitation tapes. If a length-based tape is not available, uncuffed ETT size can be estimated by the equation (age in years/4) + 4. This age-based formula has been shown to be more accurate than methods estimating ETT size based on width of the patient's fifth finger.[15] Cuffed ETT size can be calculated from the equation[16] (age in years/4) + 3 or one half size smaller than the calculated cuffed ETT diameter. Correct depth of insertion is approximately three times the uncuffed ETT size. Determining tube size for premature neonates can be challenging. **Table 2** provides an easy way to remember ETT size and depth of placement for these small infants.

Conventional teaching is that cuffed tubes should not be used in children under the age of 8 because of the risk of ischemic damage to the tracheal mucosa from compression between the cuff and the cricoid ring. This is a potential problem in young children, because the cricoid ring is the narrowest portion of the airway. However, because the design of modern ETTs has improved, it is less of a risk than previously thought.[17] ETT cuffs now are designed to be high-volume and low-pressure and produce a seal at a lower pressure. The use of cuffed tubes in young children is increasing, especially in emergency departments and pediatric ICUs.[17] Several studies have not shown an increase in postextubation stridor or reintubation rates when cuffed tubes were used in controlled settings with frequent cuff pressure monitoring.[16–18] Cuffed tubes also may provide some protection from aspiration.[19] Potential benefits of cuffed ETTs are facilitating ventilation with higher pressures, more consistent ventilation, and decreased need to exchange inappropriately sized ETTs.

Table 2
Endotrachial tube size and depth for premature newborns

Weight (kg)	Endotrachial size (mm internal diameter)	Depth of placement (cm)
Less than1	2.5	7
1-2	3.0	8
2-3	3.5	9

Care must be taken not to over inflate the cuff of a cuffed ETT.[17] A pressure of 20 mm H_2O is sufficient to provide a seal, but does not compromise mucosal blood flow.[20] Tracheal mucosal blood flow is compromised at 30 cm water pressure, and mucosal blood flow is completely obstructed at pressures of 45 cm water.[21] There is evidence that experienced physicians are unable to accurately estimate cuff pressure by palpating the pilot balloon and routinely inflate ETT cuffs to unsafe pressures in adults.[22,23] In one study of emergency medicine attending physicians, the average inflation pressure was over 90 cm water.[22] Use of an ETT cuff manometer can avoid high cuff pressures.[22–24] The advantages of uncuffed ETTs are that the risk of cuff overinflation with resultant tracheal damage does not exist, and a larger internal diameter ETT can be placed.

Choosing the correct size laryngoscope blade is critical to successful endotracheal intubation (**Table 3**). Macintosh (curved) blades primarily are used in older children and adults. The Macintosh blade is placed in the vallecula, lifting the base of the tongue and indirectly lifting the epiglottis. In infants and young children who have a larger, floppy epiglottis, this often does not provide adequate exposure of the airway. In this age group, Miller (straight) blades are preferred, because they directly lift the epiglottis and improve visualization of the vocal cords. Miller blades generally are used until about the age of 5, although they could be used in any age child. Another straight blade that can be useful in managing the pediatric airway is the Wis-Hipple blade. The Wis-Hipple blade has a widened distal tip that can be useful in controlling a large tongue and epiglottis. It is manufactured in a size 1.5, which is a convenient size for use in toddlers. Miller 0 blades should be used only in premature infants and average-sized newborns. A Miller 1 blade is appropriate for most infants beyond the immediate newborn period.

Because young children have an acute angle between the tracheal opening and epiglottis, correct placement of the laryngoscope blade is more important to ensure adequate visualization of the glottic opening. Exact depth of ETT insertion is more critical in young children than in adults, because the short trachea predisposes to accidental ETT dislodgement or right mainstem intubation. The proper depth of ETT placement is listed on the Broselow-Luten or length-based resuscitation tape.

Table 3
Laryngoscope blade size

Age	Weight (kg)	Laryngoscope Blade Size
Premature/newborn	1–3	Miller 0
1 month to 2 years	3.5–12	Miller 1, Wis–Hipple 1.5
3–6 years	15–20	Miller 2 McIntosh 2 (by age 5 years)
6–12 years	20–35	Miller 2, McIntosh 2 or 3
>12 years	>35	McIntosh 3

Alternatively, proper depth of ETT can be estimated by multiplying the size of the ETT by three; for example a 3.5 mm ETT should be placed at 10.5 cm at the lip.

The keys to successful intubation are following a standard procedure each time, choosing the correct size equipment, initially placing the laryngoscope blade in just to the base of the tongue and lifting upward, and having an assistant pass the suction and the ETT to the laryngoscopist. The assistant also can pull on the right corner of the mouth to allow more room to maneuver the ETT. Caution should be exercised with use of Sellick maneuver in young infants, as too much pressure may result in collapse of airway structures during intubation. When intubating a newly born or small infant, one trick to improve visualization during laryngoscopy is for the intubating physician to use his or her own left fifth finger to provide cricoid pressure. This avoids excessive cricoid pressure and allows the intubating physician to easily manipulate the cricoid ring. This is especially helpful in the premature neonate, because minimal pressure can alter the laryngoscopic view dramatically. A jaw thrust maneuver also may be used to aid in visualizing airway structures during intubation.

Proper ETT placement always should be confirmed by multiple methods, including clinical assessment and the used of end–tidal CO_2 detectors. Clinical assessment begins with listening for breath sounds over the stomach. In infants and small children, however, breath sounds can be transmitted easily. If breath sounds are heard in the stomach, the ETT should not be removed immediately. Breath sounds may be transmitted to the stomach from the lungs. Gurgling sounds indicate esophageal intubation, and the ETT should be removed. Next listen for two breaths over the right hemithorax and then over the left hemithorax. Decreased breath sounds over the left hemithorax may indicate that the ETT is too deep.

In addition to these clinical indicators, an end–tidal CO_2 detector should be used to confirm proper ETT placement. Pediatric end–tidal CO_2 detectors are indicated for children weighing 2 to 15 kg. Standard adult end–tidal CO_2 detectors are indicated for children weighing over 15 kg. Adult end–tidal CO_2 detectors can be used in smaller children, but cannot be left in-line, because they cause excessive dead space.[25] Pediatric end–tidal CO_2 detectors can be used in larger children in adults but should not be left in-line, because they increase resistance in the circuit. The validity of end–tidal CO_2 detectors has not been studied in infants under 2 kg. End–tidal CO_2 detectors do not detect tracheal tube placement reliably in cases of low pulmonary blood flow such as cardiac arrest and massive pulmonary embolism.[25,26] Oxygen saturation must be monitored, but an initial drop in oxygen saturation sometimes is seen immediately following intubation. If all other indicators confirm endotracheal placement of the ETT, the ETT should be left in place and ventilation continued for several breaths. Because of decreased functional residual capacity, children can take longer than adults to recover after the lack of oxygenation during laryngoscopy.

Just as in adults, close monitoring of the patient must continue after successful intubation. If an intubated patient develops problems with oxygenation or ventilation, a useful reminder of potential problems is the DOPE mnemonic: dislodgement, obstruction, pneumothorax, and equipment. Dislodgement may be more common in young children because of the short tracheal length. ETTs with a small internal diameter are more prone to obstruction than the larger tubes used in adults. The first step in troubleshooting oxygenation or ventilation problems is to remove the patient from the ventilator and hand ventilate with 100% oxygen. This serves to rule out ventilator malfunction as a cause of the problem. Auscultation over the stomach and bilateral thoraces may reveal tube dislodgement. An end–tidal CO_2 should be checked to confirm ETT position. During hand ventilation, difficulty bagging may be a clue to kinking of the ETT or obstruction with secretions. A suction catheter should pass easily down the ETT, and any secretions should be suctioned. If equipment failure, dislodgement, and obstruction are ruled out, pneumothorax must be considered. Because breath sounds can be transmitted, the presence of a pneumothorax may be more difficult to clinically diagnose in children. Poor perfusion may be the only sign of a tension pneumothorax in young children. If the child is in extremis, a needle thoracostomy can be performed. If the side of pneumothorax cannot be determined, the right side should be needled first, because the right lung is subjected to higher pressures and more likely to develop a pneumothorax from barotrauma. If the patient is not in extremis, and the cause of the problem is not obvious, a radiograph of the chest should be obtained to check for pneumothoraces or right mainstem intubation not appreciated on clinical examination.

Length-Based Resuscitation Tape

A length-based resuscitation tape should be used to determine appropriate sizes for equipment used in resuscitations. Length-based determination of ETT size has been determined to be at least as accurate as age-based calculations in normal and pathologically short children.[27]

Length-based resuscitation tapes and other resuscitation aids have other advantages over use of memory and formulas in choosing appropriate equipment and medication doses in resuscitations. Calculation of equipment sizes and medication doses and volumes is error prone, especially in a high-stress situation. The use of a length-based resuscitation aid avoids memorization of formulas and need for calculations. The other advantage is that use of resuscitation aids decreases mental effort required and allows the practitioner to focus mental effort on patient evaluation and management decisions.[3]

SUMMARY

Successful management of the pediatric airway depends on careful preparation and development of a routine that becomes automatic to the physician. The assessment and management of the airway always should proceed in a logical, orderly fashion. Knowledge of the airway differences between young children and adults will help the physician anticipate and troubleshoot difficulties that may occur. When intubation of the infant or young child is necessary, taking the time to properly position the patient, select the appropriate-sized equipment, and instruct assistants in their role will increase the likelihood of success of intubation and decrease the likelihood of potential complications. A length-based resuscitation tape will help the physician quickly select the appropriate equipment for the young child.

REFERENCES

1. Krauss BS, Harakal T, Fleisher GR. The spectrum and frequency of pediatric illnesses presenting to a pediatric emergency department. Pediatr Emerg Care 1991;7:67–71.
2. Nelson DS, Walsh K, Fleisher G. Spectrum and frequency of pediatric illnesses presenting to a general community hospital emergency department. Pediatrics 1992;90:5–10.
3. Luten R, Wears RF, Broselow J, et al. Managing the unique size-related issues of pediatric resuscitation: reducing cognitive load with resuscitation aids. Acad Emerg Med 2002;9:840–7.

4. Keens TG, Bryan AC, Levison H, et al. Developmental pattern of muscle fiber types in human ventilatory muscles. J Appl Physiol 1978;44:909–13.
5. Moss IR. Physiologic considerations. In: McMillian JA, Feigin RD, DeAngelis CD, editors. Oski's pediatrics. 4th edition. Philadelphia: Lippencott, Williams & Wilkins; 2006. p. 300–5.
6. Miller MJ, Carlo WA, Strohl KP, et al. Effect of maturation on oral breathing in sleeping premature infants. J Pediatr 1986;109:515–9.
7. Rodenstein DO, Perlmutter N, Stanescu DC. Infants are not obligatory nasal breathers. Am Rev Respir Dis 1985;131:343–7.
8. Bergeson PS, Shaw CJ. Are infants really obligatory nasal breathers? Clin Pediatr 2001;40:567–9.
9. Luten RC, Kissoon N. Approach to the pediatric airway. In: Walls RM, Murphy MF, Luten RC, editors. Manual of emergency airway management. 2nd edition. Phildadelphia: Lippincott, Williams & Wilkins; 2004. p. 263–81.
10. Sarnaik A, Heidemann SM. Respiratory pathophysiology and regulation. In: Kleigman RM, Rehrman RE, Jenson HB, editors. Nelson textbook of pediatrics. 18th edition. Philadelphia: Saunders; 2007. p. 1719–31.
11. Hislop AA, Wigglesworth JS, Desai R. Alveolar development in the human fetus and infant. Early Hum Dev 1986;13:1–11.
12. Dieckmann RA. Pediatric assessment. In: Gausche-Hill M, Fuchs S, Yamamoto L, editors. APLS: the pediatric emergency medicine resource. 4th edition. Sudbury (MA): Jones and Bartlett; 2004. p. 20–51.
13. Loughlin CE. Pulmonology. In: Robertson J, Silkofski N, editors. The Harriet Lane handbook. 17th edition. Philadelphia: Elsevier; 2005. p. 613–30.
14. Gausche-Hill M, Henderson DP, Goodrich SM, et al. Pediatric airway management for the prehospital professional DVD. Sudbury (MA): Jones and Bartlett Publishers and Unihealth Foundation; 2004.
15. King BR, Baker MD, Braitman LE, et al. Endotracheal tube selection in children: a comparison of four methods. Ann Emerg Med 1993;22:530–4.
16. Khine HH, Corddry DH, Kettrick RG, et al. Comparison of cuffed and uncuffed endotracheal tubes in young children during general anesthesia. Anesthesiology 1997;86:627–31.
17. Newth CJ, Rachman B, Patel N, et al. The use of cuffed versus uncuffed endotracheal tubes in pediatric intensive care. J Pediatr 2004;144:333–7.
18. Deakers TW, Reynolds G, Stretton M, et al. Cuffed endotracheal tubes in pediatric intensive care. J Pediat 1994;125:57–62.
19. Browning DH, Graves SA. Incidence of aspiration with endotracheal tubes in children. J Pediat 1983;102:582–4.
20. Fine GF, Borland LM. The future of the cuffed endotracheal tube. Paediatr Anaesth 2004;14:38–42.
21. Somri M, Fradis M, Malatskey S, et al. Simple on-line endotracheal cuff pressure relief valve. Ann Otol Rhinol Laryngol 2002;111:190–2.
22. Hoffman RJ, Parwani V, Hahn I. Experienced emergency medicine physicians cannot safely inflate or estimate endotracheal tube cuff pressure using standard techniques. Am J Emerg Med 2006;24:139–43.
23. Galinski M, Tréoux V, Garrigue B, et al. Intracuff pressures of endotracheal tubes in the management of airway emergencies: the need for pressure monitoring. Ann Emerg Med 2006;47:545–7.
24. Svenson JE, Lindsay MB, O'Conner JE. Endotracheal intracuff pressures in the ED and prehospital setting: is there a problem? Am J Emerg Med 2007;25:53–6.

25. Bhende MS, Thompson AE, Cook DR, et al. Validity of a disposable end-tidal CO_2 detector in verifying endotracheal tube placement in infants and children. Ann Emerg Med 1992;21:142–5.
26. Li J. Capnography alone is imperfect for endotracheal tube placement confirmation during emergency intubation. J Emerg Med 2001;20:223–9.
27. Daugherty RJ, Nadkarni V, Brenn BR. Endotracheal tube size estimation for children with pathological short stature. Pediatr Emerg Care 2006;22:710–7.

Challenges and Advances in Intubation: Airway Evaluation and Controversies with Intubation

Sharon Elizabeth Mace, MD, FACEP, FAAP[a,b,c,d,*]

KEYWORDS

- Intubation • Endotracheal intubation • Airway evaluation

THE DIFFICULT/FAILED AIRWAY

The failed airway has been defined as three failed attempts at orotracheal intubation by a skilled practitioner or failure to maintain acceptable oxygen saturations, typically 90% or above in otherwise normal individuals.[1] A failed intubation is when "placement of the endotracheal tube fails after multiple intubation attempts."[2]

A difficult airway is present whenever there is difficulty in performing any of the following: bag valve mask (BVM) ventilation, laryngoscopy and intubation, or surgical airway techniques (eg, cricothyrotomy).[1,2] Some experts also include difficulty in placement of extraglottic devices. The American Society of Anesthesiologists (ASA) also defines a difficult airway as (1) difficult BVM ventilation—the inability to maintain an adequate oxygen saturation greater than 90% or signs of inadequate ventilation (eg, cyanosis, absent breath sounds, or hemodynamic instability) with BVM ventilation[2] or (2) difficult endotracheal intubation—greater than three failed intubation attempts or failure to intubate after 10 minutes by an experienced operator.[3]

[a] Cleveland Clinic Lerner College of Medicine of Case Western Reserve, Cleveland, OH 44195, USA
[b] Observation Unit, Cleveland Clinic, 9500 Euclid Avenue, Cleveland, OH 44195, USA
[c] Emergency Services Institute, E19, Cleveland Clinic, 9500 Euclid Avenue, Cleveland, OH 44195, USA
[d] Case Western Reserve University, Metro Health Medical Center, 8500 Metro Health Drive, Cleveland, OH 44109, USA
* Emergency Services Institute, E19, Cleveland Clinic, 9500 Euclid Avenue, Cleveland, OH 44195.
E-mail address: maces@ccf.org

Emerg Med Clin N Am 26 (2008) 977–1000
doi:10.1016/j.emc.2008.09.003   emed.theclinics.com

EVALUATION OF THE AIRWAY

In emergency medicine (EM), patients in need of a definitive airway (eg, an endotracheal tube), can be categorized into two groups: (1) those who need immediate airway as soon as possible, often referred to as a crash airway,[4] and (2) those in need of an urgent airway. Those patients in need of an immediate airway, the crash airway, generally belong to the category of nearly dead or newly dead, and immediate action is taken to intervene in and secure a definitive airway by any means possible.[4] Patients in the second group may be evaluated (as with anyone needing an elective airway) for the possibility of a difficult airway.

Difficult Bag Valve Mask Ventilation

Various anatomic features associated with difficult BVM ventilation are summarized by the mnemonic, MOANS[4] (**Box 1**). MOANS refers to Mask seal, Obese, Aged, No teeth, and Snores or Stiff. Any condition that causes an inadequate seal of the mask on the face, such as facial discontinuity (as with facial trauma, including facial fractures),

---

Box 1
Difficult airway mnemonics

Difficult bag valve mask ventilation: MOANS

M = Mask seal: facial anatomic deformities, including traumatic facial injuries, or beards

O = Obese: also includes parturient women and patients who have upper airway obstruction

A = Aged (>55 years)

N = No teeth

S = Snores or Stiff

Difficult extraglottic device: RODS

R = Restricted mouth opening

O = Upper airway obstruction at the level of the larynx or below

D = Disrupted or distorted

S = Stiff lungs or cervical spine

Difficult cricothyrotomy: SHORT

S = Surgery/disrupted airway

H = Hematoma or infection

O = Obese/access problem

R = Radiation

T = Tumor

Difficult laryngoscopy and intubation: LEMON

L = Look externally

E = Evaluate 3-3-2

M = Mallampati class

O = Obstruction

N = Neck mobility

---

a beard, fluids/materials (eg, blood, emesis, or secretions), or facial anomalies (Pierre Robin syndrome, micrognathia and so forth), can lead to a poor mask seal and poor BVM ventilation (*M*). Although some clinicians suggest use of a viscous substance, such as petroleum jelly or K-Y jelly, to help create a better mask seal to the face, other experts believe this is counterproductive in that it makes the entire face too slippery to hold the mask in place.[4]

BVM frequently is difficult in obese (*O*) patients. Other patients who are especially difficult to ventilate by bag and mask include parturient women and anyone who has upper airway obstruction (*O*) from an infectious cause (including epiglottitis, retropharyngeal abscess, peritonsillar abscess, croup, or Ludwig's angina) or a noninfectious case (angioedema, allergy, hematoma, foreign body, malignancy, tumor, and so forth). Care also should be taken not to create any iatrogenic airway obstruction or turn a partial into complete obstruction by positioning or airway procedures or manipulations or by medications.

The aged (*A*), in this definition age greater than 55 years, are believed more difficult to bag and mask ventilate because of a loss of upper airway muscle and tissue tone.

Edentulous (*N*, *N*o teeth) patients, because the face caves in, may be difficult for BVM ventilation. Ideally, clinicians may leave dentures in situ while BVM ventilation is occurring and then remove them when intubating. Although some have suggested putting gauze into the cheeks to puff them out to obtain a better mask seal, the danger of possible dislodgement of the gauze into the airway makes this a less than ideal option.

The *S* in MOANS refers to snores with a need to check for sleep apnea and for stiffness of the lungs, which can occur in diseases with increased airway resistance (such as asthma) or increased pulmonary compliance (for example, pulmonary edema, heart failure, or pneumonia).

Difficult Insertion of Extraglottic Devices

In an emergency, a laryngeal mask airway (LMA) can serve as the primary rescue airway in a cannot ventilate/cannot intubate scenario or can be used as a bridge or temporary airway while completing a cricothyrotomy.[2] The LMA also is used routinely in many nonemergency settings, including operating rooms (ORs), for elective cases.

The LMA is inserted above the glottis into the laryngeal space and then a cuff is inflated to achieve the proper seal. This directs air from above the vocal cords through the glottis into the trachea. A proper seal is essential to create a channel through which oxygen is routed into the trachea. The LMA and Combitube are mentioned in the 2003 ASA difficult airway algorithm.[2] The LMA and Combitube are considered intermediate airways.

An intermediate airway refers to the use of devices that allow ventilation across the larynx but do not provide complete airway control.[5] They are in-between or intermediate between a patent airway and definitive airway control as with endotracheal intubation. Intermediate airway devices do not allow for complete airway control. They generally involve blind placement. There are many different intermediate airways. Examples of such devices include the esophageal obturator airway (EOA), esophageal gastric tube airway (EGTA), esophageal-tracheal Combitube airway, laryngotracheal airway, laryngeal airway, airway management device, cuffed oropharyngeal airway, and laryngeal mask airway (LMA). Some of these devices are placed into the esophagus (EOA and EGTA); others may be placed into the esophagus or the trachea (esophageal-tracheal Combitube); and others are inserted into the airway above the glottis (LMA). Because of the complications associated with the EOA and the EGTA and other recent advances in airway management, there has been a marked decrease in EOA/EGTA use.[5] The terms, extraglottic and supraglottic devices, also have been used to describe those intermediate airway devices that do not enter the esophagus or trachea but are placed above the glottis for the purpose of ventilation. The LMA is the prototype of the extraglottic or supraglottic devices.

The mnemonic, RODS, is used to predict difficult insertion of extraglottic devices[4] (see **Box 1**). At least some access to the oral airway is necessary for placement of an extraglottic device, so the R in RODS stands for restricted mouth opening. An extraglottic device is not feasible if there is upper airway obstruction (O). A disrupted or distorted airway (D) prevents an adequate seal, thereby resulting in unsatisfactory functioning of the extraglottic device. A stiff cervical spine or stiff lungs are the S in RODS. A proper seal in the supraglottic airway is difficult or impossible when there is a flexion deformity of the neck. A marked increase in airway resistance (as occurs in status asthmaticus) or severely decreased pulmonary compliance (for example, pulmonary edema) leads to stiff lungs.[1]

Difficult Cricothyrotomy

There are three absolute contraindications to surgical cricothyrotomy: (1) endotracheal intubation can be accomplished easily and quickly and no contraindications to endotracheal intubation are present, (2) tracheal transection with retraction of the distal end into the mediastinum, and (3) a fractured larynx or significant damage to the cricoid cartilage or larynx.[6] The relative contraindications to surgical cricothyrotomy are acute laryngeal disease, a bleeding diathesis, age less than 5 to 12 years (transtracheal ventilation is preferred instead of surgical cricothyrotomy in infants and young children), and massive neck edema (a modified technique can be used).

The mnemonic, SHORT, has been used to determine clinical characteristics that presage a difficult cricothyrotomy[4] (see **Box 1**). The S represents Surgery/disrupted airway. Any anatomic distortion, from prior surgery, trauma, congenital anomalies, or disease states, probably makes airway access and cricothyrotomy more difficult. H stands for hematoma, bleeding, or infection in the surgical area that complicates the procedure. Obese/access is the O in SHORT and represents any situation that impairs access to the cricothyroid membrane. Prior Radiation (R) to this region of the neck may cause scarring and tissue distortion and T is for Tumor in the area that may cause bleeding and distort the anatomy. Any of these conditions makes it more difficult to perform a surgical cricothyrotomy.

Difficult Laryngoscopy and Intubation

During general anesthesia, the incidence of difficult tracheal intubation has been estimated at 3% to 18% in one report[7] and from 1.5% to 8.5% in another study[8] compared with a 0.13% to 0.3% incidence of failed intubation.[8] The usual estimate for difficult intubation in anesthetic practice is cited as 1% to 3%.[9] The Australian Incident Monitoring Study reported a 4% (160/4000 patients) incidence of problems with intubation[9] and a 0.025% (5/2000) incidence of emergency transtracheal airway.[10] Various techniques or scales have been devised to predict difficult intubation in a given patient.

VISUALIZATION OF THE GLOTTIS

An inadequate view of the glottis presumes difficult laryngoscopy and intubation.

Cormack Grades of Visualization of Glottis

The traditional method for assessing the degree of visualization of the glottis is the Cormack (Cormack-Lehane) laryngeal view grade score.[11] The grades of difficulty in laryngoscopy are grade 1, full view of vocal cords/glottis; grade 2, partial view of vocal cords/glottis; grade 3, only epiglottis seen; and grade 4, no exposure of glottis, epiglottitis cannot be seen. Grades 3 and 4 imply difficult laryngoscopy (see **Box 1**; **Fig. 1**).

Percent of Glottic Opening

Other scoring systems exist that grade the percent of glottic opening (POGO) (see **Box 1**; **Fig. 2**).[12] Although POGO allows differentiation between the ranges of partial glottic visibility from small to large, the Cormack grading system is still more widely used.[7]

VISUALIZATION OF THE UPPER AIRWAY: MALLAMPATI CLASS

The ability to visualize the poster oropharyngeal structures affects the success of laryngoscopic intubation. The better the view, the more likely the intubation is successful.

The Mallampati class frequently is used to evaluate for the possibility of a difficult intubation. It originally was devised as a part of a preoperative evaluation before a controlled intubation in an OR. It is done by having a patient sit on the edge of a table or bed and lean slightly forward; then an examiner asks the patient to open his or her mouth as widely as possible without talking or vocalizing. A Mallampati class then is given based on the extent to which the base of the uvula, soft palate, and faucial pillars can be visualized.[13] The Mallampati score, as modified by Samsoon and Young, is grade I, faucial pillars, soft palate, and uvula visualized; grade II, faucial pillars and soft palate visualized but uvula masked by base of the tongue; grade III, only soft palate visualized; and grade IV, soft palate not seen (see **Box 1**; **Fig. 3**).[14] Mallampati classes I and II are associated with low intubation failure rates, whereas difficult intubation is more likely with Mallampati classes III and IV.[7] With Mallampati class IV intubation, failure rates are greater than 10%.[1]

EXTERNAL EVALUATION OF THE AIRWAY
Patil's Triangle

The thyromental distance or thyromental line has been cited as a predictor of a difficult airway.[4,7,15,16] If the thyromental distance is less than 6 cm, intubation may be impossible, and if greater than 6.5 cm conventional laryngoscopy usually is possible.[7,15,16] The thyromental line is the distance between the upper border of the thyroid cartilage (eg, superior thyroid notch or Adam's apple) to the tip of the jaw or mental

Cormack Score

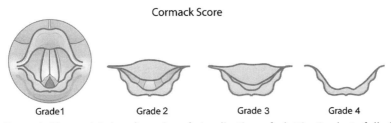

| Grade 1 | Grade 2 | Grade 3 | Grade 4 |

Fig. 1. Cormack (Cormack-Lehane) grades of visualization of glottis. Grade 1, full view of glottis, vocal cords visible; grade 2, vocal cords partly visible, only posterior aspect of glottis visible (posterior commissure view); grade 3, glottis not visible, only epiglottis is seen; and grade 4, glottis, vocal cords, and epiglottis are not visible. (*Courtesy of* Sharon E. Mace, MD, and Beth Halasz of the Cleveland Clinic Center for Medical Art and Photography, Cleveland, OH; with permission.)

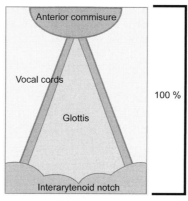

Fig. 2. POGO. (*Courtesy of* Sharon E. Mace, MD, and Beth Halasz of the Cleveland Clinic Center for Medical Art and Photography, Cleveland, OH; with permission.)

protuberance of the chin with the head extended. The thyromental line also is the hypotenuse of a right angle triangle, Patil's triangle, used to describe the anatomic relationships (see **Fig. 3**).[4,16] The axis of Patil's triangle is the length of the mandible or the floor of the mouth, which is a measure of the mandibular space. The abscissa of Patil's triangle is the distance between the base of the mandible and the top of the larynx and determines the position of the larynx with respect to the length of the mandible or the floor of the mouth. The length of the oral axis, which is the axis of Patil's triangle or the second *3* of the 3-3-2 evaluation, is important because it affects the ability to expose the glottis during laryngoscopy. With a very short oral axis, the larynx is covered by the base of the tongue which prevents visualization of the glottis, whereas an excessively long oral axis places the glottis beyond the horizon of visibility (**Box 2**; **Fig. 4**).

3-3-2 Assessment

The 3-3-2 assessment evaluates the degree of mouth opening and mandible size in relation to the position of the larynx in the neck as elements affecting the likelihood of a successful intubation (**Fig. 5**). The initial *3* represents the degree of oral access. A patient's mouth should be able to be opened at least three fingerbreadths (approximately 5 cm) between upper and lower teeth (see **Fig. 5A**).

The second *3* refers to the distance between the protuberance of the chin or mentum and the hyoid bone, which should allow three fingerbreadths (approximately 5 cm) along the floor of the mandible between the mentum and the mandible/neck junction, near the hyoid bone. The second *3* is an index of the mandibular space's ability to be large enough to have capacity for the tongue during laryngoscopy. Three fingerbreadths is ideal. Otherwise, if the mandibular space is too small (eg, <3 fingerbreadths), the mandibular space cannot accommodate the tongue, thereby obscuring the view of the glottis. Conversely, if the mandibular space is too large (eg, >3 fingerbreadths) then the elongated oral axis may impair visualization of the glottis (see **Fig. 5B**).

The *2* of the 3-3-2 refers to the position of the larynx in relation to the base of the tongue (see **Fig. 5C**). Two fingerbreadths between the hyoid bone and the upper anterior edge of the thyroid cartilage (superior laryngeal notch) is ideal. Greater than two fingerbreadths signifies the larynx is located further beyond the base of the tongue

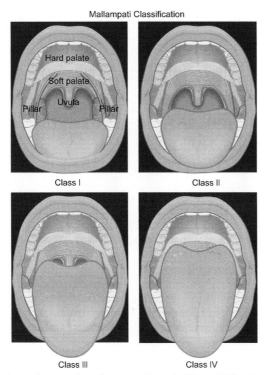

Fig. 3. Mallampati Class. Class I: soft palate, uvula and pillars visible; class II: soft palate and uvula visible; class III: soft palate and only base of uvula visible; and class IV: faucial pillars, soft palate, and uvula not visible (only hard palate visible). (*Courtesy of* Sharon E. Mace, MD, and Beth Halasz of the Cleveland Clinic Center for Medical Art and Photography, Cleveland, OH; with permission.)

and, therefore, may be positioned so far down the neck that it is beyond the visual horizon during laryngoscopy. Less than two fingerbreadths suggests an anterior larynx with the larynx located up under the base of the tongue, making it difficult to expose. Inability to attain the 3-3-2 rule implies that it will be difficult or impossible to line up the three axes (oral, pharyngeal, and tracheal axes) for intubation, thereby making intubation difficult or impossible (**Fig. 6**).

OVERALL ASSESSMENT

Another mnemonic, LEMON, has been used as an aid to recognizing risks for difficult intubation[1] (see **Box 1**). The rule of thumb is, if it looks difficult, it probably is. *L* stands for *L*ook externally. Anatomic features indicative of a likely difficult or failed intubation can be secondary to trauma or nontraumatic conditions/illnesses, which may be congenital or acquired (**Box 3**).

Evaluating 3-3-2 is the *E* in LEMON. The *M* of the LEMON refers to the Mallampati class. Obstruction is the *O* in the LEMON mneumonic. Anytime upper airway obstruction (partial or complete) is present, a difficult airway also is present. Even a small dose of a sedative or opioid (sometimes administered to relieve anxiety) relaxes the upper airway muscle tone, which can turn a partial obstruction into complete airway obstruction.

Box 2
Difficult intubation

Visualization of glottis

Cormack laryngeal view score

    Grade 1: Full view of glottis and vocal cords

    Grade 2: Vocal cords and glottis are partly visible

    Grade 3: Only epiglottis seen, glottis is not visible

    Grade 4: No exposure of glottis, the glottis and epiglottis are not visible

Percent of glottic opening

Visualization of upper airway

Mallampati class

    Class I: Faucial pillars, soft palate, and uvula visualized

    Class II: Faucial pillars and soft palate visualized, uvula not seen (masked by tongue)

    Class III: Only soft palate visualized

    Class IV: Faucial pillars, soft palate, and uvula not visualized (only hard palate visualized)

External evaluation of the airway

Patil's triangle

    Hypotenuse: thyromental line equals distance between the protuberance of the chin (mentum) and the angle of the superior thyroid notch (Adam's apple) (eg, upper border of the thyroid cartilage)

    Axis: distance between the protuberance of the chin (mentum) and the angle of the mandible equals length of the mandible, measures mandibular space or floor of the mouth

    Abscissa: distance between the angle of the superior thyroid notch and the base of the mandible

Overall evaluation

Intubation difficulty scale

    N1: Number of supplementary attempts at endotracheal intubation

    N2: Number of supplementary additional operators

    N3: Number of alternative techniques used

    N4: Cormack grade minus 1 (eg, N4 = 0, with Cormack grade = 1)

    N5: Lifting force applied during laryngoscopy (N5 = 0 little effort, N5 = 1 increased effect)

    N6: Is external laryngeal manipulation required (N6 = 0 no, N6 = 1 yes)

    N7: Position of vocal cords (N7 = 0 abduction, N7 = 1 abduction)

Elements for best attempt at conventional laryngoscopy

    Performance by a reasonably experienced practitioner

    No significant muscle tone

    Optimal "sniffing" position

    Blade length

    Blade type

    Use of laryngeal manipulation

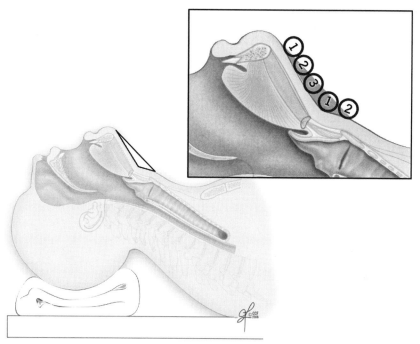

Fig. 4. Patil's triangle. (*Courtesy of* Sharon E. Mace, MD, and Beth Halasz of the Cleveland Clinic Center for Medical Art and Photography, Cleveland, OH; with permission.)

Neck mobility is the *N* component of LEMON. Positioning the head and neck in the sniffing position to obtain the best view of the glottis is considered one of the key elements in successful laryngoscopic intubation (see **Fig. 6**). Inability to do so for any reason, including cervical spine immobilization in a trauma patient, makes intubation more difficult.

SPECIFIC VARIABLES ASSOCIATED WITH FAILED/DIFFICULT AIRWAY

Specific conditions/injuries associated with a difficult or failed airway are listed in **Box 3**. Obesity, limited neck mobility, and mouth opening are the most frequently noted anatomic features leading to difficult intubation or a failed airway according to a review of more than 4000 patients in the Australian Incident Monitoring Study.[9]

Variables associated with a difficult or failed airway according to some experts include interincisor distance less than or equal to 3 cm, thyromental distance less than or equal to 6 cm, maxillary dentition interfering with jaw thrust, Mallampati class IV, neck in fixed flexion, and extreme head or neck changes secondary to masses, scarring, radiation, and so forth.[15] Other elements that are associated with a difficult or failed airway in some reports (but not in other studies) are increased age, male gender, obstructive sleep apnea, high body mass index, and pretracheal soft tissue.[15]

There have been other attempts to predict difficult intubation. The combination of a high modified Mallampati class and a thyromental distance less than 7 cm has been suggested as a predictor of a difficult intubation.[17] The triad of decreased atlanto-occipital extension, decreased mandibular space, and increased tongue thickness presages a difficult intubation according to a retrospective radiographic study.[18]

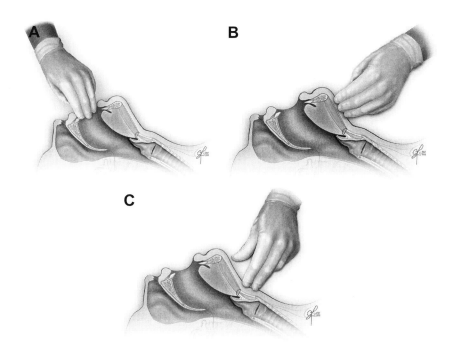

Fig. 5. Evaluate 3-2-2. (*A*) Oral access: mouth opening (three fingerbreadths) between upper and lower teeth. (*B*) Mentum and hyoid bone (three fingerbreadths). (*C*) Thyroid notch and hyoid bone (two fingerbreadths). (*Courtesy of* Sharon E. Mace, MD, and Beth Halasz of the Cleveland Clinic Center for Medical Art and Photography, Cleveland, OH; with permission.)

Another study using mouth opening, chin protrusion, and atlanto-occipital extension had 86.8% sensitivity and 96% sensitivity in predicting difficult intubation.[19]

Intubation Difficulty Scale

The intubation difficulty scale (IDS), suggested by the ASA in 1997, uses seven variables to grade an intubation.[20]

Higher scores are significantly correlated with longer intubation times and an operator's subjective rating of intubation difficulty. The seven IDS variables are N1, number of supplementary attempts at endotracheal intubation; N2, number of supplementary/additional operators; N3, number of alternative techniques used; N4, Cormack grade minus one (eg, N4 = 0 with Cormack grade = 1); N5, lifting force applied during laryngoscopy (N5 = 0, little effort, and N5 = 1, increased effort); N6, is external laryngeal manipulation required (N6 = 0, no, and N6 = 1, yes); and N7, position of vocal cords (N7 = 0, abduction, and N7 = abduction)[20] (see **Box 2**).

In the 2003 ASA report on management of the difficult airway, 11 airway examination components along with nonreassuring findings were listed as part of the preoperative airway physical examination[2] (**Table 1**).

Use of Scales and Techniques to Predict Difficult Intubation in Emergency Departments

Whether or not these various scales and techniques to predict difficult intubation are applicable to emergency department (ED) settings has been questioned for several reasons. First, most of the scales and techniques, including the Mallampati classes, were developed as part of a preoperative anesthesia evaluation or in the controlled

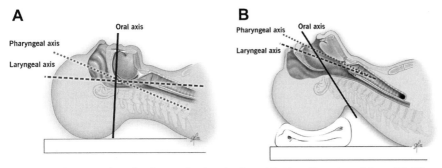

Fig. 6. Oral-pharyngeal-tracheal axes for intubation. (*A*) Nonaligned position. (*B*) Aligned sniffing position with neck flexed and head extended. (*Courtesy of* Sharon E. Mace, MD, and Beth Halasz of the Cleveland Clinic Center for Medical Art and Photography, Cleveland, OH; with permission.)

environment of an OR, in which there is time to assess cooperative patients. They were not developed in the chaotic, uncontrolled, usually time-limited urgent or emergency conditions of EDs, which generally involve uncooperative, unfasted, critically ill, or unstable patients. This is underscored by an ED study using three variables, Mallampati class, neck mobility, and thyromental distance, to predict difficult intubation.[21] According to this study, these three physical examination techniques could not be performed on two thirds of ED patients for various reasons, including inability to follow commands or cervical spine immobilization, thereby nullifying its use for emergent airway assessment in the ED.[21]

Even in the 2003 ASA report, there is the acknowledgment that in a patient who does not have obvious pathology, there is no evidence indicating that a difficult airway can be predicted by physical examination, but it is still recommended to do a physical examination to "improve detection of a difficult airway."[2]

INTUBATION: SUCCESS RATE AND COMPLICATIONS
Non–Emergency Department Intubations

A prospective multicenter study of ICUs found at least one severe complication in 28% of all intubations.[22] Comorbidity (eg, shock and acute respiratory failure) was a risk factor for intubation complications, with supervision by a senior physician having a protective effect with fewer complications occurring.[22]

These results are consistent with findings in another ICU study of unplanned endotracheal extubations in which difficulty with reintubation (multiple or prolonged attempts or need for a fiberoptic bronchoscope) was common, occurring in 20% of patients.[23] Another study of the airway management of ICU patients noted major complications in a significant number of patients, including difficult intubations (8%), esophageal intubations (8%), and pulmonary aspiration (4%).[24] Of intubations in an acute care military hospital, 7.9% (22/278) had one or more significant endotracheal tube misplacements of which 23% had serious complications.[25]

Emergency Department Intubations

According to the National Emergency Airway Registry (NEAR), a prospective multicenter registry of ED intubations with more than 6000 patients, the intubation success rates for EM residents were first attempt 83% and first intubator 90% with a 0.9% cricothyrotomy rate.[26] The rate of successful intubation increased with

---

Box 3
Specific conditions associated with a difficult or failed airway

Traumatic injuries

Facial bone fractures

- Le Fort fractures
- Mandibular fractures

Cervical spine fractures/injuries

- Limit neck mobility

Burns

Oral trauma: loose/broken teeth, gum/palatal injuries

Neck injuries

- Laryngotracheal trauma

Injuries that impair visibility of the laryngx

- Bleeding
- Hematoma
- Edema/swelling of soft tissue

Nontraumatic conditions/illnesses

Congenital: osseous abnormalities

- Micrognathia
- Limited cervical spine mobility (restricted neck movement)
- Limited temporomandibular joint mobility (restricted mouth opening)
- Small mouth (restricted mouth opening)
- Cleft palate, high arched bony palate

Congenital: nonosseous/soft tissue abnormalities

- Macroglossia
- Protruding upper incisors (buck teeth)
- Cleft palate, high arched soft palate
- Small mouth (restricted mouth opening)

Acquired

- Upper airway tumors/malignancies
- Angioedema
- Foreign body in extrathoracic airway
- Upper airway infections: epiglottis, retropharyngeal abscess, peritonsillar abscess, Ludwig's angina, others
- Hematemesis
- Vomiting

Table 1
Components of the preoperative airway physical examination

Airway Examination Component	Nonreassuring Findings
1. Length of upper incisors	Relatively long
2. Relation of maxillary and mandibular incisors during normal jaw closure	Prominent overbite (maxillary incisors anterior to mandibular incisors)
3. Relation of maxillary and mandibular incisors during voluntary protrusion	Patient mandibular incisors anterior to (in mandible front of) maxillary incisors
4. Interincisor distance	Less than 3 cm
5. Visibility of uvula	Not visible when tongue is protruded with patient in sitting position (eg, Mallampati class greater than II)
6. Shape of palate	Highly arched or very narrow
7. Compliance of mandibular space	Stiff, indurated, occupied by mass, or nonresilient
8. Thyromental distance	Less than three ordinary fingerbreadths
9. Length of neck	Short
10. Thickness of neck	Thick
11. Range of motion of head and neck	Patient cannot touch tip of chin to chest or cannot extend neck

This table displays some findings of the airway physical examination that may suggest the presence of a difficult intubation. The decision to examine some or all of the airway components shown in this table depends on the clinical context and judgment of the practitioner. The table is not intended as a mandatory or exhaustive list of the components of an airway examination. The order of presentation in this table follows the line of sight that occurs during conventional oral laryngoscopy.

Reprinted from Caplan RA, Benumof JL, Berry FA, et al. Practice guidelines for the management of the difficult airway: an updated report by the American Society of Anesthesiologists task force on management of the difficult airway. Anesthesiology 2003;98:1269–77; with permission.

experience: postgraduate year 1 (PG1), 80%; PG2, 89%; PG3, 94%; and attending physicians, 98%.[26]

There was a 2.7% need for a rescue airway with a 0.0056% (N = 43/7712) incidence of cricothyrotomy in the NEAR study.[27]

A study of ED intubations found a success rate of 74% for EM PG1 versus 100% for EM attending physicians and a cricothyrotomy rate of 1.2% (4/324).[28] Higher first-attempt intubation success rates from 80% to 90% were noted in other ED intubation studies in which the ED intubators were not restricted to first-year residents.[27,29–32] This is consistent with the NEAR study[26] and the ICU study,[22] which found the intubation success rate increased with the level of experience.

A study of ED intubations in which rapid sequence intubation (RSI) was used in only 33% of patients noted success rates for ED physicians of 90% for the first attempt and 97% overall success, with only 3% needing airway management by anesthetists and only one cricothyrotomy needed.[32] In another study of ED intubations, EM physicians successfully intubated 99% of patients (321/324), with anesthesia intubating only 1% (3/324) and with cricothyrotomies done in only four patients.[28] In another report of 610 ED patients needing tracheal intubation in which RSI was used in 84% of patients,

93% were intubated by EM residents or attending physicians; 98.7% were successfully intubated; and seven patients underwent cricothyrotomy (7/610 = 0.01%).[30]

A large, prospective, multicenter study of pediatric ED intubations from the NEAR registry (in which RSI was used in 81%) noted a 77% first-attempt success and an 85% success rate for the first intubator.[33] As with the other ED studies, the vast majority (88%) of the initial intubators were in training (residents or fellows). This percent of first success rate is slightly lower than other studies of ED intubations, which suggests that intubations of ED pediatric patients may be more difficult with a lower successful intubation rate[33] than ED adult patients.[28–32] This pediatric ED intubation study also found that the age of the pediatric patient was a critical factor in determining intubation success with only a 60% first-attempt success in infant/toddlers and preschoolers, 71% in school-aged children, and 85% in adolescents. The first intubator's success rate showed a similar trend: infant/toddler 79%, preschool-aged 74%, school-aged 86%, and adolescents 94%.[33]

With ED intubations, the need for a rescue airway occurred in 2.7% of emergency intubations[27] and the need for cricothyrotomy ranged from 0.006% to 1.2%,[26–32] with the highest incidence of cricothyrotomy (1.2%) noted in PG1 residents[27] and the lowest incidence in the NEAR registry database.[26]

The ED incidence of difficult intubations and cricothyrotomies compares favorably with that for anesthesiology.[7–10] The reported incidence of difficult intubation in anesthesia practice is 1.5% to 18%,[7–10] with a usual cited rate of 1% to 3%, and 4% according to the Australian Incident Monitoring Study,[9] and need for emergent transtracheal airway at 0.003%.[10] The ED rates in the NEAR study were need for a rescue airway 2.7% and incidence of cricothyrotomy 0.006%.[26]

Intubation Success Rates: Emergency Physicians and Anesthesiologists

A comparison of EM resident intubations versus anesthesia-managed intubations at a level 1 training center showed no significant difference between the two groups with first-attempt success rates of 73.7% (EM) versus 77.2% (anesthesia) and overall success rates (three attempts) of 97.0% (EM) versus 98.0% (anesthesia).[34]

In another study of RSI performed outside ORs on emergency patients, there were no significant differences in the complication rate between three types of intubating teams comprised of anesthetists, nonanesthetists, or both.[35]

According to one report, the mean complication rate for ED RSI patients was less for emergency physicians (EPs) than anesthetists. The complication rates (mean) were for anesthetists, trauma patients 17% and nontrauma patients 22%, versus for EPs, trauma patients 14% and nontrauma patients 4%.[36]

Another large prospective study of ED trauma patient intubations found "no differences in laryngoscopy performance and intubation success in trauma airways managed...by emergency medicine versus anesthesia residents" (86.4% versus 89.7% first-attempt success, respectively).[31]

In contrast to these studies,[30–32,34–36] there is one report with slightly different findings. In this study from Scotland, anesthetists had a significantly higher initial success rate (91.8% versus 83.8%) and a better laryngoscopic view (Cormack grades 1 and II) (94.0% versus 89.3%) with a trend to fewer complications (8.7% versus 12.7%) than EPs.[37] EPs, however, intubated a significantly greater number of patients within 15 minutes of arrival (32.6% versus 11.3%).[37] Their conclusion was anesthetists obtained better laryngoscopic views with higher initial success rates during RSI, although EPs performed RSI on a greater percentage of critically ill patients within 15 minutes of arrival.[37]

A best evidence review of studies comparing EPs with anesthetists found "little or no difference in the rates of success and complications" for RSI.[38]

Rapid Sequence Intubation Versus Non–Rapid Sequence Intubation Techniques

The NEAR study indicated that intubation using RSI had higher success rates than non-RSI techniques.[26] First-attempts/first-intubator success rates were RSI 85%/91% versus oral, no medication 76%/86%. Furthermore, some of the non-RSI techniques were successful on repeat attempts after switching to an alternative technique, most commonly RSI.[26]

The pediatric NEAR data registry also found higher success rates for RSI than for non-RSI techniques. Successful intubation on the first attempt was RSI 78%, without medication 47% (P<.01), and sedation without neuromuscular blockage 44% (P<.05). First intubator success rates were RSI 85%, without medication 75%, and sedation without neuromuscular blockage 89% (not significant).[33]

Other studies collaborate higher rates of successful intubation, fewer complications, and faster intubation completion times with RSI compared with non-RSI endotracheal intubations.[39–41] In a study of physicians working on board ambulances, significant differences were found when succinylcholine was added to the intubation protocols.[39] The results of presuccinylcholine versus postsuccinylcholine for tracheal intubation were first-attempt success 55% versus 74%, duration of intubation (minutes) 4.1 versus 1.4, and incidence of complications (hypoxemia, laryngospasm, and bronchospasm) 31% versus 15%.[39] After the introduction of RSI using etomidate and succinycholine, an air medical transport program with nurses and paramedics as the intubators reported a significant increase in the first intubation success rate from 65.7% to 79.3%, a decrease in the number of intubation attempts from 105 to 87 or an average from 1.5 to 1.2, and a decrease in the duration of intubation (minutes) from 5.1 to 2.1.[40]

A prospective study compared ED intubation with RSI (N = 166 patients) and without RSI (N = 67).[41] They found complications were greater in number and severity in the non-RSI group. Complications observed in the non-RSI group included aspiration (15%), airway trauma (12.8%), and death (3%). None of these complications occurred in the RSI group (P<.0001).[41]

Intubation success rates may depend on a patient's underlying condition, eg, medical versus trauma, vital signs absent (with absent airway reflexes) versus vital signs present (with airway reflexes present) and whether oral or nasal intubation is done.[42] A prehospital study of paramedic intubations reported first-attempt/overall success rates for medical emergencies 60.4%/74.3%, trauma patients 66.6%/71.4%, and patients who had vital signs absent 80.1%/96% and for nasal compared with oral intubations (63% versus 94%). Whether or not the significant differences for medical or trauma patients compared with patients who had absent vital signs are related to preserved airway reflexes in the former versus absent reflexes in the later or to other factors (training, experience, technical difficulties, and so forth) remains to be determined.[42]

Complications of Intubation

Many complications are associated with intubation. In one report, oxygen desaturation was reported as the most common complication of emergency RSI followed by hypotension.[35] Immediate complications of emergency RSI noted in one study from Britain included hypoxemia (19.2%), hypotension 17.8%, and dysrhythmia 3.4%.[35] The probability of complications was significantly associated with patients' underlying conditions, with hypoxemia occurring more frequently in patients who had underlying respiratory or cardiovascular conditions.[36] An ICU study also correlated an increased risk for complications during intubations with pre-existing shock or acute respiratory failure.[22]

A study of ED intubations in the United States found that 8.0% (49/610) of patients had an immediate complication with a total of 9.3% (57/610) immediate complications (some patients had more than one complication).[30] When inadvertent esophageal placement did occur (5.4% = 33/616), it was quickly recognized and corrected. There were three postintubation cardiac arrests; two patients had agonal rhythms before intubation and one likely had a succinylcholine-induced hyperkalemic cardiac arrest.[30]

Similar findings were reported in another study of ED intubations in which complications occurred in 10.3% of patients (22/214) with a total complication rate of 14.9% (32/214).[32] Complications included esophageal intubation 6.1% (13/214), soft tissue damage 3.3% (7/214), oxygen desaturation 1.9% (4/214), hypotension 1.4% (3/214), bronchial intubation 1.4% (3/214), dental trauma (1/214), and dysrhythmia (1/214).[32]

Elements for Best-Attempted Conventional Laryngoscopy

According to some experts, the best attempt at conventional laryngoscopy is predicated on six elements: performance by a reasonably experienced practitioner, no significant muscle tone, an optimal sniffing position, blade length, blade type, and use of laryngeal manipulation. Unfortunately, in the ED setting, optimizing all six variables may not be possible. For example, for a trauma patient who has suspected or known cervical spine injury, positioning in a sniffing position is not possible.

CONTROVERSIES WITH RAPID SEQUENCE INTUBATION

Although RSI is standard of care,[41,43–45] several issues and controversies have arisen.

Step 2: Preoxygenation

Ideally, preoxygenation (step 2) is accomplished by having patients breathe 100% oxygen via a tight fitting facemask for 3 to 5 minutes and avoiding BVM to prevent gastric distention. Unfortunately, in the ED allowing time, even 3 to 5 minutes may not be feasible.[45] Furthermore, many ED patients have ineffective breathing or are apneic so BVM is necessary. Although adults who have normal functional residual capacity (FRC) can tolerate up to 5 minutes of apnea before they desaturate,[46] many if not most ED patients undergoing RSI do not have a normal FRC. Patients who have a limited FRC may desaturate within 2 minutes if apneic. Patients who have a limited FRC in danger of rapidly becoming hypoxic include infants, children, pregnant females, obese adults, patients who have an elevated diaphragm (eg, bowel obstruction), and patients who have underlying lung disease (eg, interstitial lung disease). A recent study documented that patients who have respiratory failure as a result of underlying cardiopulmonary disease frequently do not respond to the standard mode of preoxygenation.[47] Only half of such patients had an increase in PaO_2 greater than 5% above baseline with the standard 4-minute preoxygenation.[47] Another prospective randomized study of ICU patients found better PaO_2 and pulse oximetry values using noninvasive positive pressure ventilation (NIPPV) than with conventional preoxygenation before endotracheal intubation.[48]

In summary, the preoxygenation phase (step 2) should allow adequate oxygenation for most patients such that BVM ventilation should be avoided if possible during RSI because of an increased risk for regurgitation and aspiration from gastric distention secondary to BVM. Some patients who have hypoxemia, apnea, inadequate ventilation, or respiratory distress/failure, however, may need BVM before, during, and after RSI. BVM should not be withheld from such patients.

Step 3: Pretreatment

With the pretreatment phase (step 3), questions include which drugs should be given and in what doses? The routine use of atropine for pediatric RSI has been questioned recently[49] although the two cited studies had methodologic flaws[50,51] (eg, insufficient power and design).[49] It has been theorized that a component of the bradycardia noted during pediatric RSI with succinylcholine may be the result of the hypoxia and underlying diseases or conditions and not just to the administered medication. Whether or not this is the case may be irrelevant because symptomatic bradycardia, whatever the cause, is treated with atropine.[52,53] The current consensus for pretreatment in RSI suggests (1) lidocaine and fentanyl for patients who have significant central nervous system trauma or disease (eg, elevated intracranial pressure), (2) fentanyl in patients who have vascular dissection/rupture or ischemic heart disease or anyone who would be affected negatively by reflex sympathetic nervous system–mediated discharge of catecholamines that leads to a transient but significant rise in blood pressure and heart rate, (3) lidocaine if acute asthma or bronchospasm (wheezing) is present, and (4) atropine if a pediatric patient ($\leq$ 10 years old) or any patient who has significant bradycardia when succinylcholine is to be given.[54]

Step 4: Paralysis with Induction

Decisions that arise with step 4—paralysis with induction—include the sedative choice, whether or not to use succinylcholine or a nondepolarizing neuromuscular blocking agent, and doses of the drugs. When succinylcholine is the paralytic agent, which pretreatment drugs should be used and when to use them has been controversial. In view of the associated risks and complications with a defasciculating dose of a nondepolarizing neuromuscular blocking agent is not widely used in ED RSI,[55] in view of the associated risks and complications associated with defasciculating doses of these drugs, although lidocaine, fentanyl, and atropine are used in some cases.[54]

Step 5: Protection and Positioning—Cricoid Pressure

The use of cricoid pressure[56] in step 5 (protection and positioning) has been questioned. Although cricoid pressure is routinely recommended in RSI, problems can occur and there are no outcome studies documenting the clinical advantages of the Sellick maneuver.[57–59] Because of these concerns, some experts have suggested that the use of the Sellick maneuver during RSI and bag mask ventilation be considered optional, noting that "there is little evidence to support the widely held belief that application of cricoid pressure reduces the incidence of aspiration during RSI" and cricoid pressure may actually "worsen the quality of laryngeal exposure" thereby making endotracheal intubation more difficult.[57]

The purpose of cricoid pressure is to prevent regurgitation of gastric contents into the lungs. Whether or not cricoid pressure actually accomplishes this has been challenged recently. The esophagus was lateral to the larynx in over 50% of the awake volunteers in a recent MRI study.[60] Furthermore, cricoid pressure increased (not decreased) the incidence of an unoccluded esophagus by 50% and caused airway compression (>1 mm) in 81% of the subjects studied.[60] This report, however, differs from the results of two studies (a cadaver study and a clinical study) that documented decreased gastric insufflation with air during mask ventilation when cricoid pressure was applied.[61,62] This raises the question or whether or not studies with mask ventilation can be applied to endotracheal intubation and what effect, if any, cricoid pressure has on preventing gastric aspiration during endotracheal intubation. A literature review of 241 articles dealing with cricoid pressure concluded there was little evidence to support the view that cricoid pressure decreases the risk for aspiration.[58]

There are data suggesting that cricoid pressure may worsen the degree of laryngeal exposure. A study compared cricoid pressure with backward, upward, and rightward pressure (BURP) on the thyroid cartilage and bimanual laryngoscopy by an endoscopist.[63] The Sellick maneuver and BURP actually worsened the larygnoscopic view.[63] Other studies also have found that cricoid pressure may worsen the laryngeal/glottic view.[64,65] This may be why there have been instances of regurgitation and aspiration in spite of appropriate use of cricoid pressure. Some reports have indicated that use of the Sellick maneuver may cause airway obstruction and increase the difficulty of intubation.[66–68] Furthermore, cricoid pressure may cause unwanted significant increases in the heart rate and blood pressure.[69]

Disadvantages cited with use of cricoid pressure include visualization of the larynx/glottis is more difficult and airway obstruction can occur, making intubation more difficult; movement of the cervical spine can occur; and possible esophageal injury in actively vomiting patients.

Furthermore, a review of the Sellick maneuver indicated that cricoid pressure may be applied inconsistently and incorrectly during an emergency, even by health care workers who often perform the procedure.[70,71]

Currently, although the effectiveness of the Sellick maneuver in preventing regurgitation has been questioned, and its use considered optional by some, occasionally it may be beneficial. Therefore, cricoid pressure may be used at least initially with RSI. If the use of cricoid pressure obscures the view of the glottis, hampers endotracheal tube passage, or impairs adequate BVM ventilation, however, then cricoid pressure should be immediately decreased or eliminated. It may be that a variant of the Sellick maneuver, however, optimal external laryngeal manipulation, may be beneficial in improving the laryngeal/glottic view.[63]

Step 5: Protection and Positioning—Positioning of Patients

The classic teaching is to place patients in the sniffing position with the neck flexed and the head slightly extended about the atlantooccipital joint before intubation to align the three axes: oral, pharyngeal, and laryngeal (see **Fig. 6**). A recent randomized MRI study in general surgery patients in ORs questioned the use of the sniffing position.[72] Another randomized study in ORs found that simple head extension was as effective as the sniffing position in facilitating endotracheal intubation.[73] Similar studies in ED patients are lacking so whether or not these reports in ORs can be generalized to ED patients is unknown.

ED patients who have known or possible cervical spine injury needing intubation pose a special challenge. The best mode of endotracheal intubation in such patients is a controversial topic.[74] Several studies suggest, however, that removing the anterior part of the cervical collar, while maintaining manual in line cervical spine immobilization, is acceptable and may cause less cervical spine movement than cervical collar immobilization during laryngoscopy for endotracheal intubation.[75,76]

Nontrauma patients associated with a decreased range of neck motion include patients who have degenerative disc disease and patients' status post cervical spine surgery/instrumentation. Among those who have degenerative disk disease are the elderly (age >70 years) and patients who have rheumatoid arthritis, osteoarthritis, and ankylosing spondylitis.

In morbidly obese patients, a better view of the larynx was obtained with ramped positions using blankets underneath a patient's body and head to obtain a horizontal alignment between the external auditory meatus and the sternal notch rather than with the sniffing position.[77] Although this study was done in morbidly obese patients undergoing elective bariatric surgery, it seems logical that this also may apply to morbidly obese patients undergoing intubation in the ED.[77] Because of physiology with decreased expiratory reserve volume, forced vital capacity, forced expiratory volume in 1 second, and maximum voluntary ventilation, the morbidly obese are more susceptible to hypoxemia than normal weight individuals. Furthermore, the body habitus of morbidly obese patients may make repositioning difficult or impossible during endotracheal intubation.[57]

CLINICAL RESPONSES TO INTUBATION

There are many negative clinical responses to intubation. The goal of RSI is to minimize or prevent some of these detrimental clinical responses. A review of the clinical responses to intubation and the pathophysiology is useful to understand RSI.

The cardiovascular reflexes to intubation are initiated by proprioceptors in the supraglottic region and trachea. Afferent neural impulses travel via the vagal (cranial nerve [CN] X) and glossopharyngeal (CN IX) nerves to the nucleus tractus solitarius (NTS) in the medulla with efferent activation of both divisions of the autonomic nervous system. In infants and small children, bradycardia, bradypnea, and even apnea can occur during laryngoscopy or intubation. This is secondary to increased parasympathetic (vagal) tone, including at the sinoatrial node. Upper airway reflexes; including laryngospasm (eg, the glottic closure reflex) and the sneeze, cough, and swallow reflexes, are essentially monosynaptic responses to an irritant stimulus in the airway.[78]

Conversely, in adults and adolescents, increased heart rate and blood pressure are the typical responses to airway manipulation.[79] This response is mediated via postganglionic cardioacceleratory nerves from the paravertebral sympathetic chain ganglia, which includes norepinephrine release from adrenergic nerve terminals and the secretion of norephinephrine from the adrenal medulla. Stimulation of the β-adrenergic nerves to the renal juxtaglomerular apparatus activates the renin-angiotensin system resulting in the release of renin, which further raises the blood pressure.

Stimulation of the central nervous system caused by activation of the autonomic nervous system leads to elevations in the cerebral metabolic rate, oxygen consumption, and cerebral blood flow. This could have disastrous consequences in patients who hve impaired CNS autoregulation or elevated intracranial pressure from illness or trauma.

Any rise in heart rate or blood pressure causes an increase in myocardial oxygen demand, which in turn, could lead to myocardial ischemia in patients who have coronary artery insufficiency. Patients who have any vascular dissection/rupture or a vascular aneurysm/arteriovenous malformation could be adversely affected by a rise in arterial blood pressure.

Airway reflexes, such as coughing or vomiting, can lead to elevated intrathoracic and intra-abdominal pressure, which could worsen many conditions (such as decreased cardiac output secondary to impaired venous return from increased intrathoracic pressure or abdominal distention/rupture) and create new problems (eg, Mallory-Weiss tear or Boerhaave's syndrome or aspiration). Increased cerebrospinal fluid pressure secondary to an elevated intrathoracic and intra-abdominal pressure results in increased intracranial pressure.

PATHOPHYSIOLOGY OF INTUBATION

CN IX (glossopharyngeal) and CN X (vagus) innervate the upper airway and digestive tract mucosa. Afferents from the CN IX and X project to the solitary tract-nucleus (NTS) in the medulla.

The NTS serves as the visceral sensory (visceral afferent) nuclei of the brainstem. The NTS receives the afferent fibers from CN IX, X, and VII (facial) nerves. Nerve impulses originating in the pharynx, larynx, intestinal tract, respiratory tract, heart, and large blood vessels are processed in the NTS. The NTS receives sensory input from all the viscera of the thorax and abdomen.

The vomiting or emetic center, an anatomically indistinct group of receptor and effector nuclei in the NTS coordinates the efferent (autonomic, respiratory, and gastro-intestinal) activity related to vomiting. The area postrema, located in the floor of the fourth ventricle, can react to stimuli in the blood or cerebrospinal fluid and provides afferent input to the vomiting center in the NTS.

The upper airway reflexes include the glottic closure reflex (laryngospasm), cough, sneeze, and swallow reflex. The function of the various upper airway reflexes is to pro-tect the respiratory system and gas exchange surface from foreign or noxious sub-stances. This is why there is a profusion of sensory nerve endings in the airway and rapid motor responses to any stimuli in the airway.

The glossopharyngeal (CN IX) and the vagus (CN X) nerves serve as the afferent nerve pathways for these upper airway reflexes and for the cardiovascular responses to endo-tracheal intubation. When the airway stimuli are located superior to the anterior epiglottic surface, then the afferents travel via the glossopharyngeal nerve to the NTS. When the stimuli are at or below the posterior epiglottic surface, continuing interiorly into the lower airway, the vagus nerve serves as the afferent pathway to the NTS. Stimulation of the air-way mechanoreceptors or nociceptors can trigger any of these airway reflexes.

Parasympathetic nerves innervate the airway smooth muscle, vasculature, and the mucus glands of the airway. Parasympathetic (vagal) stimulation causes mucus secre-tion, and dilatation of airway blood vessels. The sympathetic nerves also innervate the airway vasculature. Sympathetic stimulation causes vasoconstriction of airway blood vessels. Upper airway sympathetic efferent nerves arise from the trigeminal ganglion.

Activation of the NTS causes stimulation of the sympathetic nervous system with an increase in heart rate and blood pressure than can foster dysrhythmias and a rise in intracranial pressure and intraocular pressure.

Bronchospasm also can occur as a reflex response to endotracheal intubation and may occur even in patients who have no history of asthma or obstructive lung disease. Efferent parasympathetic fibers travel to the bronchial smooth muscle and stimulate the M_3 cholinergic fibers on the bronchial smooth muscle, causing a cholinergically mediated bronchoconstriction. Stimulation of the laryngeal and upper tracheal airway receptors can cause airway constriction in the large and smaller peripheral airways, which results in a reflex mediated increase in airway resistance.

SUMMARY

Management of the airway is the first priority in any patient. Dealing with a difficult air-way can be a challenge, whether or not it involves BVM ventilation, an intermediate airway device, laryngoscopy and intubation, or a surgical airway. Various scales have been devised to predict which patients are likely to have a difficult airway. Irrespective of the location, ED, ICU, or OR, the issues regarding intubation, including complications and success rates, are somewhat similar. The goal of RSI is to eliminate or mitigate the untoward reflex responses to intubation. Knowing the pathophysiology and negative clinical responses associated with intubation is useful in understanding the procedure of RSI. Although controversy has arisen regarding the various steps in RSI, it remains an essential component of EM practice.

REFERENCES

1. Murphy M, Walls RM. Identification of the difficult and failed airway. In: Walls RM, Murphy MF, Luten R, editors. Manual of emergency airway management. Philadelphia: Lippincott, Williams & Wilkins; 2004. p. 70–81 [chapter 6].
2. Caplan RA, Benumof JL, Berry FA, et al. Practice guidelines for the management of the difficult airway: an updated report by the American Society of Anesthesiologists task force on management of the difficult airway. Anesthesiology 2003;98: 1269–77.
3. Anonymous. Practice guidelines for the management of the difficult airway: a report by the American Society of Anesthesiologists task force on management of the difficult airway. Anesthesiology 1993;78:597–602.
4. Murphy MF, Doyle DJ. Airway evaluation. In: Hung OR, Murphy MF, editors. Management of the difficult and failed airway. New York: McGraw-Hill; 2008. p. 1–14 [chapter 1].
5. Vrocher D, Hopson LR. Basic airway management and decision-making. In: Roberts JR, Hedges JR, editors. Clinical procedure in emergency medicine. 4th edition. Philadelphia: Saunders; 2004. p. 53–68 [chapter 3].
6. Herbert RB, Bose S, Mace SE. Cricothyrotomy and transtracheal jet ventilation. In: Roberts JR, Hedges JR, editors. Procedures in emergency medicine. Philadelphia: Elsevier Publishing Co; 2008 [chapter 6].
7. Wilson IH, Kopf A. Prediction and management of difficult tracheal intubation. Practical Procedures 1998;9:37–45.
8. Crosby ET, Cooper RM, Douglas MJ, et al. The unanticipated difficult airway with recommendations for management. Can J Anaesth 1998;45:757–76.
9. Paix AD, Williamson JA, Runciman WB. Crisis management during anaesthesia: difficult intubation. Qual Saf Health Care 2005;14:e5. Available at: (http://www.qshc.com/cgi/content/full/14/3/e5). Accessed August 14, 2008.
10. Williamson JA, Webb RK, Szekely S, et al. Difficult intubation: an analysis of 2000 incident reports. Anaesth Intensive Care 1993;21:602–7.
11. Cormack RS, Lehane J. Difficult tracheal intubation in obstetrics. Anesthesia 1984;39:1105–11.
12. Levitan RM, Ochrock EA, Kush S, et al. Assessment of airway visualization: validation of the percentage of glottic opening (POGO) scale. Acad Emerg Med 1998;5:919–23.
13. Mallampati SR, Gatt SP, Gugino LD. A clinical sign to predict difficult tracheal intubation: a prospective study. Can J Anaesth 1985;32:429–34.
14. Samsoon GLT, Young JRB. Difficult tracheal intubation: a retrospective study. Anaesthesia 1987;42:487–90.
15. Liess BD, Scheidt RD, Templer JW. The difficult airway. Otolaryngol Clin North Am 2008;41:567–80.
16. Patil VU, Stehling LC, Zaunder HL. Fiberoptic endoscopy in anesthesia. Chicago: Year Book Medical Publishers; 1983.
17. Frerk CM. Predicting difficult intubation. Anaesthesia 1991;46:1005.
18. Bellhouse CP, Dore C. Criteria for estimating likelihood of difficult endotracheal intubation with the macintosh laryngoscope. Anaesth Intensive Care 1988;16:329.
19. Karkouti K, Rose KD, Wigglesworth D, et al. Predicting difficult intubation: a multivariable analysis. Can J Anaesth 2000;47:730–9.
20. Adnet F, Barron SW, Racine SX, et al. The intubation difficult scale (IDS): proposal and evaluation of a new score characterizing the complexity of endotracheal intubation. Anesthesiology 1997;87:1290.

21. Levitan RM, Everett WW, Ochrock EA. Limitations of difficult airway prediction in patients intubated in the emergency department. Ann Emerg Med 2004;44:307–13.

22. Jaber S, Amraoui J, Lefrant JY, et al. Clinical practice and risk factors for immediate complications of endotracheal intubation in the intensive care unit: a prospective, multi-center study. Crit Care Med 2006;34:2355–61.

23. Christie JM, Dethlefsen M, Cane RD. Unplanned endotracheal extubation in the intensive care unit. J Clin Anesth 1996;8:289–93.

24. Schwartz DE, Matthay MA, Cohen NH. Death and other complications of emergency airway management in critically ill adults: a prospective investigation of 297 tracheal intubations. Anesthesiology 1995;82:367–76.

25. Kollef MH, Legare EJ, Damiano M. Endotracheal tube misplacement: incidence, risk factors, and impact of a quality improvement program. South Med J 1994;87: 248–54.

26. Sagarin MJ, Barton ED, Chung YM, et al. Airway management by US and Canadian emergency medicine residents: a multicenter analysis of more than 6,000 endotracheal intubation attempts. Ann Emerg Med 2005;46(4):328–36.

27. Bair AE, Filbin MR, Kulkarni RG, et al. The failed intubation attempt in the emergency department: analysis of prevalence, rescue techniques and personnel. J Emerg Med 2002;23(2):131–40.

28. Calderon Y, Gennis P, Martinez C, et al. Intubations in an emergency medicine residency: the selection and performance of intubators. Acad Emerg Med 1995;2:411–2.

29. Tayal VS, Riggs RW, Marx JA, et al. Rapid-sequence intubation at an emergency medicine residency: success rate and adverse events during a two-year period. Acad Emerg Med 1999;6:31–7.

30. Sakles JC, Laurin EG, Rantapaa AA, et al. Airway management in the emergency department: a one-year study of 610 tracheal intubations. Ann Emerg Med 1998; 31(3):325–32.

31. Levitan RM, Rosenblatt B, Meiner EM, et al. Alternating day emergency medicine and anesthesia resident responsibility for management of the trauma airway: a study of laryngoscopy performance and intubation success. Ann Emerg Med 2004;43:48–53.

32. Tam AY, Lau FL. A prospective study of tracheal intubation in an emergency department in Hong Kong. Eur J Emerg Med 2001;8(4):305–10.

33. Sagarin MJ, Chiang V, Sakles JC, et al. Rapid sequence intubation for pediatric emergency airway management. Pediatr Emerg Care 2002;18(6):417–23.

34. Omert L, Yeaney W, Mizikowski S, et al. Role of the emergency physician in the airway management of the trauma patient. J Trauma 2001;51(6):1065–8.

35. Reid C, Chan L, Tweedale M. The who, where, and what of rapid sequence intubation: prospective observational study of emergency RSI outside the operating theatre. Emerg Med J 2004;21(3):296–301.

36. Simpson J, Munro PT, Graham CA. Rapid sequence intubation in the emergency department: a 5-year trend. Emerg Med J 2006;23:54–6.

37. Graham CA, Bear D, Henry JM, et al. Rapid sequence intubation of trauma patients in Scotland. J Trauma 2004;56:1123–6.

38. Dibble C, Maloba M. Best evidence topic report. Rapid sequence induction in the emergency department by emergency medicine personnel. Emerg Med J 2006; 23(1):62–4.

39. Ricard-Hibon A, Chollet C, Leroy C, et al. Succinylcholine improves the time of performance of a tracheal intubation in prehospital critical care medicine. Eur J Anaesthesiol 2002;19:361–7.

40. Pearson S. Comparison of intubation attempts and completion times before and after the initiation of a rapid sequence intubation program in an air medical transport program. Air Med J 2003;22(6):28–33.
41. Li J, Murphy-Lavoie H, Bugas C, et al. Complications of emergency intubation with and without paralysis. Am J Emerg Med 1999;17(2):141–3.
42. Rocca B, Crosby E, Maloney J, et al. An assessment of paramedic performance during invasive airway management. Prehosp Emerg Care 2000;4(2):164–7.
43. Rapid sequence intubation. ACEP policy statement. Available at: www.ACEP. ORG/practres. Accessed August 5, 2008.
44. Walls RM. Rapid sequence intubation. In: Walls RM, Murphy MF, editors. Manual of airway management. Philadelphia: Lippincott Willias & Wilkins; 2004. p. 22–32 [chapter 3].
45. Hopson LR, Dronen SC. Pharmacologic adjuncts to intubation. In: Roberts JR, Hedges JR, editors. Clinical procedures in emergency medicine. 4th edition. Philadelphia: Saunders; 2004. p. 100–14 [chapter 5].
46. Benumof JL, Dagg R, Benumof R. Critical hemoglobin desaturation will occur before return to an unparalyzed state following 1 mg/kg intravenous succinylcholine. Anesthesiology 1997;87(4):979–82.
47. Mort TC. Preoxygenation in critically ill patients requiring emergency tracheal intubation. Crit Care Med 2005;33:2672–5.
48. Baillard C, Fosse JP, Sebbane M, et al. Noninvasive ventilation improves preoxygenation before intubation of hypoxic patients. Am J Respir Crit Care Med 2006;174:171–7.
49. Beam A. Atropine: re-evaluating its use during paediatric RSI. Emerg Med J 2007;24:361–2.
50. McAuliffe G, Bissonnette B, Boutin C. Should the routine use of atropine before succinycholine in children be reconsidered? Can J Anaesth 1995;42:724–9.
51. Fastle RK, Roback MG. Pediatric rapid sequence intubation: incidence of reflex bradycardia and effects of pretreatment with atropine. Pediatr Emerg Care 2004; 20:651–5.
52. American Heart Association. Recognition and management of bradyarrhythmias and tachyarrhythmias. In: Ralston M, Hazinski MF, Zaritsky AL, et al, editors. Pediatric advanced life support provider manual. Dallas (TX): American Heart Association; 2006. p. 115–52 [chapter 6].
53. American Heart Association. Bradycardia case. In: Field JM, Gonzalez L, Hazinski MF, editors. Advance cardiovascular life support provider manual. Dallax, (TX): American Heart Association; 2006. p. 78–86 [part 4].
54. Schneider RE, Caro DA. Pretreatmetn agents. In: Walls RM, Murphy MF, editors. Manual of emergency airway management. 2nd edition. Philadelphia: Lippincott, Williams & Wilkins; 2004. p. 183–8 [chapter 16].
55. Decker JM, Lowe DA. Rapid sequence induction. In: Henretig FM, King C, editors. Textbook of pediatric emergency procedures. Baltimore: Williams & Wilkins; 1997. p. 141–60 [chapter 15].
56. Sellick BA. Cricoid pressure to control regurgitation of stomach contents during induction of anaesthesia. Lancet 1961;2:404–6.
57. Walz JM, Zayaruzny M, Heard SO. Airway management in critical illness. Chest 2007;131(2):608–20.
58. Butler J, Sen A. Cricoid pressure in emergency rapid sequence induction. Emerg Med J 2005;22:815–6.
59. Ellis DY, Harris T, Zideman D. Cricoid pressure in emergency department rapid sequence tracheal intubation: a risk benefit analysis. Ann Emerg Med 2007;50:653–65.

60. Smith KJ, Dobranowski J, Yip G, et al. Cricoid pressure displaces the esophagus: an observational study using magnetic resonance imaging. Anesthesiology 2003; 99:60–4.

61. Salem M, Joseph N, Heyman H, et al. Cricoid compression is effective in obliterating the esophageal lumen in the presence of a nasogastric tube. Anesthesiology 1985;63:443–6.

62. Lawes EG, Campbell I, Mercer D. Inflation pressure, gastric insufflation and rapid sequence induction. Br J Anaesth 1987;59:315–8.

63. Levitan RM, Kinkle WC, Levin WJ, et al. Laryngeal view during laryngoscopy: a randomized trial comparing cricoid pressure, backwar-upward-rightward pressure, and bimanual laryngoscopy. Ann Emerg Med 2006;47:548–55.

64. Noguchi T, Koga K, Shiga Y, et al. The gum elastic bougie eases tracheal intubation while applying cricoid pressure compared to a stylet. Can J Anaesth 2003; 50:712–7.

65. Haslam N, Parker L, Duggan JE. Effect of cricoid pressure on the view at laryngoscopy. Anaesthesia 2005;60:41–7.

66. Ho AM, Wong W, Ling E, et al. Airway difficulties cause by improperly applied cricoid pressure. J Emerg Med 2001;20:29–31.

67. Lyons G. Failed intubation. Six years' experience in a teaching maternity unit. Anaesthesia 1985;40:759–62.

68. Williamson R. Cricoid pressure. Can J Anaesth 1989;36:601.

69. Saghaei M, Masoonifar M. The pressor response and airway effects of cricoid pressure during induction of general anaesthesia. Anesth Analg 2001;93(3): 787–90.

70. Clark RK, Trethewy CE. Assessment of cricoid pressure application by emergency department staff. Emerg Med Australas 2005;17:376–81.

71. Meek T, Gittins N, Duggen JE. Cricoid pressure: knowledge and performance amongst anaesthetic assistants. Anaesthesia 1999;54:59–62.

72. Adnet F, Borron SW, Dumas JL, et al. Study of the "sniffing position" by magnetic resonance imaging. Anesthesiology 2001;94:83–6.

73. Adnet F, Baillard C, Borron SW, et al. Randomized study comparing the "sniffing position" with simple head extension for laryngoscopic view in elective surgery patients. Anesthesiology 2001;95:836–41.

74. Crosby ET. Airway management in adults after cervical spine trauma. Anesthesiology 2006;104:1293–318.

75. Majernick TG, Bieniek R, Houston JB, et al. Cervical spine movement during orotracheal intubation. Ann Emerg Med 1986;15:417–20.

76. Watts AD, Gelb AW, Bach DB, et al. Comparison of the Bullard and Macintosh laryngoscopes for endotracheal intubation of patents with a potential cervical spine injury. Anesthesiology 1997;87:1335–42.

77. Collins JS, Lemmens HJ, Brodsky JB, et al. Laryngoscopy and morbid obesity: a comparison of the "sniff" and "ramped" positions. Obes Surg 2004;14:1171–5.

78. Deem SA, Bishop MJ, Bedford RF. Physiologic and pathophysiologic responses to intubation. In: Hagberg CA, editor. Benumof's airway management. 2nd edition. Philadelphia: Mosby Elsevier; 2007. p. 193–214 [chapter 6].

79. Mort TC. Complications of emergency tracheal intubation: hemodynamic alterations—part 1. J Intensive Care Med 2007;22(3):157–65.

Tracheal Intubation: Tricks of the Trade

Michael F. Murphy, MD, FRCPC[a,b,c],*, Orlando R. Hung, MD, FRCPC[a,c,d,e],
J. Adam Law, MD, FRCPC[a,e,f]

KEYWORDS

• Tracheal intubation • Larynscopy • Intubation

In 1878, William Macewen[1] was the first to use endotracheal intubation for a patient who had cancer of the base of the tongue rather than tracheostomy, as was routine at that time. Subsequently, Macewen guided metal tubes into the airway with his fingers, honing his skills on cadavers, and then packed the pharynx with oil-soaked gauze to achieve a seal.

The first direct laryngoscope was described by Kirstein[2] in 1895. It was a straight blade design with a light electrically powered and positioned at the tip. The original laryngoscopic technique with a straight blade was no different than it is today. The tip of the laryngoscope blade was passed posterior to the epiglottis, which was then elevated directly to expose the vocal cords. Chevalier Jackson[3] is credited as being the first to place batteries in the handle of the laryngoscope. Jackson[3] also recommended that the head be placed on a pillow in full extension rather than in the "sniffing position" (flexion of the neck and extension of the head) now recommended and that the tip of the laryngoscope be inserted sufficiently beyond the tip of the epiglottis to elevate it out of the line of sight (LOS). He postulated that the epiglottis must be identified for successful intubation, cautioned against using the teeth as a fulcrum, and emphasized that the force applied to the laryngoscope was designed to lift the hyoid and epiglottis.[4] He recommended that the laryngoscope blade be advanced along the right side of the tongue (ie, paraglossal approach).

Magill[5] also recommended a paraglossal approach, particularly if laryngoscopy proved difficult. He postulated (correctly) that positioning the laryngoscope blade as

[a] Department of Anesthesiology, Dalhousie University, Halifax, Nova Scotia, Canada
[b] Department of Emergency Medicine, Dalhousie University, Halifax, Nova Scotia, Canada
[c] Department of Anesthesia, Dalhousie University, Capital District Health Authority, 1278 South Park Street, 10 West, Halifax, Nova Scotia, Canada B3H 2Y9
[d] Department of Pharmacology, Dalhousie University, Halifax, Nova Scotia, Canada
[e] Department of Surgery, Dalhousie University, Halifax, Nova Scotia, Canada
[f] Department of Anesthesia, Dalhousie University, Queen Elizabeth II Health Science Centre, 1796 Summer Street, Halifax, Nova Scotia, Canada B3H 3A7
* Corresponding author. Department of Anesthesia, Dalhousie University, Capital District Health Authority, 1278 South Park Street, 10 West, Halifax, Nova Scotia, Canada B3H 2Y9.
E-mail address: murphymf1@gmail.com (M.F. Murphy).

Emerg Med Clin N Am 26 (2008) 1001–1014
doi:10.1016/j.emc.2008.07.009
0733-8627/08/$ – see front matter © 2008 Elsevier Inc. All rights reserved.

emed.theclinics.com

far lateral as possible improved the laryngeal view.[6] Bonfils[7] later described this technique as "retromolar," although the terminology is inaccurate because the laryngoscope is almost never passed posterior to the molar teeth. Henderson[8] maintains that the key feature of the techniques of Magill and Bonfils is passage of the laryngoscope along the paraglossal gutter, a position that facilitates optimum lateral displacement of the entire tongue. He also states that "paraglossal" is a more accurate description for this technique. Even today, moving the blade from the midline to the paraglossal position during laryngoscopy may rapidly convert an intubation failure to a success, particularly with adjunctive use of an endotracheal tube introducer (ETI), such as an Eschmann introducer (EI). It is a maneuver that may improve the laryngeal view so substantially that every airway manager ought to be aware of it.[9]

Sir Robert Macintosh[10] described the curved laryngoscope blade in 1943, in large measure, to subvert the addition of bulky balloons to rubber endotracheal tubes (ETTs) in the 1940s, which hindered, or even made impossible, their passage through the flange of the Magill blade. This blade was designed to control the tongue and sweep it to the left side of the mouth, creating sufficient room to pass the bulky tube-balloon combination. Macintosh's key innovation was not the curved blade design but the technique, which involved inserting the blunt tip of the blade into the vallecula and actively depressing the hyoepiglottic ligament to flip the epiglottis anteriorly to expose the glottis. The importance of the technique is often overlooked, but it is the key to understanding the success of the Macintosh laryngoscope—and its limitation.[8] By the late 1940s, Macintosh tired of his design and reverted to the Magill blade, having invented the intubating stylet (gum elastic bougie, EI) to get around the problem. Macintosh inserted the EI down the flange of the paraglossally inserted Magill blade into the trachea and then moved the blade to the center of the mouth and guided the ETT into the trachea over the EI.[9]

LARYNGOSCOPY AND INTUBATION

Laryngoscopic oral intubation is a difficult skill to master. Using a statistical model to study the learning curve of novice intubators, Mulcaster and colleagues[11] determined that 47 intubations were required to ensure a 90% probability that a laryngoscopic intubation would be successful. Laryngoscopy is a multifaceted procedure that requires a solid knowledge of the relevant anatomy in addition to dexterity and creativity to align the oral, pharyngeal, and laryngeal axes of the airway so that the laryngoscopist gains the best possible view of the glottis.

Benumof[12] describes a "best attempt" at laryngoscopy as having six components: (1) performance by a reasonably experienced laryngoscopist, (2) no significant muscle tone (paralysis), (3) optimal positioning of the airway (eg, sniff position), (4) the use of external laryngeal manipulation, (5) appropriate length of blade, and (6) type of blade. With this definition and no other confounding considerations, the optimal attempt at laryngoscopy and intubation may be achieved on the first attempt and should take no more than three attempts.[9] Because there are different techniques of laryngoscopy, the laryngoscopist needs to choose one method that works best and use or practice it often, although not to the exclusion of the others.

The laryngoscopist must recognize the anatomy of the laryngeal inlet revealed at direct laryngoscopy. Beneath the epiglottis, a view is sought of the whitish vocal cords in their triangular orientation (**Fig. 1**). Below the cords, the rounded paired posterior (corniculate) cartilages may be seen. Between and slightly beneath these cartilages, the small vertical interarytenoid notch appears, and in a restricted view situation, it may be the only landmark identifying the more superiorly located glottic opening. When

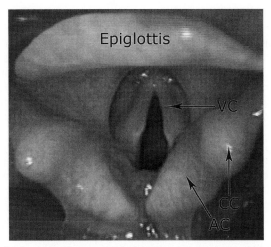

Fig. 1. Anatomy of the laryngeal inlet revealed at direct laryngoscopy. Beneath the epiglottis (E), a view is sought of the whitish vocal cords (VC) in their triangular orientation. The rounded paired posterior (corniculate) cartilages (CC) and arytenoid cartilages (AC) are also shown.

seen and recognized, an endotracheal introducer can easily be placed above the notch or cartilages to gain access to the trachea.

Cormack and Lehane[13] devised a scoring system that, although limited by an element of intra- and interobserver variability, provided an objective descriptive measure of the glottic view during laryngoscopy. The definitions they used are as follows:

Grade 1: most of the glottis is visible.
Grade 2: only the posterior extremity of the glottis is visible.
Grade 3: no part of the glottis but only the epiglottis is visible.
Grade 4: not even the epiglottis can be seen.

Perhaps the most useful modification of this basic system is one that parses a grade 3 view into a grade 3a, in which the epiglottis can be lifted off the posterior pharyngeal wall, and grade 3b, in which it cannot be lifted (**Fig. 2**).[14] Persistent attempts to intubate a patient with a grade 3b view while using a curved blade and intubating stylet cannot be justified.

Although there are many different types of laryngoscopic blades, they are all essentially straight or curved. Typically, the straight blades are intended to pick up the epiglottis to optimize visualization of the glottic opening. The curved blades are used to

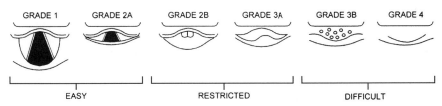

Fig. 2. Modified Cormack and Lehane's classification of laryngeal grade. (*From* Cook TM. A new practical classification of laryngeal view. Anaesthesia 2000;55:274–9; with permission.)

negotiate around the base of the tongue to make contact with the hyoepiglottic ligament. Depressing this ligament with the blunt (and usually beaded) tip of a curved blade produces elevation of the epiglottis and exposure of the glottis. Although these devices are effective and safe, they all have limitations. Straight blades seem to provide better visualization of the larynx, whereas tracheal intubation seems to be easier with curved blades.[15] The choice of these blades largely depends on the airway manager's training, experience, and the clinical situation. Airway managers need to be familiar with both techniques so that if one fails, the other can be used.

Positioning of the Head and Neck for Laryngoscopy and Intubation

Laryngoscopy is more successful if the laryngoscopist assumes or creates a comfortable intubating position that allows in-line visualization of the airway. This can be accomplished by adjusting the height of the patient or the height of the intubator (eg, stool, kneeling) to bring the airway into the laryngoscopist's central field of vision. Uncomfortable contorted body positions lead to fatigue and unnecessarily complicate laryngoscopy.[9]

The optimal position for direct laryngoscopy and intubation is controversial. Jackson[3] advocated full head extension, and Magill[16] recommended the "sniff" position, whereby the neck is flexed on the torso and the head is slightly extended on the neck (the flex-extend position). The triple-axis alignment was first proposed by Bannister (an anesthetist) and MacBeth[17] (an ear, nose, and throat surgeon) in 1944.

There is clinical evidence of the value of the sniff position.[18] Head extension facilitates insertion of the laryngoscope, reduces contact between the laryngoscope and the maxillary teeth, improves the view of the larynx, and is essential for full mouth opening.[19] Adnet and colleagues[20] compared the view achieved during laryngoscopy in patients in the sniff position (neck flexion) with simple head extension. They concluded that the sniff position was particularly beneficial in patients who are obese or have limited neck mobility. The sniff position improved glottic visualization in 18% of patients and worsened it in 11%. In those patients in whom the sniff position improved the view, the grade was improved from 4 to 3 in 2 patients, from 3 to 2 in 16 patients, and from 2 to 1 in 66 patients. These improvements are clinically important.

Although there has been some controversy as to whether or not the sniffing position is best, it is generally accepted that when not contraindicated by cervical spine precautions, this is the best starting position. It is crucial that the airway manager treat laryngoscopy as a two-handed procedure. Holding the laryngoscope in the left hand, the right hand can be used to lift and tilt the patient's head back during laryngoscopy or to manipulate the thyroid cartilage externally in an attempt to visualize the glottis optimally. Once the airway manager has obtained the "best view" of the glottis, the assistant is asked to reproduce the corresponding maneuver while the laryngoscopist passes the ETT.

Laryngoscopy

The purpose of direct laryngoscopy is to facilitate tracheal intubation under vision. Successful direct laryngoscopy depends on achieving an LOS from the maxillary teeth to the larynx. Management of the tongue and epiglottis is crucial to successful direct laryngoscopy. While holding the laryngoscope in the left hand, the right hand is used to extend the head on the neck, provided there are no contraindications to moving the cervical spine. This motion causes the mouth to open a moderate amount. The blade is inserted into the partially open mouth, and the little finger of the left hand then retracts the lower lip from between the mandibular teeth and the blade. This maneuver prevents injury to the lower lip and also serves to open the mouth more fully. The laryngoscope blade is further advanced into the right side of the mouth and then moved to the middle of the mouth to displace the tongue to the left and into the mandibular space. The tip of the blade is used to move the epiglottis out of the LOS. A straight blade is ordinarily inserted to the point where the epiglottis can be picked up ("look as you go" or "insert and withdraw"), whereas the curved blades are designed to be inserted into the vallecula to contact the underlying hyoepiglottic ligament, which flips the epiglottis forward out of the LOS. Forward movement of the hyoid bone and epiglottis out of the LOS with both types of blades is achieved by applying a significant lifting force along the long axis of the handle.

The amount of lifting force required to expose the glottis maximally is related to some known variables: the heavier the patient, the greater is the force required;[21] the McCoy laryngoscope blade[22] requires less lifting force; and the lifting force required is 30% less with a straight blade than with a curved one.[23] The amount of lifting force required to expose the larynx optimally while minimizing the risk for trauma to fragile tissues is gained with experience.

The key differences between the curved and straight laryngoscope blade techniques relate to better tongue control by the broader curved blade together with indirect epiglottis elevation achieved by stretching the hyoepiglottic ligament, as opposed to the direct elevation of the epiglottis with the straight blade.

Many factors may cause difficulty with direct laryngoscopy. Failure to displace some of the tongue to the left of the blade occurs when there is increased tongue size, reduced volume of the mandibular space, reduced volume of the mouth (eg, "high arched palate"), or a fibrotic postinflammatory tongue (eg, postradiation therapy).[24] Additionally, reduced access to the oral cavity (ie, mouth opening) is postulated to lead to trapping of the tongue between the blade and the hyoid. In the event that one is using a curved blade, this prevents the tip of the blade from entering the vallecula and depressing the hyoepiglottic ligament. This is probably the final common pathway of many causes of failure to see the vocal cords with the Macintosh laryngoscope.[25]

The Macintosh laryngoscope blade works well in most patients. Insertion is usually easy, because the curved blade follows the natural curve of the tongue through the mouth and into the vallecula with a sliding radial wrist deviation ("rocking") kind of motion. The laryngoscope is inserted to the right of the tongue, moving it to midline as it is advanced, helping to locate the epiglottis and glottis in most patients. Nevertheless, there are the inherent limitations as described, and it is necessary to be skilled in alternative techniques.[26]

The straight blade has the potential to provide glottic visualization in most patients for whom a curved blade has failed to do so. Some researchers have suggested that the mechanism of the greater efficacy of the straight laryngoscope is an improved LOS, because there is no laryngoscope curve to intrude into the LOS.[27,28] Further, the paraglossal approach reduces the distance from the near point (the teeth) to the far point (the glottis), improving the LOS. This is akin to moving an object just beyond the visual horizon closer so as to bring it into view. Additional mechanisms include more effective displacement of the tongue and more reliable elevation of the epiglottis. Coupling this technique with an ETI further improves intubation success rates.

There is evidence to support the contention that the straight blade provides tracheal intubation success when the curved blade has failed. The first series that defined the efficacy of the straight laryngoscope in patients in whom the larynx could not be visualized with the Macintosh laryngoscope was published in 1983.[7] Six further series were reviewed by Henderson[8] in 1997.

Many variations of the curved laryngoscope blade have been described, most without significant data about their efficacy, and few have stood the test of time. The levering tip McCoy curved blade deserves special mention, however. This Macintosh-type laryngoscope blade was introduced by McCoy and Mirakhur[29] in 1993 and features a hinged tip that flexes when a lever on the handle is depressed. The mechanism of displacement of the tongue and elevation of the epiglottis is similar to that of the Macintosh laryngoscope in that the tip of the laryngoscope blade is inserted into the vallecula and the epiglottis is elevated indirectly by stretching the hyoepiglottic ligament. There have been many reports of conversion of grade 3 views to grade 1 or 2,[30–33] particularly in series of patients with applied neck immobilization.[34–36] There have also been reports of failures, however.[37–40]

A variety of prisms and mirror modifications of the curved blade have come and gone over the years. For the most part, prisms and mirrors have been superseded by alternative devices that give better views and are easier to use. Nevertheless, the Truview EVO2 blade (Truphatek International Ltd., Netanya, Israel) (**Fig. 3**) and the Viewmax (Rusch Inc., Duluth, Georgia) (**Fig. 4**), the recent players in this field, are relatively easy to use and may find a place in the armamentarium of some practitioners. Although these devices may provide an improved view of the larynx compared with Macintosh blade laryngoscopy, clinical experience with these devices is presently limited.[41,42]

A variety of straight laryngoscope blades have been introduced over the years, but only three bear elaboration: Miller, Phillips, and Henderson. Two early straight laryngoscopes were designed by Jackson and Magill. Others include the Flagg, Guedel, Wisconsin, Wisconsin-Forreger, and other straight blades. Generally speaking, the design modifications (reduced proximal cross section,[43,44] angulation,[28,45,46] or others) are intended to reduce contact with the maxillary teeth.

The Miller[47] laryngoscope blade is the most popular straight laryngoscope blade. It has a lower cross-sectional dimension than other straight-blade laryngoscopes, facilitating its insertion and positioning features. This design advantage is also its major disadvantage in that an ETT cannot easily and safely (without lacerating the balloon) be passed through its channel. One's inability to see the tip of the blade hinders the ability to ensure precise placement on the epiglottis. This factor, coupled with the sharpness of the tip, has the potential to lead to tissue trauma and unstable epiglottic

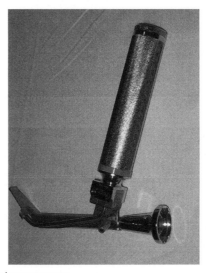

Fig. 3. The Truview EVO2 laryngoscope.

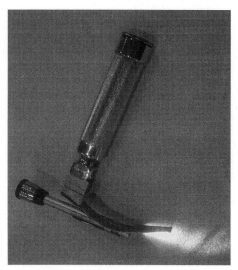

Fig. 4. The Viewmax laryngoscope.

elevation.[25] Additionally, there is a tendency for its light source to become obscured by tissues or secretions.[48] This problem has been resolved in some of the most recent fiberlight models.[49]

The other two straight blades (Phillips and Henderson) are specifically designed to be used with a paraglossal technique and to permit introduction of an ETT through the channel of the blade. The Phillips laryngoscope blade[50] has a semitubular cross section that tapers, with the wider diameter being proximal. The tip is similar to the tip of the Miller laryngoscope. The Henderson blade[51] was designed to overcome the drawbacks of the Miller laryngoscope by incorporating several important design modifications. The cross section of the laryngoscope allows steering of the tip of the tracheal tube during passage so that the tip emerges at the larynx. The illumination site from the fiberlight lies within the lumen of the laryngoscope so that it cannot be easily obscured by soft tissue or secretions. The blade has an atraumatic tip that remains in vision during passage and positioning of the laryngoscope. Finally, the uniform semitubular cross section of the Henderson laryngoscope is slightly wider than that of the Miller laryngoscope and is designed to facilitate visualization of the larynx and passage of an 8-mm (internal diameter [ID]) tracheal tube down the lumen of the laryngoscope. To date, no head-to-head comparisons of the Henderson blade with older established straight blades have been published.

Optimizing the Laryngoscopic View

The most important maneuver used to bring more of the glottic opening into view during direct laryngoscopy is external laryngeal manipulation, which should be an integral part of direct laryngoscopy. Wilson and colleagues[52] were the first to quantify the value of laryngeal pressure (**Fig. 5**) when they used it to reduce the incidence of grade 3 and 4 views from 9.3% to 5.9%. Benumof and Cooper[53] found that the technique, which they called optimal external laryngeal manipulation (OELM), could consistently improve the laryngeal view by one Cormack-Lehane grade. They stressed the importance of the manipulation being performed with the right hand of the airway practitioner, who then guides an assistant to provide identical manipulation. Knill[54] termed the maneuver *BURP* (backward upward right pressure), and Levitan and

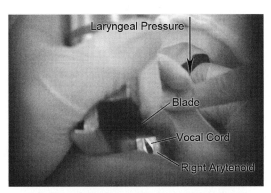

Fig. 5. Improved laryngeal view with the application of laryngeal pressure during direct laryngoscopy with a curved (Macintosh) blade.

colleagues[55] coined the term *bimanual laryngoscopy*, although, conventionally, the term *bimanual laryngoscopy* has been used to describe the use of one hand to manipulate the laryngoscope while the other manipulates the head and neck into an optimal position. External laryngeal manipulation should be an integral part of direct laryngoscopy and should be the first maneuver used to improve the view of the larynx.[25]

Alternative maneuvers that have been demonstrated to improve the laryngeal view include the following:

- Increased neck flexion, achieved by head elevation, can make intubation under vision possible in some patients who initially have a Cormack-Lehane grade 3 view of the glottis.[56]
- Laryngeal lift by an assistant may improve the view.[57]
- Manual forward displacement of the mandible by an assistant can improve the view of the vocal cords.[58]

Intubating the Trachea

A malleable ETT stylet ought to be used for all emergency intubations. Although the angle to which the ETT-stylet combination is bent is an individualized decision, it has been shown that an angle of less than 35° seems to facilitate passage of the ETT beyond the glottis.[9]

Once the glottis has been identified, it is important that the laryngoscopist not lose sight of the target. In preparation for passing the ETT, the individual assisting the airway manager, standing at the patient's right side, should pull open the right side of the patient's mouth with the left index finger, providing generous access to the oropharynx and, most importantly, providing room for unimpeded passage of the ETT. The ETT should be inserted into the right side of the mouth and advanced with the tip of the ETT in gentle contact with the hard and soft palates to keep it in the periphery of the LOS. It is positioned just posterior to the glottic opening, and with a "pill-rolling" counterclockwise motion, the ETT is then rotated 90° from a horizontal to a vertical plane and up into the glottic opening. The narrowest dimension of the bevelled ETT tip is now aligned with the vocal cords.[9,59] Alternatively, if a Phillips or Henderson straight blade is used, the ETT may be guided directly through the channel of the blade into the trachea.

Endotracheal Tube Introducers

ETIs are devices that are passed (introduced) into the trachea and then used as a guide over which the tube is advanced ("railroaded") into the trachea.[60] They are a fundamental piece of airway management equipment that must be part of every airway manager's skill set.

These introducers are ordinarily used in two circumstances in which direct laryngoscopy is undertaken: when a poor grade 2 or grade 3a view (see **Fig. 2**) is obtained with a curved blade or when a Miller blade passed paraglosally exposes a portion of the glottis but there is insufficient room to pass the ETT because it cannot be passed down the narrow channel of the Miller blade. They are also commonly used with video-assisted techniques, such as the video larynscope, or in blind techniques, such as digital intubation. For most of these approaches (except the video larynscope), a blind technique is used (the ETT is not seen directly to enter the trachea).

ETIs are ordinarily plastic or spun nylon, are 60 to 70 cm in length, and incorporate a 30° deflection of the distal tip ("coudé tip") (**Fig. 6**). The tip deflection enhances the anterior movement of the distal tip underneath the epiglottis, maximizing the chance of it passing into the glottis, and hence the trachea; it also permits the tactile appreciation of tracheal rings once placed in the trachea. Seventy-centimeter devices are easier to use than those 60 cm in length. A standard ETT is 30 cm in length, such that 60 cm is exactly twice the length of an ETT; the added 10 cm of the 70-cm device facilitates grasping the proximal end of the ETI as the ETT is advanced into the trachea. One manufacturer supplies a device with a hollow lumen to permit some degree of oxygenation in the event that tube passage over the ETI fails (Frova Intubation Introducer; Cook Critical Care, Bloomington, Indiana). Some ETIs are reusable, whereas others are intended as single-use devices.[9]

The ETIs are labeled in centimeters, depicting the distance from the tip. The print on the ETI is aligned on the same side of the ETI as the tip deflection. Positioning the 25-cm mark of the ETI at the patient's lip correlates with the tip of the ETI at midtrachea. It is important to keep the writing, and hence the deflected tip, up (anterior), because the ETT is passed over the ETI to minimize the chance of forcing the ETT posteriorly in the trachea, risking a posterior tracheal perforation.

When using the ETI, some laryngeal structure (epiglottis or better [grade 2 or 3]) must be visible. Under direct vision, the ETI is inserted beneath the epiglottis (**Fig. 7**) and an attempt is made to insert the tip through the glottis into the trachea. In a grade 2 view, the ETI may be seen to enter the glottis. In a grade 3 view, the tip of the ETI is not seen to enter the glottis or trachea. Once in the trachea, the ETI tip can often transmit a subtle "click, click, click" sensation to the practitioner's fingers, generated by rubbing the tracheal rings as it is moved gently in and out of the airway.[61] A more horizontal (rather than vertical) insertion angle enhances the chance of the

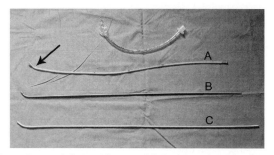

Fig. 6. Intubating introducers. (A) EI with a coudé tip (*arrow*) at the distal end. (B) Frova intubation introducer is an intubating catheter with a hollow lumen and a coudé tip at the distal end. (C) ETI is similar to the EI in size and shape with a coudé tip, but it is 10 cm longer.

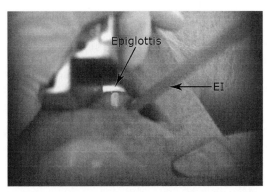

Fig. 7. When using the ETI, some laryngeal structure, such as the epiglottis, must be visible. Under direct vision, the EI is inserted beneath the epiglottis.

coudé tip "rubbing" against the anterior tracheal rings. Feeling this sensation enhances confidence that the ETI is in the trachea; failing to sense it does not mean that the ETI is not in the trachea. The tongue or other airway structures contacting the shaft of the ETI may insulate against the transmission of the corrugated vibrations. In the case in which tracheal rings cannot be felt, the ETI should be gently advanced. If it is in the trachea, it should "hold up" at some point, usually when the 30-cm mark is adjacent to the lips.[61] Hold up does not occur if the ETI is in the esophagus. In the study by Kidd and colleagues,[61] the hold-up sign seemed to more reliable than clicks, because hold up was observed in 100% of tracheal placements of the ETI, whereas the clicks were present in only 90%. In the event that hold up occurs, the ETI should be withdrawn to 25 cm at the lips before advancing the ETT over the ETI.

Failure of the ETT to pass easily over the ETI into the trachea is most often attributable to the failure to maintain a "best laryngoscopic view" during the ETT insertion. Keeping the laryngoscope in place minimizes the angle the ETT-ETI combination must negotiate and enhances the chance of successfully intubating the trachea **(Fig. 8)**.[62]

With an assistant holding the ETI, the ETT is passed over the ETI. A gentle clockwise or counterclockwise twist of the ETT as the bevel of the ETT reaches the glottis

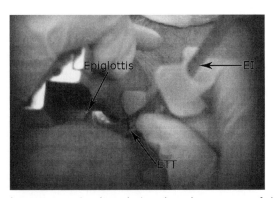

Fig. 8. Keeping the laryngoscope in place during the advancement of the ETT over the EI minimizes the angle the ETT-EI combination must negotiate and enhances the placement of the ETT.

enhances passage. Should the ETT get hung up, the tube should be rotated through 90°, first counterclockwise (ETT bevel faces downward) and then clockwise (ETT bevel faces upward) if necessary. The tip of the ETT may be caught on the posterior commissure of the glottis, the anterior commissure of the cords, the cord or aryepiglottic fold, or the cricoid cartilage, although it is impossible to know the exact location. A similar experience may occur when the ETI is passed. The possibilities and remedies are identical.

Once the ETT is in place, the intubating ETI is removed and tube position is confirmed.

The ETI is not a failsafe device and there are case reports[63,64] of failure of this technique. It does enjoy a high success rate, however. Among the 2000 incidents reviewed by the Australian Incident Monitoring Study, 85 (4%) indicated problems with endotracheal intubation.[65] The most successful intubation aid in this series was the EI. In a prospective study, Latto and colleagues[66] reported a high success rate of tracheal intubation using the EI (99.5%, or 199 of 200 intubations), with most achieved in a single attempt (89%, or 178 of 200 intubations). In another prospective study, Combes and colleagues[67] reported a 90% success rate for tracheal intubation using the EI in unanticipated difficult airways after two attempts. The technique works less well when the laryngeal view grade is 3b or only the tip of the epiglottis can be seen.

Complications related to the use of this device are rare, although mediastinitis after use of the introducer technique has been reported in closed claims analyses of anesthetic cases[68] and in a review of emergency medicine cases.[69] These studies identify the association of persistent intubation attempts with pharyngeal and esophageal perforation, mediastinitis, and death. Persistent attempts at tracheal intubation can lead to increasing difficulty with mask ventilation[70] and to pharyngeal or esophageal perforation that results in mediastinitis.[71]

SUMMARY

Although they are not truly "tricks" so much as maneuvers basic to successful orotracheal laryngoscopic intubation, the following ought to be incorporated into the skill sets of individuals called on to manage the airway in an emergency:

- Use both hands when performing laryngoscopy: one to hold the laryngoscope and the other first to manipulate the head into position and then to perform external laryngeal manipulation (BURP).
- Gain familiarity with curved and straight blade (particularly by a paraglossal approach) techniques.
- Ensure that batteries are charged and that illumination is adequate.
- Place a malleable stylet in all ETTs to be used.
- Do not obscure the LOS when the ETT is inserted.
- Have an ETI immediately available and know how to use it; most importantly, remember to leave the laryngoscope in place while railroading the ETT into place over the ETI.

REFERENCES

1. Macewen W. Clinical observations on the introduction of tracheal tubes by the mouth instead of performing tracheotomy or laryngotomy. Br Med J 1880;1: 163–5.
2. Kirstein A. Autoskopie des larynx und der trachea. Berlin Klinische Wochenschrift 1895;32:476–8 [in German].

3. Jackson C. The technique of insertion of intratracheal insufflation tubes. Surg Gynecol Obstet 1913;17:507–9.

4. Jackson C. Bronchoscopy and esophagoscopy. Gleanings from experience. J Am Med Assoc 1909;13:1009–13.

5. Magill IW. An improved laryngoscope for anaesthetists. Lancet 1926;1:500.

6. Magill IW. Technique in endotracheal anaesthesia. Br Med J 1930;2:817–20.

7. Bonfils P. Difficult intubation in Pierre-Robin children, a new method: the retromolar route. Anaesthesist 1983;32:363–7.

8. Henderson JJ. The use of paraglossal straight blade laryngoscopy in difficult tracheal intubation. Anaesthesia 1997;52:552–60.

9. Schneider RE, Murphy MF. Bag/mask ventilation and endotracheal intubation. In: Walls RM, Murphy MF, Luten RC, et al, editors. Manual of emergency airway management. 2nd edition. Philadelphia: Lippincott Williams and Wilkins; 2004. p. 43–69.

10. Macintosh RR. A new laryngoscope. Lancet 1943;1:205.

11. Mulcaster JT, Mills J, Hung OR, et al. Laryngoscopic intubation: learning and performance. Anesthesiology 2003;98:23–7.

12. Benumof JL. Difficult laryngoscopy: obtaining the best view. Can J Anaesth 1994; 41:361–5.

13. Cormack RS, Lehane J. Difficult tracheal intubation in obstetrics. Anaesthesia 1984;39:1105–11.

14. Cook TM. A new practical classification of laryngeal view. Anaesthesia 2000;55: 274–9.

15. Arino JJ, Velasco JM, Gasco C, et al. Straight blades improve visualization of the larynx while curved blades increase ease of intubation: a comparison of the Macintosh, Miller, McCoy, Belscope and Lee-Fiberview blades. Can J Anaesth 2003; 50:501–6.

16. Magill IW. Endotracheal anesthesia. Am J Surg 1936;34:450–5.

17. Bannister FB, MacBeth RG. Direct laryngoscopy and tracheal intubation. Lancet 1944;2:651–4.

18. Horton WA, Fahy L, Charters P. Defining a standard intubating position using "angle finder". Br J Anaesth 1989;62:6–12.

19. Calder I, Picard J, Chapman M, et al. Mouth opening: a new angle. Anesthesiology 2003;99:799–801.

20. Adnet F, Baillard C, Borron SW, et al. Randomized study comparing the "sniffing position" with simple head extension for laryngoscopic view in elective surgery patients. Anesthesiology 2001;95:836–41.

21. Bishop MJ, Harrington RM, Tencer AF. Force applied during tracheal intubation. Anesth Analg 1992;74:411–4.

22. McCoy EP, Mirakhur RK, Rafferty C, et al. A comparison of the forces exerted during laryngoscopy. The Macintosh versus the McCoy blade. Anaesthesia 1996;51: 912–5.

23. Hastings RH, Hon ED, Nghiem C, et al. Force and torque vary between laryngoscopists and laryngoscope blades. Anesth Analg 1996;82:462–8.

24. Pauloski BR, Rademaker AW, Logemann JA, et al. Speech and swallowing in irradiated and nonirradiated postsurgical oral cancer patients. Otolaryngol Head Neck Surg 1998;118:616–24.

25. Henderson JJ. Direct laryngoscopy and intubation of the trachea. In: Hung OR, Murphy MF, editors. Management of the difficult and failed airway. New York: McGraw Hill; 2007. p. 103–22.

26. Henderson JJ. Tracheal intubation of the adult patient. In: Calder IA, Pearce AC, editors. Core topics in airway management. Cambridge (UK): Cambridge University Press; 2004.

27. Arai T, Nagaro T, Nitta K. Management of the difficult endotracheal intubation; advantages of the Miller blade and a facilitated nasotracheal intubation with a fiberoptic bronchoscope. Masui 1987;36:1112–6.

28. Bellhouse CP. An angulated laryngoscope for routine and difficult tracheal intubations. Anesthesiology 1988;69:126–9.

29. McCoy EP, Mirakhur RK. The levering laryngoscope. Anaesthesia 1993;48:516–9.

30. Chadwick IS, McCluskey A. Another trachea intubated with the McCoy laryngoscope. Anaesthesia 1995;50:571.

31. Farling PA. The McCoy levering laryngoscope blade. Anaesthesia 1994;49:358.

32. Johnston HML, Rao U. The McCoy levering laryngoscope blade. Anaesthesia 1994;49:358.

33. Ward M. The McCoy levering laryngoscope blade. Anaesthesia 1994;49:357–8.

34. Uchida T, Hikawa Y, S aito Y, et al. The McCoy levering laryngoscope in patients with limited neck extension. Can J Anaesth 1997;44:674–6.

35. Gabbott DA. Laryngoscopy using the McCoy laryngoscope after application of a cervical collar. Anaesthesia 1996;51:812–4.

36. Laurent SC, de Melo AE, Alexander-Williams JM. The use of the McCoy laryngoscope in patients with simulated cervical spine injuries. Anaesthesia 1996;51:74–5.

37. Asai T, Hirose T, Shingu K. Failed tracheal intubation using a laryngoscope and intubating laryngeal mask. Can J Anaesth 2000;47:325–8.

38. Haridas RP. The McCoy levering laryngoscope blade. Anaesthesia 1996;51:91.

39. Leary JA. Mechanical failure of the McCoy laryngoscope during a difficult intubation. Anaesthesia 2001;56:88–9.

40. Sheeran P, Maguire T, Browne G. Mechanical failure of the McCoy laryngoscope during difficult intubation. Anaesthesia 2000;55:184–5.

41. Leung YY, Hung CT, Tan ST. Evaluation of the new Viewmax laryngoscope in a simulated difficult airway. Acta Anaesthesiol Scand 2006;50:562–7.

42. Barak M, Philipchuck P, Abecassis P, et al. A comparison of the Truview blade with the Macintosh blade in adult patients. Anaesthesia 2007;62:827–3.

43. Gould RB. Modified laryngoscope blade. Anaesthesia 1954;9:125.

44. Portzer M, Wasmuth CE. Endotracheal anesthesia using a modified Wis-Foregger laryngoscope blade. Cleve Clin Q 1959;26:140–3.

45. Choi JJ. A new double-angle blade for direct laryngoscopy. Anesthesiology 1990; 72:576.

46. Schapira M. A modified straight laryngoscope blade designed to facilitate endotracheal intubation. Anesth Analg 1973;52:553–4.

47. Miller RA. A new laryngoscope. Anesthesiology 1940;2:317–20.

48. Bruin G. The Miller blade and the disappearing light source. Anesth Analg 1996; 83:888.

49. Raw D, Skinner A. Miller laryngoscope blades. Anaesthesia 1999;54:500.

50. Phillips OC, Duerksen RL. Endotracheal intubation. A new blade for direct laryngoscopy. Anesth Analg 1973;52:691–8.

51. Henderson JJ. Solutions to the problem of difficult tracheal tube passage associated with the paraglossal straight laryngoscopy technique. Anaesthesia 1999;54: 601–2.

52. Wilson ME, Spiegelhalter D, Robertson JA, et al. Predicting difficult intubation. Br J Anaesth 1988;61:211–6.

53. Benumof JL, Cooper SD. Quantitative improvement in laryngoscopic view by optimal external laryngeal manipulation. J Clin Anesth 1996;8:136–40.

54. Knill RL. Difficult laryngoscopy made easy with a "BURP." Can J Anaesth 1993; 40:279–82.

55. Levitan RM, Mickler T, Hollander JE. Bimanual laryngoscopy: a videographic study of external laryngeal manipulation by novice intubators. Ann Emerg Med 2002;40:30–7.

56. Schmitt HJ, Mang H. Head and neck elevation beyond the sniffing position improves laryngeal view in cases of difficult direct laryngoscopy. J Clin Anesth 2002;14:335–8.

57. Krantz MA, Poulos JG, Chaouki K, et al. The laryngeal lift: a method to facilitate endotracheal intubation. J Clin Anesth 1993;5:297–301.

58. Tamura M, Ishikawa T, Kato R, et al. Mandibular advancement improves the laryngeal view during direct laryngoscopy performed by inexperienced physicians. Anesthesiology 2004;100:598–601.

59. Smith M, Buist RJ, Mansour NY. A simple method to facilitate difficult intubation. Can J Anaesth 1990;37:144–5.

60. Hung OR, Stewart RD. Intubating stylets. In: Hagberg C, editor. Benumof's airway management. 2nd edition. Philadelphia: Mosby, Inc.; 2007. p. 463–75.

61. Kidd JF, Dyson A, Latto IP. Successful difficult intubation. Use of the gum elastic bougie. Anaesthesia 1988;43:437–8.

62. Dogra S, Falconer R, Latto IP. Successful difficult intubation. Tracheal tube placement over a gum-elastic bougie. Anaesthesia 1990;45:774–6.

63. Boys JE. Failed intubation in obstetric anaesthesia. A case report. Br J Anaesth 1983;55:187–8.

64. Christian AS. Failed obstetric intubation. Anaesthesia 1990;45:995.

65. Williamson JA, Webb RK, Szekely S, et al. The Australian Incident Monitoring Study. Difficult intubation: an analysis of 2000 incident reports. Anaesth Intensive Care 1993;21:602–7.

66. Latto IP, Stacey M, Mecklenburgh J, et al. Survey of the use of the gum elastic bougie in clinical practice. Anaesthesia 2002;57:379–84.

67. Combes X, Le Roux B, Suen P, et al. Unanticipated difficult airway in anesthetized patients: prospective validation of a management algorithm. Anesthesiology 2004;100:1146–50.

68. Peterson GN, Domino KB, Caplan RA, et al. Management of the difficult airway: a closed claims analysis. Anesthesiology 2005;103:33–9.

69. Mort TC. Emergency tracheal intubation: complications associated with repeated laryngoscopic attempts. Anesth Analg 2004;99:607–13.

70. Caplan RA, Posner KL, Ward RJ, et al. Adverse respiratory events in anesthesia: a closed claims analysis. Anesthesiology 1990;72:828–33.

71. Domino KB, Posner KL, Caplan RA, et al. Airway injury during anesthesia: a closed claims analysis. Anesthesiology 1999;91:1703–11.

Airway Adjuncts

Catherine A. Marco, MD*, Alan P. Marco, MD, MMM

KEYWORDS

- Airway • Emergency airway management

Airway management is an essential component of the emergency medicine skill set. Management of the difficult airway may include airway adjuncts, including variants of laryngoscopic blades, supraglottic devices, stylets, and optical or video laryngoscopy. A PubMed literature search in January 2008 identified 4461 indexed publications using the term *airway device* published in the past 10 years. Several recent studies demonstrated widespread availability of airway adjuncts in academic centers, including cricothyrotomy kits, transtracheal jet ventilation systems, fiberoptic scopes, bougies, laryngeal mask airways, lighted stylets, retrograde intubation kits, Combitube (Tyco Healthcare, Mansfield, Massachusetts), and esophageal obturator airways. Despite the widespread availability of equipment in these environments, such airway adjuncts are rarely used, however.[1,2] Because of the wide variety of types of products currently available, and the likely expansion of products in the near future, careful consideration of the advantages and disadvantages of airway adjuncts and the selection of a small number of products with which to maintain a high degree of quality clinical experience are important.

Numerous proprietary products are available for airway management. This article focuses on several broad categories of airway adjuncts and their indications, advantages, and disadvantages. Although several proprietary products are mentioned as examples, this article is not intended to be an inclusive review of available products or an endorsement of a particular product or device.

As additional innovative airway adjuncts continue to be developed, knowledge and skills of their use in airway management should be important to the competent emergency physician.

Since the introduction of direct laryngoscopy by Alfred Kirstein in 1895, physicians have sought to improve the instrumentation used to visualize the larynx while minimizing trauma to the tissues. The introduction of the Miller and Macintosh style blades in the 1940s heralded the widespread acceptance of these designs and the quest for better ones. The development of fiberoptics and miniaturized cameras has led to

---

This article describes multiple airway devices currently available. Discussion of these devices within classes requires the use of their respective proprietary names. However, the authors and publishers have made every effort to avoid bias in this manuscript and the use of proprietary names does not constitute endorsement of any specific product.

University of Toledo College of Medicine, 3045 Arlington Avenue, Toledo, OH 43614, USA
* Corresponding author.
E-mail address: catherine.marco@utoledo.edu (C. Marco).

Emerg Med Clin N Am 26 (2008) 1015–1027
doi:10.1016/j.emc.2008.07.005
0733-8627/08/$ – see front matter © 2008 Elsevier Inc. All rights reserved.

emed.theclinics.com

the design of numerous additional airway adjuncts. Although flexible fiberoptic laryngoscopes and bronchoscopes have been used for decades as aids in the difficult intubation setting, their use is limited by the high degree of skill necessary, high acquisition cost, skilled care in cleaning and disinfecting, and high maintenance costs.

There are two main reasons for the interest in these adjunct airway devices: to aid in dealing with the difficult airway, whether anticipated or not, and to minimize movement of the cervical spine in cases of known or suspected cervical spine injury. When choosing which device or devices to use at a particular institution, it is important to consider the skills of the user, the anticipated frequency of use, any special training needed to acquire or maintain facility with the device, ease of assembly of the device, and the care and maintenance of the device. It is advisable to choose one or a few devices with which to become facile rather than attempt to maintain skills with a multitude of devices. Larger institutions, especially teaching centers, may wish to maintain a broader range of devices if their use is frequent enough to maintain skills with each. Finally, to enhance systems-based practice, the emergency physician should consider the economic aspects of choosing a device. Single-use devices may be comparable in cost to the total cost of use of reusable devices when the cost of disposables, cleaning, and maintenance is considered. Using advanced devices on every patient may result in excess resource use and violate the emergency physician's responsibility to be a wise steward of the community's health care resources.

Airway adjunct devices fall into several categories, including special blade designs that are modifications of the standard laryngoscope, stylets (traditional and lighted), and devices using optical pathways to give a direct view of the glottic opening.

LARYNGOSCOPY BLADES

The first type of device intended to improve visualization of the vocal cords during laryngoscopy (other than fundamental blade design) was the addition of the prism. These prisms refract light approximately 30° so that the direct "line of sight" usually needed would no longer be necessary. Prisms are commercially available and have the advantage that they are relatively inexpensive, are easy to clean, and are a simple modification of an existing technique, such that little or no training is needed. Disadvantages include use and storage of a small piece of equipment and the fact that the prism may actually interfere with the passage of the endotracheal tube (ETT). Some researchers have found that the Belscope blade, which incorporates an acrylic prism, may actually lead to longer intubation times in some trainees.[3] Similarly, small telescopes that enhance the field of view can be attached to conventional laryngoscope blades; these have similar advantages and disadvantages as the prisms in addition to a higher acquisition cost.

Special blades have been developed to aid in intubation. The Lee-Fiberview Blade (LF; Anesthesia Medical Specialties, Beaumont, California), available in several blade styles, incorporates a telescope into the blade to improve the view of the glottic opening. The Viewmax (Rusch, Duluth, Georgia) incorporates a lens system that refracts the image approximately 20° to improve visualization of the vocal cords, much like the clip-on prisms do. Although the Viewmax may have improved visualization, use of this device may take longer than that of traditional blades with similar rates of successful intubation.[4] Another conventional laryngoscope blade modified with an optic bundle is the TruView EVO2 laryngoscope (Truphatek International Ltd., Netanya, Israel). Although visualization is better, time to intubate may be longer when compared with standard Macintosh blades.[5,6] The McCoy blade has a lever that allows the tip of the blade to flex to improve the view. The Flexiblade levering laryngoscope

(Arco-Medic Ltd., Omer, Israel) similarly has a lever to flex the blade to improve visualization and may lead to shorter intubation times in patients with poor initial views.[7,8]

SUPRAGLOTTIC DEVICES

Several supraglottic devices for airway management are available. Advantages of these devices include ease of insertion, success rate, low rates of cervical spine movement, and low rates of airway trauma. Potential disadvantages include inappropriate placement in airway anatomic abnormalities, lower oxygen delivery, risk for dislodgement, and long-term airway pressure damage.

The laryngeal mask airway (LMA) is an example of a supraglottic airway device. It is easy to insert and is easily used with cervical spine immobilization. Other periglottic (or supraglottic) devices include the Cobra Perilaryngeal Airway (Engineered Medical Systems, Indianapolis, Indiana), Soft Seal laryngeal mask (SS-LM; Portex Ltd., Hythe, United Kingdom), and the Ambu laryngeal mask (Ambu, St. Ives, Cambridgeshire, United Kingdom).

The esophageal-tracheal Combitube (ETC) is a double-lumen double-balloon supraglottic airway device that is inserted blindly and is functional in esophageal or tracheal placement. It is relatively easy to insert, is easy to learn, and has good success rates of ventilation in the emergency department and prehospital settings.[9–12] This device may be less successful with cervical spine immobilization.[13] Potential disadvantages are relatively common and include vomiting; aspiration; oral, tracheal, or esophageal trauma; subcutaneous emphysema; and inadequate oxygenation.[14–18]

The laryngeal tube (King laryngeal tube; King Systems Corp., Noblesville, Indiana) is a similar device with a double cuff that is inserted blindly. Ease of use and short time to successful intubation have been demonstrated with this device.[19–21]

STYLETS

Various types of stylets are commonly available as adjuvants to endotracheal intubation. Types of stylets available include the traditional ETT malleable stylet, the gum elastic bougie, lighted stylets, and optical stylets.

Beyond the simple malleable stylet that helps to shape the traditional ETT, there is the simplest of all adjuvants, the gum-elastic bougie (Eschmann stylet). This stylet is flexible but has a tip angled at approximately 30°. It is commonly used when only the epiglottis can be visualized (Cormack and Lehane grade 3 view) (see the article by Murphy and colleagues elsewhere in this issue for further exploration of this topic) by gently feeling with the tip for the glottic opening and passing the bougie through it, feeling for the characteristic "bumping" as the angled tip passes over the tracheal rings. An ordinary ETT can then be passed over the bougie. The gum elastic bougie is superior to a stylet in tracheal intubation while applying cricoid pressure.[22] Although the bougie is flexible, it is still stiff enough to serve as a reliable guide for the ETT. Multiple-use bougies have a higher intubation success rate compared with single-use bougies and are less likely to cause tissue trauma.[23,24] Although other catheters can be used, such as tube-change catheters, they may become overly flexible when warmed to body temperature and the catheter can be forced out of the trachea by the relatively stiff room-temperature ETT, leading to an inadvertent esophageal intubation. One advantage of using a tube-exchanging catheter or endotracheal tube introducer (ETI) (see the article by Murphy and colleagues elsewhere in this issue for further exploration of this topic) as a stylet is that these are typically hollow and oxygen can be insufflated into the trachea after placement (**Fig. 1**). Some manufacturers offer tube changers with standard 15-mm adapters so that a manual resuscitator can be used to insufflate

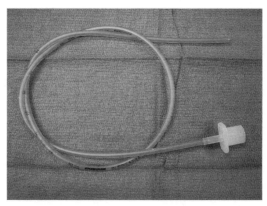

Fig. 1. Sheridan tracheal tube exchanger.

oxygen into the trachea. Other catheters can be readily adapted by press-fitting the connecter from an appropriately sized ETT onto the end. Advantages of stylets include low price, availability, minor modification of existing technique, and simple cleaning (reusable) or no cleaning (single-use devices).

Other types of stylets include lighted stylets, such as the Vital Light and Light Wand (Vital Signs), Trachlight (TL; Laerdal Corporation, New York, New York), and others. These devices rely on the principle of transillumination and do not require direct visualization of the glottis for successful use. Lighted stylets have demonstrated improved success rates compared with traditional stylets.[25–27] Some investigators suggest that for novices, conventional laryngoscopy may be superior to the use of transillumination, however.[28,29] For practitioners experienced in its use, transillumination can be as reliable as conventional laryngoscopy.[30] Transillumination may also be associated with less cervical spine movement compared with other techniques, such as the intubating laryngeal mask or even video laryngoscopes.[31,32] In situations in which access to the head and neck is limited, use of a lightwand in conjunction with intubating laryngeal masks has been shown to be successful.[33] Although the use of transillumination is safe and effective, practice is required to become familiar with the technique and it is optimized by decreasing the amount of ambient light. Because of the size of the bulbs, these devices may not be suitable for use with pediatric tubes. The Trachlight's malleable stylet can be withdrawn from the assembly, allowing it to be used as an aid to blind nasal intubation. Advantages of lighted stylets include ease of use, utility in obstructed conditions, low acquisition costs, and disposable components that eliminate the need for disinfection of the equipment. Disadvantages include size limits on ETTs and moderate training requirements in the technique of transillumination.

Optical stylets offer certain advantages. These devices incorporate an optical viewing system (fiberoptic in most modern systems) within a stylet that may be malleable or preshaped. These may be configured for direct viewing through an eyepiece, or the image may be displayed on a video system. Universal camera adapters offer the advantage of ease of use (no camera) for individual use and a remote viewing screen for the teaching setting. The advantage of using the video system is that the practitioner can be in a more comfortable position, minimize personal risk from the patient's body fluids, and, in teaching settings, provide a ready means for observers to view the procedures. Examples of optical stylets include the Shikani Optical Stylet (previously known as the Shikani Seeing Stylet; Clarus Medical, Minneapolis Minnesota), the Bonfils Intubation Fiberscope (Karl Storz Endoscopy Ltd., Tuttlingen, Germany), the

SensaScope (Accutronic Medical Systems, Switzerland), and the Levitan FPS (Clarus Medical), which is a modification of the Shikani Optical Stylet.

The Shikani Optical Stylet has specific advantages, including cost, oxygen delivery during the procedure, and ease of loading the ETT on the stylet before its use.[34] Although providing a direct view of the oral, pharyngeal, and glottic structures, these devices do not require the upward and forward thrust of the jaw that conventional laryngoscopy does. In the difficult intubation setting, the optical stylet may be superior to the gum elastic bougie.[35–38] Others have found no reason to recommend an optical stylet over the bougie.[39] Some investigators have found that the optical stylet is simpler and more effective than rigid video laryngoscopes.[40] Optical stylets are made in pediatric sizes; these can be useful in the unexpected difficult airway in children.[41,42] Although various techniques of use have been described, the two most commonly used are to pull up on the mandible to allow space for the optical stylet and then advance under direct vision, or the retromolar approach, in which the stylet is introduced behind the third molar and advanced under vision to the target. Extending the head may aid laryngoscopy, as may the use of a conventional laryngoscope to lift the tongue and epiglottis off of the posterior pharynx to aid in initial introduction of the device. Even with the head in a neutral position, use of the Shikani Optical Stylet may result in less cervical spine movement, although at the cost of a small increase in intubation times.[43] Advantages of these devices include easier learning, less expense, and lower maintenance than flexible fiberoptic devices, in addition to less complicated processing and cleaning requirements after use. Disadvantages include the need for specific training, somewhat longer intubation times, inability to suction material that may obscure the view, and bulkiness of the device–tracheal tube combination that may hinder manipulation.

The Levitan FPS stylet is a short malleable optical stylet similar to the Shikani Optical Stylet. It is designed for augmentation of traditional laryngoscopy and requires trimming and positioning of the ETT onto the device before use.[44]

VIDEO LARYNGOSCOPY

Fiberoptic visualization of the airway has several distinct advantages, including direct visualization of the airway and oral and nasal pathways in addition to minimal movement of the cervical spine.[45] Equipment cost, availability, potentially obscured visualization with blood or secretions, and limitations in physician training are important considerations with the use of traditional fiberoptic laryngoscopy, however.

Rigid fiberoptic laryngoscopy has several important advantages. These devices also allow direct visualization of the airway and, in theory, allow for minimal cervical spine movement. Similar to traditional fiberoptic laryngoscopy, disadvantages may include physician training (although typically less than that required for flexible fiberoptic scopes), cost, availability, and obscured views with blood or secretions. These vary in design from devices that incorporate a fiberoptic scope into a metal holder or guide, such as the Bullard laryngoscope (Circon Corporation, Stamford, Connecticut), Wu laryngoscope (Achi Corp, Fremont, California), and Upsher scopes (UpsherScope; Upsher Laryngoscope Corporation, Foster City, California), to compact single- or limited-use designs that use traditional optics or cameras (Airtraq; Prodol Meditec S.A. and Airway Scope AWS-S100; Pentax), to systems that incorporate miniaturized video cameras into a more traditional laryngoscope design, such as the GlideScope Video Laryngoscope (GVL) System (Saturn Biomedical System Inc., Burnaby, British Columbia, Canada) and the McGrath Video Laryngoscope (LMA North America). These devices have the advantage of eliminating the need to align the axes of the larynx and oropharynx to achieve glottic visualization and successful endotracheal intubation. They are not passive devices, however, and, typically, some degree of suspension laryngoscopy is needed.

The Bullard laryngoscope has been found to be as effective or potentially faster than the intubating laryngeal mask by some researchers.[46,47] In simulations of immobile cervical spines, the Bullard laryngoscope seems to be readily learned.[48] In a model of cervical in-line stabilization with cricoid pressure, the Bullard laryngoscope was found to be superior to flexible fiberoptic laryngoscopy.[49]

The Wu scope is a similar design, incorporating a rigid metal laryngoscope with fiberoptic bundles.[50] The UpsherScope was not found to offer advantages in difficult airways by some investigators.[51] Although these devices are useful, they are fairly complicated to assemble, require some experience to master, and also have similar cleaning and maintenance limitations.

With the advent of miniaturized cameras, incorporation of video systems into otherwise conventional laryngoscopes became possible. Initially, this was accomplished through the placement of the camera on the blade of a fixed handle-blade assembly. Devices like the Storz DCI Video Laryngoscope and the GVL have a clear advantage in teaching and visualizing the vocal cords.

In simulations and in actual patients, the GVL has been shown to be useful in the difficult airway and may provide superior views in some cases, but at a modest increase in intubation time.[52–59] The GVL is somewhat large, with a maximum width of 1.8 cm; thus, it may be difficult to position in a patient with limited mouth opening. Connected to a large (7–10-inch) video display by a cable, these devices offer excellent image quality. One disadvantage, however, is that the video display needs to be placed on a cart or other support, making the device less convenient and less portable. The GVL and Storz products require cold sterilization, which can affect per-use cost and turn-around time.

A newer development is the McGrath video laryngoscope. It is a self-contained device, with the video display attached to the handle. Shaped much like a traditional Macintosh laryngoscope, the McGrath video laryngoscope has a 1.7-inch display attached to the handle (**Fig. 2**). Both the light-emitting diode (LED) light source and display are powered by an AA battery in the handle, making the device portable and familiar in use. The effective length of the blade can be adjusted by positioning the "camera stick" on the handle assembly; single-use sterile blades cover the camera stick and eliminate cleaning issues. One disadvantage of the McGrath video laryngoscope over the other video laryngoscopes is the relatively small size of the display; however, this is offset by its excellent portability. The McGrath video laryngoscope has been used for

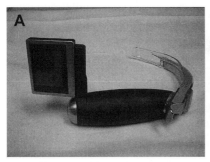 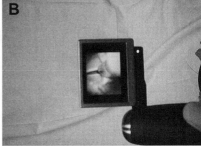

Fig. 2. (*A*) McGrath video laryngoscope. (*B*) Laryngoscopic view from the McGrath video laryngoscope.

rescue from the unexpected difficult airway and in cases of known or suspected difficult airways.[60,61] Although these devices require less training and experience than flexible fiberoptic laryngoscopes, their use is not exactly like that of traditional direct laryngoscopes. The video system does improve the visualization of the glottic opening, but because the axes of the larynx and pharynx are not aligned as in direct laryngoscopy, it can be difficult to advance the ETT into the trachea. Adjusting the bend of the tube ("hockey stick") on the stylet may help, and withdrawing the stylet a few centimeters from the tip may make the tube flexible enough to bend and follow the tracheal lumen while advancing the tube under direct vision. Because these angles are most awkward in the patient with a difficult airway, this difficulty of advancing the tube can occur when least desired. Therefore, it is essential with these devices, as with all devices and techniques, that appropriate expertise with patients and simulations with normal anatomy be developed before critical situations.

Some devices attempt to combine ease of use, cost savings, and portability. For example, the Airtraq is a simple single-use device with an optical channel and a channel for an ETT (**Fig. 3**). It is a single-use device, eliminates processing issues, and has the advantage that if left somewhere, little is lost as compared with the much more expensive portable video laryngoscope. A self-contained light source and antifogging system ensure a good view. It is easy to use and requires little training.[62–65] A similar device, the Airway Scope AWS-S100, relies on a small camera and disposable blades. The base unit is weather resistant, and the manufacturer states that it can be used in foul weather, making it an option for wet or rainy conditions. It is simple to use and requires little training.[66,67] It may also be useful in minimizing cervical spine movement compared with traditional techniques.[68,69] It may be easier to use than rigid fiberoptic laryngoscopes and other techniques.[70,71]

SUMMARY

A wide variety of airway adjuncts are available to the emergency physician to aid in the management of difficult airways. An understanding of the appropriate use, indications and contraindications, and advantages and disadvantages of airway adjuncts is

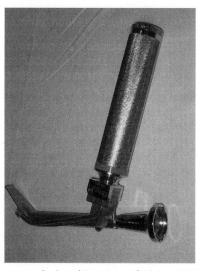

Fig. 3. The Airtraq laryngoscopy device. (*Courtesy of* Airtraq LLC, Bonita Springs, FL; with permission.)

Table 1
Summary of airway adjuncts

Device	Clinical Indications	Advantages	Disadvantages
Laryngoscopic blades			
Traditional laryngoscopy	Most clinical settings	Ease of use, rapid time to intubation, high success rate	Inadequate view in difficult airways and cervical spine movement
Laryngoscopy prisms	Moderately difficult airway	Ease of use, inexpensive, easy to clean	Small, easy to lose, and may be cumbersome
Optical laryngoscope (eg, Viewmax, Lee Fibreview, TruView, McCoy)	Moderately difficult airway	Improved visualization	Increased time to successful intubation
Supraglottic devices			
LMA and similar devices	Suspected cervical spine trauma, difficult airway	Ease of use	Risks for aspiration, inadequate oxygenation, and difficulty with ventilation if poor seal
Combitube	Prehospital difficult intubations	Ease of use	Risks for airway trauma, aspiration, and inadequate oxygenation
Laryngeal tube	Prehospital difficult intubations	Ease of use	Inadequate evidence to support widespread use
Stylets			
Gum elastic bougie	Moderately difficult airways, cervical spine trauma	Ease of use, inexpensive	Blind insertion
Lighted stylets (eg, Trachlight, VitalLight, Trach Wand)	Moderately difficult airways, cervical spine trauma	Ease of use	Blind insertion
Optical stylets (eg, Shikani, Levitan, Bonfils, SensaScope)	Difficult airways, cervical spine trauma	Direct visualization	Airway trauma, cost, and training and experience requirements
Video laryngoscopy			
Traditional laryngoscope design with video (eg, GlideScope)	Difficult airways, cervical spine trauma	Direct visualization, ease of use	Cost, storage, cleaning, maintenance, and difficulty advancing tube

(*continued on next page*)

Device	Clinical Indications	Advantages	Disadvantages
Table 1 *(continued)*			
Rigid with fiberoptics eg, Bullard, WuScope, Upsher Scope)	Difficult airways, cervical spine trauma	Direct visualization, less training needed than with flexible fiberoptics	Complex assembly, training requirements, cost, storage, cleaning, and maintenance
Rigid scope with optics or cameras (eg, Airtraq, Airway Scope)	Difficult airways, cervical spine trauma	Direct visualization, ease of use	Cost, storage, cleaning, and maintenance
Portable video laryngoscopy (eg, McGrath)	Difficult airways, cervical spine trauma	Direct visualization, ease of storage, portability	Cost, cleaning, maintenance, and difficulty in advancing tube

This table displays representative examples of airway adjuncts, indications, advantages, and disadvantages. It is not intended to be an inclusive information source.

essential to the effective management of the difficult airway (**Table 1**). The appropriate selection of a small number of adjunct devices allows greater clinical experience, judgment, and expertise with those devices.

REFERENCES

1. Reeder TJ, Brown CK, Norris DL. Managing the difficult airway: a survey of residency directors and a call for change. J Emerg Med 2005;28(4):473–8.
2. Levitan RM, Kush S, Hollander JE. Devices for difficult airway management in academic emergency departments: results of a national survey. Ann Emerg Med 1999;33(6):694–8.
3. Hodges UM, O'Flaherty D, Adams AP. Tracheal intubation in a manikin: comparison of the Belscope with the Macintosh laryngoscope. Br J Anaesth 1993;71:905–7.
4. Leung YY, Hung CT, Tan ST. Evaluation of the new Viewmax laryngoscope in a simulated difficult airway. Acta Anaesthesiol Scand 2006;50:562–7.
5. Li JB, Xiong YC, Wang XL, et al. An evaluation of the TruView EVO2 laryngoscope. Anaesthesia 2007;62:940–3.
6. Barak M, Philipchuck P, Abecassis P, et al. A comparison of the TruView blade with the Macintosh blade in adult patients. Anaesthesia 2007;62:827–31.
7. Beilin B, Yardeni IZ, Smolyarenko V, et al. Comparison of the Flexiblade levering laryngoscope with the English Macintosh laryngoscope in patients with a poor laryngoscopic view. Anaesthesia 2005;60:400–5.
8. Cheung RW, Irwin MG, Law BC, et al. A clinical comparison of the Flexiblade™ and Macintosh laryngoscopes for laryngeal exposure in anesthetized adults. Anesth Analg 2006;102:626–30.
9. Rabitsch W, Schellongowski P, Staudinger T, et al. Comparison of a conventional tracheal airway with the Combitube in an urban emergency medical services system run by physicians. Resuscitation 2003;57:27–32.
10. Gaitini LA, Vaida SJ, Agro F. The esophageal-tracheal Combitube. Anesthesiol Clin North America 2002;20(4):893–906.
11. Weksler N, Tarnopolski A, Klein M, et al. Insertion of the endotracheal tube, laryngeal mask airway and oesophageal-tracheal Combitube. A 6-month comparative

prospective study of acquisition and retention skills by medical students. Eur J Anaesthesiol 2005;22(5):337–40.

12. Mort TC. Laryngeal mask airway and bougie intubation failures: the Combitube as a secondary rescue device for in-hospital emergency airway management. Anesth Analg 2006;103:1264–6.

13. Mercer MH, Gabbott DA. Insertion of the Combitube airway with the cervical spine immobilized in a rigid cervical collar. Anaesthesia 1998;53(10):971–4.

14. Davis DP, Valentine C, Ochs M, et al. The Combitube as a salvage airway device for paramedic rapid sequence intubation. Ann Emerg Med 2003;42(5): 697–704.

15. Lefrancois DP, Dufour DG. Use of the esophageal tracheal Combitube by basic emergency medical technicians. Resuscitation 2002;52(1):77–83.

16. Vezina D, Lessard MR, Bussieres J, et al. Complications associated with the use of the esophageal-tracheal Combitube. Can J Anaesth 1998;45(1):76–80.

17. Calkins TR, Miller K, Langdorf MI. Success and complication rates with prehospital placement of an esophageal-tracheal Combitube as a rescue airway. Prehosp Disaster Med 2006;21(2 Suppl 2):97–100.

18. Vezina MC, Trepanier CA, Nicole PC, et al. Complications associated with the esophageal-tracheal Combitube in the pre-hospital setting. Can J Anaesth 2007;54(2):124–8.

19. Russi CS, Wilcox CL, House HR. The laryngeal tube device: a simple and timely adjunct to airway management. Am J Emerg Med 2007;25(3):263–7.

20. Asai T, Hidaka I, Kawachi S. Efficacy of the laryngeal tube by inexperienced personnel. Resuscitation 2002;55(2):171–5.

21. Russi CS, Miller L, Hartley MJ. A comparison of the King-LT to endotracheal intubation and Combitube in a simulated difficult airway. Prehosp Emerg Care 2008; 12(1):35–41.

22. Noguchi T, Koga K, Shiga Y, et al. The gum elastic bougie eases tracheal intubation while applying cricoid pressure compared to a stylet. Can J Anaesth 2003; 50:712–7.

23. Annamaneni R, Hodzovic I, Wilkes AR, et al. A comparison of simulated difficult intubation with multiple-use and single-use bougies in a manikin. Anaesthesia 2003;58(1):45–9.

24. Hodzovic I, Wilkes AR, Latto IP. Bougie-assisted difficult airway management in a manikin—the effect of position held on placement and force exerted by the tip. Anaesthesia 2004;59(1):38–43.

25. MacNab AJ, PacPhail I, MacNab MK, et al. A comparison of intubation success for paediatric transport team paramedics using lighted vs regular tracheal tube stylets. Paediatr Anaesth 1998;8(3):215–20.

26. Harvey K, Davies R, Evans A, et al. A comparison of the use of Trachlight® and Eschmann multiple-use introducer in simulated difficult intubation. Eur J Anaesthesiol 2007;24:76–81.

27. Agro F, Hung OR, Cataldo R, et al. Lightwand intubation using the Trachlight: a brief review of current knowledge. Can J Anaesth 2001;48(6):592–9.

28. Soh CR, Kong CF, Kong CS, et al. Tracheal intubation by novice staff: the direct vision laryngoscope or the lighted stylet (Trachlight). Emerg Med J 2002;19(4):292–4.

29. Berns SD, Patel RI, Chamberlain JM. Oral intubation using a lighted stylet vs direct laryngoscopy in older children with cervical immobilization. Acad Emerg Med 1996;3(1):34–40.

30. Inoue Y. Lightwand intubation can improve airway management. Can J Anaesth 2004;51(10):1052–3.

31. Inoue Y, Koga K, Shigematsu A. A comparison of two tracheal intubation techniques with Trachlight™ and Fastrach™ in patients with cervical spine disorders. Anesth Analg 2002;94:667–71.
32. Turkstra P, Eng M, Eng P, et al. Cervical spine motion: a fluoroscopic comparison during intubation with lighted stylet, GlideScope, and Macintosh laryngoscope. Anesth Analg 2005;101:910–5.
33. Dimitriou V, Voyagis GS, Grosomanidis V, et al. Feasibility of flexible lightwand-guided tracheal intubation with the intubating laryngeal mask during out-of-hospital cardiopulmonary resuscitation by an emergency physician. Eur J Anaesthesiol 2006;23(1):76–9.
34. Kovacs G, Law AJ, Petrie D. Awake fiberoptic intubation using an optical stylet in an anticipated difficult airway. Ann Emerg Med 2007;49(1):81–3.
35. Evans A, Morris S, Petterson J, et al. A comparison of the Seeing Optical Stylet and the gum elastic bougie in simulated difficult tracheal intubation: a manikin study. Anaesthesia 2006;61:478–81.
36. Kovacs G, Law JA, McCrossin C, et al. A comparison of a fiberoptic stylet and a bougie as adjuncts to direct laryngoscopy in a manikin-simulated difficult airway. Ann Emerg Med 2007;50(6):676–85.
37. Biro P, Weiss M, Gerber A, et al. Comparison of a new video-optical intubation stylet versus the conventional malleable stylet in simulated difficult tracheal intubation. Anaesthesia 2000;55(9):886–9.
38. Biro P, Battig U, Henderson J, et al. First clinical experience of tracheal intubation with the SensaScope, a novel steerable semirigid video stylet. Br J Anaesth 2006; 97(2):255–61.
39. Greenland KB, Liu G, Tan H, et al. Comparison of the Levitan FPS Scope™ and the single-use bougie for simulated difficult intubation in anaesthetized patients. Anaesthesia 2007;62:509–15.
40. Weiss M, Schwarz U, Gerber AC. Difficult airway management: comparison of the Bullard laryngoscope with the videooptical intubation stylet. Can J Anaesth 2000; 47(3):280–4.
41. Shukry M, Hanson RD, Koveleskie JR, et al. Management of the difficult pediatric airway with Shikani Optical Stylet™. Paediatr Anaesth 2005;15:342–5.
42. Pfitzner L, Cooper MG, Ho D. The Shikani Seeing Stylet for difficult intubation in children: initial experience. Anaesth Intensive Care 2002;30(4):462–6.
43. Turkstra TP, Pelz DM, Shaikh AA, et al. Cervical spine motion: a fluoroscopic comparison of Shikani Optical Stylet vs Macintosh laryngoscope. Can J Anaesth 2007;54(6):441–7.
44. Levitan RM. Design rationale and intended use of a short optical stylet for routine fiberoptic augmentation of emergency laryngoscopy. Am J Emerg Med 2006;24: 490–5.
45. Brimacombe J, Keller C, Künzel KH, et al. Cervical spine motion during airway management: a cinefluoroscopic study of the posteriorly destabilized third vertebrae in human cadavers. Anesth Analg 2000;91(5):799–801.
46. Nileshwar A, Thudamaladinne A. Comparison of intubating laryngeal mask airway and Bullard laryngoscope for oro-tracheal intubation in adult patients with simulated limitation of cervical movements. Br J Anaesth 2007;99(2):292–6.
47. Shin O, Taro K, Mayumi T. A comparison of Bullard laryngoscope and intubating laryngeal mask using fiberoptic guidance for tracheal intubation. The Japanese Journal of Anesthesiology 2000;49(7):736–9.
48. Wackett A, Anderson K, Thode H. Bullard laryngoscopy by naive operators in the cervical spine immobilized patient. J Emerg Med 2005;29(3):253–7.

49. Shulman GB, Connelly NR. A comparison of the Bullard laryngoscope versus the flexible fiberoptic bronchoscope during intubation in patients afforded inline stabilization. J Clin Anesth 2001;13(3):182–5.

50. Smith CE, Pinchak AB, Sidhu TS, et al. Evaluation of tracheal intubation difficulty in patients with cervical spine immobilization: fiberoptic (WuScope) versus conventional laryngoscopy. Anesthesiology 1999;91(5):1253–9.

51. Fridrich P, Frass M, Krenn CG, et al. The UpsherScope™ in routine and difficult airway management: a randomized, controlled clinical trial. Anesth Analg 1997; 85:1377–81.

52. Rai MR, Dering A, Verghese C. The GlideScope system: a clinical assessment of performance. Anaesthesia 2005;60:60–4.

53. Xue F, Zhang G, Liu J, et al. A clinical assessment of the GlideScope videolaryngoscope in nasotracheal intubation with general anesthesia. J Clin Anesth 2006;18(8):611–5.

54. Lai HY, Chen IH, Chen A, et al. The use of the GlideScope for tracheal intubation in patients with ankylosing spondylitis. Br J Anaesth 2006;97(3):419–22.

55. Benjamin FJ, Boon D, French RA. An evaluation of the GlideScope®, a new video laryngoscope for difficult airways: a manikin study. Eur J Anaesthesiol 2006;23:517–21.

56. Fun WL, Lim Y, Teoh WH. Comparison of the GlideScope video laryngoscope vs. the intubating laryngeal mask for females with normal airways. Eur J Anaesthesiol 2007;24:486–91.

57. Cooper RM, Pacey JA, Bishop MJ, et al. Early clinical experience with a new videolaryngoscope (GlideScope®) in 728 patients. Can J Anaesth 2005;52(2):191–8.

58. Sun DA, Warriner CB, Parsons DG, et al. The GlideScope video laryngoscope: randomized clinical trial in 200 patients. Br J Anaesth 2005;94:381–4.

59. Lim Y, Yeo SW. A comparison of the GlideScope with the Macintosh laryngoscope for tracheal intubation in patients with simulated difficult airway. Anaesth Intensive Care 2005;33(2):243–7.

60. Shippey B, Ray D, McKeown D. Use of the McGrath videolaryngoscope in the management of difficult and failed tracheal intubation. Br J Anaesth 2008; 100(1):116–9.

61. Shippey B, Ray D, McKeown D. Case series: the McGrath videolaryngoscope— an initial clinical evaluation. Can J Anaesth 2007;54(4):307–13.

62. Norman A, Date A. Use of the Airtraq laryngoscope for anticipated difficult laryngoscopy. Anaesthesia 2007;62:533–4.

63. Woollard M, Mannion W, Lighton D, et al. Use of the Airtraq laryngoscope in a model of difficult intubation by prehospital providers not previously trained in laryngoscopy. Anaesthesia 2007;62:1061–5.

64. Maharaj CH, Higgins BD, Harte BH, et al. Evaluation of intubation using the Airtraq or Macintosh laryngoscope by anaesthetists in easy and simulated difficult laryngoscopy—a manikin study. Anaesthesia 2006;61(5):469–77.

65. Woollard M, Lighton D, Mannion W, et al. Airtraq vs standard laryngoscopy by student paramedics and experienced prehospital laryngoscopists managing a model of difficult intubation. Anaesthesia 2008;63(1):26–31.

66. Miki T, Inagawa G, Kikuchi T, et al. Evaluation of the airway scope, a new video laryngoscope, in tracheal intubation by naive operators: a manikin study. Acta Anaesthesiol Scand 2007;51(10):1378–81.

67. Hirabayashi Y. Airway scope versus Macintosh laryngoscope: a manikin study. Emerg Med J 2007;24(5):357–8.

68. Maruyama K, Yamada T, Kawakami R, et al. Upper cervical spine movement during intubation: fluoroscopic comparison of the airway scope, McCoy laryngoscope, and Macintosh laryngoscope. Br J Anaesth 2008;100(1):120–4.
69. Hirabayashi Y, Fujita A, Seo N, et al. Cervical spine movement during laryngoscopy using the airway scope compared with the Macintosh laryngoscope. Anaesthesia 2007;62(10):1050–5.
70. Hirabayashi Y. Ease of use of the airway scope vs the Bullard laryngoscope: a manikin study. Can J Anaesth 2007;54(5):397–8.
71. Koyama Y, Inagawa G, Miyashita T, et al. Comparison of the airway scope, gum elastic bougie and fibreoptic bronchoscope in simulated difficult tracheal intubation: a manikin study. Anaesthesia 2007;62(9):936–9.

Retrograde Intubation

David Burbulys, MD, FACEP[a],*, Kianusch Kiai, MD[b]

KEYWORDS

• Intubation • Retrograde • Tracheal • Guidewire • Fiberoptic

Airway management in the emergency department is a critical skill that must be mastered by emergency physicians.[1–3] It is one of the most vital initial steps in pediatric and adult resuscitation. Failure to obtain and maintain an adequate and protected airway for oxygenation and ventilation results in poor outcome. Rapid-sequence induction with oral-tracheal intubation performed by way of direct laryngoscopy is generally the preferred initial method of airway control. It has been shown to be highly successful in the hands of skilled practitioners.[4,5]

In approximately 1% to 6% of cases, initial oral-tracheal intubation may be difficult if not impossible due to a variety of circumstances,[6–38] including acquired or congenital anatomic abnormalities or distortions, traumatic facial or neck injuries, uncontrolled hemorrhage or emesis, and foreign bodies. When these limitations cannot be overcome by technique or experience, an alternative method or device must be used for a rescue airway. These alternative methods and devices have been well described in the literature and include numerous alternative laryngoscope designs (direct, flexible, fiberoptic), various endotracheal tubes and guides, lighted wands, laryngeal mask airways (LMAs), esophageal tracheal tubes, hollow stylet or transtracheal jet ventilators, retrograde guided intubation, and percutaneous or surgical cricothyrotomy or tracheostomy.[6,8,12,21,37,39–69]

Many courses and texts have been developed to address the use of the growing numbers of airway adjuncts. It is unlikely that anyone is able to become expert in the use of all of these devices; however, it is essential that all practitioners have a repertoire of techniques or equipment immediately available to them in the event of the failed airway. Percutaneous or surgical cricothyrotomy has generally been accepted as the definitive method of airway management in this situation.[70–88] Retrograde guided oral or nasal intubation is an easily learned and maintained skill set and may be a rapid, less invasive alternative to a surgical airway in many settings.[6,8,30,57,63,70,89–95]

[a] David Geffen School of Medicine at UCLA, Department of Emergency Medicine, Harbor–UCLA Medical Center, 1000 West Carson Street, Box 21, Torrance, CA 90504, USA
[b] David Geffen School of Medicine at UCLA, Department of Anesthesiology, Ronald Regan Medical Center, 757 Westwood Boulevard, Suite 3325, Box 957403, Los Angeles, CA 90095-7403, USA
* Corresponding author.
E-mail address: burbulys@emedharbor.edu (D. Burbulys).

Emerg Med Clin N Am 26 (2008) 1029–1041
doi:10.1016/j.emc.2008.08.007
0733-8627/08/$ – see front matter © 2008 Elsevier Inc. All rights reserved.

emed.theclinics.com

INDICATIONS AND CONTRAINDICATIONS

Retrograde intubation is a well-described technique. It encompasses several methods of translaryngeal guided nonsurgical airway access to facilitate orotracheal or nasotracheal intubation. It has been used in awake, sedated, obtunded, or apneic patients when other methods have been unsuccessful, unavailable, or contraindicated.[91,96] It has been used in the management of anticipated and unanticipated difficult airway scenarios.[8,30,35,57,63,70,91,92,97–102] It has also been shown to be successful in adult and pediatric patient populations.[30,103,104] It has been performed in the supine, prone, and sitting positions with the neck extended or in neutral position.[105]

Retrograde intubation is contraindicated in the presence of unfavorable anatomy in the area of the cricothyroid (nonpalpable landmarks, pretracheal mass, severe flexion deformity of the neck), laryngotracheal pathologic conditions (tracheal stenosis, malignancy, upper airway mass or foreign body), significant coagulopathy, and infection.

CLASSIC TECHNIQUE

Retrograde endotracheal intubation was first described by Butler and Cirillo[106] in 1960 as a means to remove the tracheotomy tube from the operative field in neck surgery. A catheter was passed cephalad through the tracheostomy site and out through the mouth and was sutured to an endotracheal tube. The tube was then simply pulled into position. Waters,[107] in 1963, described passing small plastic tubing through the cricothyroid membrane in a similar retrograde fashion and then using it as a guide to intubate patients who had deformities of the jaw.

Since then, there have been several variations proposed for primary airway management. The most common involves the use of a commercially available retrograde intubation kit (Cook Retrograde Intubation Set with Rapi-Fit Adapters, Cook Critical Care, Bloomington, Indiana). The kit contains a syringe with an 18-gauge introducer needle and the needle catheter sheath, a 50-cm flexible J-tipped wire, a radiopaque guiding catheter, and a needle holder (**Fig. 1**). Following sterile preparation of the anterior neck, lidocaine is administered in the inferior area of the cricothyroid membrane in appropriate patients. Transtracheal anesthesia should also be used. A small amount of liquid is drawn up into the syringe, and an initial percutaneous puncture through the cricothyroid membrane is made with the introducer needle and catheter at a 30° to 40° angle to the skin in a cephalad direction. The free flow of air bubbles in the syringe confirms entry into the trachea. Holding the catheter in place, the needle and syringe are removed and the J-tip of the wire is passed up the trachea until it can be retrieved from the mouth or nose with fingers or forceps. A black proximal positioning mark on the wire should be visible at the skin access site, ensuring that enough is exposed orally or nasally to facilitate the subsequent passage of the guiding catheter and endotracheal tube from the other end. The catheter sheath at the skin is removed and the wire is clamped at this site to stabilize its entry into the skin at the cricothyroid membrane. The guiding catheter is advanced anterograde over the wire, by way of the mouth or nose, into the trachea until tenting is noted at the cricothyroid access site. The endotracheal tube is then passed over the wire and guiding catheter into position below the level of the vocal cords. The needle holder is unclamped, and the wire and guiding catheter are removed from above the endotracheal tube. As the last portion of the wire is removed, the endotracheal tube is further advanced into final position. The balloon cuff is inflated, and endotracheal tube placement is verified in the standard fashion (**Fig. 2**).

This procedure may be undertaken without the benefit of the Cook Retrograde Intubation Set, using standard supplies found in most emergency departments,

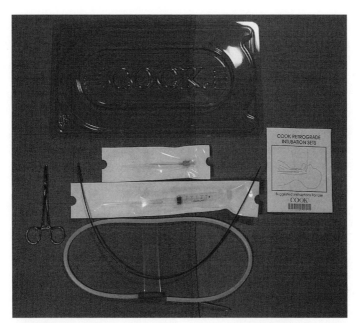

Fig. 1. Cook Retrograde Intubation Kit (Cook Critical Care, Bloomington, Indiana).

although it is helpful to preassemble the needed supplies in one location. The guiding catheter facilitates the movement of the endotracheal tube past the vocal cords and into the trachea and, although it is not essential, may offer some protection from injury to these structures. Alternatives that have been used include various catheters, modified endotracheal tube exchangers, bougies, ureteral stents, and fiberoptic intubating scopes. It should also be noted that the guidewire commonly supplied in most central line kits is not long enough to facilitate this procedure. Guidewires should be at least 70 to 100 cm in length. Longer wires are commonly available in most radiology suites.

MODIFIED TECHNIQUES

This basic procedure has been modified by various authors to improve its success rate, to adapt its use to specific patients or situations, or to make use of supplies available. Some of the more notable modifications are described in the following paragraphs.

Bourke and Levesque[108] described a minor modification in which the guiding catheter or wire was fed through the side hole at the distal end of the endotracheal tube. The guide was then passed into the lumen and out the proximal end of the endotracheal tube before its passage down the wire (**Fig. 3**). As the tube was moved into final position, an extra 1 cm of endotracheal tube could be placed below the level of the vocal cords before the guide removal, which was believed to help prevent the dislodgement of the tip of the tube into the esophagus as the guide and wire were removed. The investigators showed an improved procedure success rate with this modification, but others have suggested that this technique may lead to more trauma of the vocal cords.[109]

Lenfant and colleagues[90] described another technique of removing the guiding catheter, but not the wire, near the completion of the procedure. The guiding catheter was then passed anterograde down the endotracheal tube into the trachea (**Fig. 4**). As

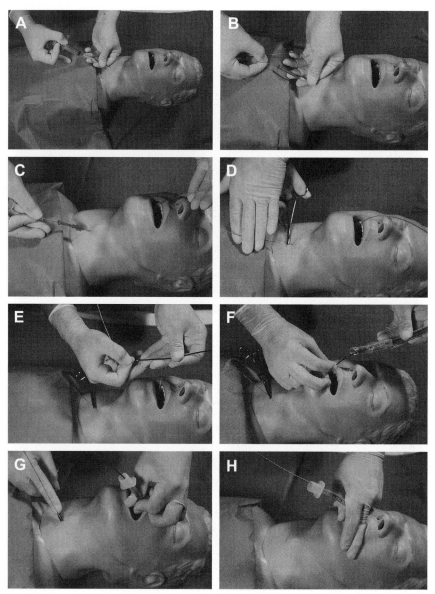

Fig. 2. Retrograde intubation using the guidewire technique. (*A*) Initial percutaneous puncture at the cricothyroid membrane into the trachea with the introducer needle/catheter sheath. (*B*) The needle is removed and the J-tip of the wire is passed through the catheter sheath into the trachea and to the mouth or nares. (*C*) The wire is recovered from the mouth or nares with fingers or forceps. (*D*) The wire is advanced until the black positioning mark is visible at the skin access site. The catheter sheath is removed. The wire is clamped at the insertion site to stabilize its entry into the cricothyroid area. (*E*) The guiding catheter sheath is advanced anterograde over the wire by way of the mouth or nares until it tents the skin at the cricothyroid access site. (*F*) The endotracheal tube is passed over the wire/guiding catheter sheath into position below the vocal cords to the skin puncture site. (*G*) The needle holder is unclamped. (*H*) The wire/guiding catheter sheath is removed by way of the mouth, and the endotracheal tube is advanced into final position.

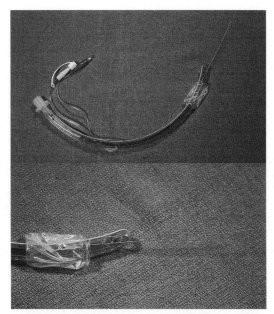

Fig. 3. The Bourke and Levesque modification. The guidewire is fed through the distal side hole of the endotracheal tube during placement, allowing the tip of the endotracheal tube to be placed further below the level of the vocal cords before the removal of the wire/guiding catheter sheath.

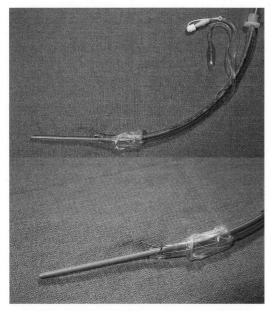

Fig. 4. The Lenfant and colleagues modification. To prevent esophageal displacement, the guiding catheter is removed from the wire and passed anterograde down the endotracheal tube into the trachea prior to the removal of the wire.

the wire was removed and the endotracheal tube was passed into final position, the guide helped direct the tube further down the trachea and prevented esophageal displacement. This method also showed an enhanced success rate in their study.

Shantha[110] suggested that an infracricoid region approach might offer a higher success rate. In this modification, the initial puncture takes place at the level of the first or second tracheal ring rather than at the cricothyroid membrane. It is believed that this modification also allows the endotracheal tube to be passed further below the vocal cords before removal of the wire to prevent esophageal dislodgement. Other investigators, however, have suggested that this technique may lead to a higher bleeding and complication rate.[109]

Hung and al-Qatari[96] described a technique of light wand–guided retrograde intubation. In their description, the standard procedure was followed; however, prior to passage of the endotracheal tube, a light wand was inserted to its tip. As the tube was advanced down the guide and wire, a bright circumscribed glow was readily seen in the anterior neck. They believed that this helped verify placement of the end of the tube in the trachea below the vocal cords rather than in the esophagus. They too described an improved procedural success rate using this modification.

Harvey and colleagues[111] published a unique modification of retrograde intubation through an LMA. Generally, LMAs are replaced by an endotracheal tube following the antegrade passage of an airway exchange catheter, flexible wire, or fiberoptic bronchoscope. These investigators believed that the potential existed for the unsecured distal portion of these devices to become dislodged when passed antegrade into the trachea, and they thought that this might occur during removal of the LMA or by the attempted passage of the endotracheal tube. In their description, they avoided this dislodgement by passing a retrograde guidewire up the airway, through the LMA aperture bars, and out the mouth. They then passed a guide catheter anterograde down the wire and removed the LMA. An endotracheal tube was then placed in the usual fashion over the wire and guide to the skin puncture site at the cricothyroid membrane.

The most common modification of retrograde intubation involves the use of fiberoptic-assisted direct visualization of the tracheal intubation. Several investigators have described this technique.[30,35,63,70,97,112–118] This method may be limited by the presence of excessive airway secretions or bleeding. A retrograde wire is placed in the standard fashion. The cephalad portion of the wire is fed through the suction port of a standard intubating bronchoscope that has been previously loaded with an endotracheal tube. The bronchoscope is advanced past the vocal cords and the wire is withdrawn (**Fig. 5**). The bronchoscope is further advanced, and the endotracheal tube is placed at the appropriate depth in the trachea under direct visualization. This method has been extremely successful in patients who have various types of partially obstructing laryngopathology.

COMPLICATIONS

The most common complication of retrograde intubation is a sore throat, seen in approximately 60% of patients. More significant complications are rare and may include failure to obtain an airway, soft tissue infections, hematoma or hemorrhage, subcutaneous emphysema, pneumomediastinum, and injury to the larynx, vocal cords, and upper airway.[8,96,99,101,119–122] These complications may be minimized by the use of an antegrade sheath over the guidewire, removal of the guidewire by way of the mouth or nose rather than the neck, and puncture of the cricothyroid membrane at the inferior portion.

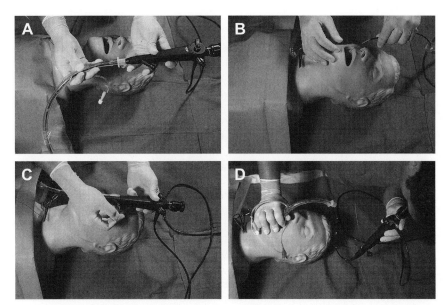

Fig. 5. Fiberoptic-assisted retrograde intubation. (*A*) Following standard placement of the guidewire, the endotracheal tube is loaded on the fiberoptic scope. (*B*) The guidewire is advanced up the working channel of the fiberoptic scope. (*C*) When the wire exits the port of the fiberoptic scope, the endotracheal tube is passed into position below the vocal cords to the skin puncture site. (*D*) Under direct visualization, the wire is removed by an assistant, and the tube is visually guided into final position, ensuring passage down the trachea.

SUMMARY

Retrograde intubation requires little equipment and has few contraindications. This technique is easy to learn and has a high level of skill retention. Familiarity with this technique is a valuable addition to the airway-management armamentarium of emergency physicians caring for ill or injured patients. Variations of the technique have been described, and their use depends on the individual circumstances.

REFERENCES

1. Thomas HA, Beeson MS, Binder LS, et al. The 2003 model of the clinical practice of emergency medicine: the 2005 update. Acad Emerg Med 2006;13(10):1070–3.
2. Hockberger RS, Binger LS, Chisholm CD, et al. The model of the clinical practice of emergency medicine: a 2-year update. Ann Emerg Med 2005;45(6):659–74.
3. Perina DG, Collier RE, Thomas HA, et al. Report of the task force on residency training information (2004–2005), American Board of Emergency Medicine. Ann Emerg Med 2005;45(5):532–47.
4. Dibble C, Maloba M. Best evidence topic report. Rapid sequence induction in the emergency department by emergency medicine personnel. Emerg Med J 2006;23(1):62–4.
5. Clancy M, Nolan J. Airway management in the emergency department. Emerg Med J 2002;19(1):2–3.
6. El-Orbany M. New airway devices and the management of the difficult airway. Anaesth Intensive Care 2008;36(3):456–7 [author reply 456–7].

7. Lavery GG, McCloskey BV. The difficult airway in adult critical care. Crit Care Med 2008;36(7):2163–73.

8. Warner KJ, Sharar SR, Copass MK, et al. Prehospital management of the difficult airway: a prospective cohort study. J Emerg Med 2008.

9. Liess BD, Scheidt TD, Templer JSW. The difficult airway. Otolaryngol Clin North Am 2008;41(3):567–80.

10. Kuduvalli PM, Jervis A, Tighe SQ, et al. Unanticipated difficult airway management in anaesthetised patients: a prospective study of the effect of mannequin training on management strategies and skill retention. Anaesthesia 2008;63(4): 364–9.

11. Gandy WE. Conquering the difficult airway. Emerg Med Serv 2008;37(1):46, 48, 53–6 passim.

12. Guarino A. Difficult airway management: is there a limit in the selection of the proper device and procedure? Minerva Anestesiol 2007;73(11):555–7.

13. Boseley ME, Hartnick CJ. A useful algorithm for managing the difficult pediatric airway. Int J Pediatr Otorhinolaryngol 2007;71(8):1317–20.

14. Rosen P, Sloane C, Ban KM, et al. Difficult airway management. Intern Emerg Med 2006;1(2):139–47.

15. Ezri T, Szmuk P. Recent trends in tracheal intubation: emphasis on the difficult airway. Curr Opin Anaesthesiol 2004;17(6):487–90.

16. Yarrow S. Trends in tracheal intubation: emphasis on the difficult airway. Curr Opin Anaesthesiol 2004;17(6):485–6.

17. Heidegger T, Gerig HJ. Algorithms for management of the difficult airway. Curr Opin Anaesthesiol 2004;17(6):483–4.

18. Schwartz AJ. Difficult-airway management need not be difficult! Curr Opin Anaesthesiol 2004;17(6):477–8.

19. Frova G, Guarino A, Petrini F, et al. Recommendations for airway control and difficult airway management in paediatric patients. Minerva Anestesiol 2006;72(9):723–48.

20. Connelly NR, Ghandour K, Robbins L, et al. Management of unexpected difficult airway at a teaching institution over a 7-year period. J Clin Anesth 2006;18(3): 198–204.

21. Lim MS, Hunt-Smith JJ. Difficult airway management in the intensive care unit: alternative techniques. Crit Care Resusc 2003;5(1):53–62.

22. Lim MS, Hunt-Smith JJ. Difficult airway management in the intensive care unit: practical guidelines. Crit Care Resusc 2003;5(1):43–52.

23. Morley P. Plan A, plan B and plan C: management of the difficult airway in the critically ill. Crit Care Resusc 2003;5(1):8–9.

24. Heidegger T, Gerig HJ, Henderson JJ. Strategies and algorithms for management of the difficult airway. Best Pract Res Clin Anaesthesiol 2005;19(4):661–74.

25. Helm M, Gries A, Mutzbauer T. Surgical approach in difficult airway management. Best Pract Res Clin Anaesthesiol 2005;19(4):623–40.

26. Petrini F, Axxorsi A, Adrario E, et al. Recommendations for airway control and difficult airway management. Minerva Anestesiol 2005;71(11):617–57.

27. Mulcahy AJ, Yentis SM. Management of the unexpected difficult airway. Anaesthesia 2005;60(11):1147–8.

28. Maier WR, Cunningham PS. A new approach to securing a difficult airway. J Clin Anesth 2005;17(4):286–9.

29. Heringlake M, Ocker H. Seldinger approach to the difficult airway. J Clin Anesth 2005;17(4):239–40.

30. Reeder TJ, Brown CK, Norris DL. Managing the difficult airway: a survey of residency directors and a call for change. J Emerg Med 2005;28(4):473–8.

31. Baraka A. Difficult Airway Society guidelines. Anaesthesia 2005;60(4):415.
32. Russell L. Difficult airway management. Anaesthesia 2005;60(2):202–3 [author reply 203].
33. Watts JC, Price SR. Difficult Airway Society guidelines. Anaesthesia 2004; 59(12):1246 [author reply 1247].
34. Henderson JJ, Popat MT, Latto IP, et al. Difficult Airway Society guidelines for management of the unanticipated difficult intubation. Anaesthesia 2004;59(7):675–94.
35. Ezri T, Szmuk P, Warters RD, et al. Difficult airway management practice patterns among anesthesiologists practicing in the United States: have we made any progress? J Clin Anesth 2003;15(6):418–22.
36. Stasiuk RB. The difficult airway paradigm revisited. Can J Anaesth 2003;50(7): 753–4.
37. Butler KH, Clyne B. Management of the difficult airway: alternative airway techniques and adjuncts. Emerg Med Clin North Am 2003;21(2):259–89.
38. Practice guidelines for management of the difficult airway: an updated report by the American Society of Anesthesiologists task force on management of the difficult airway. Anesthesiology 2003;98(5):1269–77.
39. Youngquist S, Gausche-Hill M, Burbulys D. Alternative airway devices for use in children requiring prehospital airway management: update and case discussion. Pediatr Emerg Care 2007;23(4):250–8 [quiz 259–61].
40. Krafft P, Schebesta K. Alternative management techniques for the difficult airway: esophageal-tracheal combitube. Curr Opin Anaesthesiol 2004;17(6):499–504.
41. Gravenstein D, Liem EB, Bjoraker DG. Alternative management techniques for the difficult airway: optical stylets. Curr Opin Anaesthesiol 2004;17(6):495–8.
42. Truhlar A, Ferson DZ. Use of the laryngeal mask airway supreme in pre-hospital difficult airway management. Resuscitation 2008;78(2):107–8.
43. Hagberg CA, Vogt-Harenkamp CC, Iannucci DG. Successful airway management of a patient with a known difficult airway with the direct coupler interface video laryngoscope. J Clin Anesth 2007;19(8):629–31.
44. Hirabayashi Y, Seo N. Use of a new videolaryngoscope (airway scope) in the management of difficult airway. J Anesth 2007;21(3):445–6.
45. Farooq M. Is endoscope-assisted intubation a useful addition to difficult airway management? Anesth Analg 2007;105(2):540–1.
46. Mchugh R, Kumar M, Sprung J, et al. Transtracheal jet ventilation in management of the difficult airway. Anaesth Intensive Care 2007;35(3):406–8.
47. Timmermann A, Russo SG, Rosenblatt WH, et al. Intubating laryngeal mask airway for difficult out-of-hospital airway management: a prospective evaluation. Br J Anaesth 2007;99(2):286–91.
48. Mastakar S, Leschinskiry D. A response to airway rescue in acute upper airway obstruction using a ProSeal laryngeal mask airway and an Aintree catheter: a review of the ProSeal laryngeal mask airway in the management of the difficult airway. Anaesthesia 2006;61(6):618–9.
49. Abbasi S, Hamid M. Fibreoptic bronchoscopic intubation for difficult airway management. J Coll Physicians Surg Pak 2006;16(3):239–41.
50. Cook TM, Silsby J, Simpson TP. Airway rescue in acute upper airway obstruction using a ProSeal laryngeal mask airway and an Aintree catheter: a review of the ProSeal laryngeal mask airway in the management of the difficult airway. Anaesthesia 2005;60(11):1129–36.
51. Winterhalter M, Kirchhoff K, Groschel W, et al. The laryngeal tube for difficult airway management: a prospective investigation in patients with pharyngeal and laryngeal tumours. Eur J Anaesthesiol 2005;22(9):678–82.

52. Thienthong S, Horatanarung D, Wongswadiwat M, et al. An experience with intubating laryngeal mask airway for difficult airway management: report on 38 cases. J Med Assoc Thai 2004;87(10):1234–8.

53. Doyle DJ, Zura A, Ramachandran M. Videolaryngoscopy in the management of the difficult airway. Can J Anaesth 2004;51(1):95 [author reply 95–6].

54. Hodzovic I, Wilkes AR, Latto IP. Bougie-assisted difficult airway management in a manikin—the effect of position held on placement and force exerted by the tip. Anaesthesia 2004;59(1):38–43.

55. Cooper RM. Use of a new videolaryngoscope (GlideScope) in the management of a difficult airway. Can J Anaesth 2003;50(6):611–3.

56. Bahk JH, Ryu HG, Park C. Use of gum elastic bougie during difficult airway management. Anesth Analg 2003;96(6):1845 [author reply 1845–6].

57. Khan MA, Shafaq M, Manzoor T. Management of difficult airway by retrograde tracheal intubation. J Coll Physicians Surg Pak 2003;13(5):284–6.

58. Leoni A, Crescenzi G, Landoni G, et al. Use of the laryngeal mask airway and a modified sequential intubation technique for the management of an unanticipated difficult airway in a remote location. Can J Anaesth 2003;50(5):523–4.

59. Langeron O, Semjen F, Bourgain JL, et al. Comparison of the intubating laryngeal mask airway with the fiberoptic intubation in anticipated difficult airway management. Anesthesiology 2001;94(6):968–72.

60. Saruki N, Saito S, Sato J, et al. Difficult airway management with the combination of a fibreoptic stylet and McCoy laryngoscope. Can J Anaesth 2001;48(2):212.

61. Park W, Kim S, Choi H. The two different-sized fibreoptic bronchoscope method in the management of a difficult paediatric airway. Anaesthesia 2001;56(1):90–1.

62. Weiss M, Schwarz U, Gerber AC. Difficult airway management: comparison of the Bullard laryngoscope with the video-optical intubation stylet. Can J Anaesth 2000;47(3):280–4.

63. Levitan RM, Kush S, Hollander JE. Devices for difficult airway management in academic emergency departments: results of a national survey. Ann Emerg Med 1999;33(6):694–8.

64. McGuire GP, Wong DT. Airway management: contents of a difficult intubation cart. Can J Anaesth 1999;46(2):190–1.

65. Shikani AH. New "seeing" stylet-scope and method for the management of the difficult airway. Otolaryngol Head Neck Surg 1999;120(1):113–6.

66. Fridrich P, Frass M, Krenn CG, et al. The UpsherScope in routine and difficult airway management: a randomized, controlled clinical trial. Anesth Analg 1997;85(6):1377–81.

67. Brimacombe JR. Difficult airway management with the intubating laryngeal mask. Anesth Analg 1997;85(5):1173–5.

68. Wulf H, Brinkmann G, Rautenberg M. Management of the difficult airway. A case of failed fiberoptic intubation. Acta Anaesthesiol Scand 1997;41(8):1080–2.

69. Gottschalk A. Jet ventilation in management of the difficult airway. Can J Anaesth 1997;44(3):337.

70. Hatton KW, Price S, Craig L, et al. Educating anesthesiology residents to perform percutaneous cricothyrotomy, retrograde intubation, and fiberoptic bronchoscopy using preserved cadavers. Anesth Analg 2006;103(5):1205–8.

71. Melker JS, Gabrielli A. Melker cricothyrotomy kit: an alternative to the surgical technique. Ann Otol Rhinol Laryngol 2005;114(7):525–8.

72. Borg P. Emergency cricothyrotomy. Anaesthesia 2005;60(4):412–3 [author reply 413].

73. Keane MF, Brinsfield KH, Dyer KS, et al. A laboratory comparison of emergency percutaneous and surgical cricothyrotomy by prehospital personnel. Prehosp Emerg Care 2004;8(4):424–6.

74. Hodgson R. A response to 'Emergency cricothyrotomy: a randomised crossover trial comparing the wire-guided and catheter-over-needle techniques', Fikkers BG, van Vugt S, van der Hoeven JG, van den Hoogen FJA, Marres HAM, Anaesthesia 2004;59:1008–11. Anaesthesia 2005;60(1):105.

75. Marcolini EG, Burton JH, Bradshaw JR, et al. A standing-order protocol for cricothyrotomy in prehospital emergency patients. Prehosp Emerg Care 2004;8(1): 23–8.

76. DiGiacomo C, Neshat KK, Angus LD, et al. Emergency cricothyrotomy. Mil Med 2003;168(7):541–4.

77. Bair AE, Panacek EA, Wisner DH, et al. Cricothyrotomy: a 5-year experience at one institution. J Emerg Med 2003;24(2):151–6.

78. Dubey PK, Kumar A. A device for cricothyrotomy and retrograde intubation. Anaesthesia 2000;55(7):702–4.

79. Davis DP, Bramwell KJ, Hamilton RS, et al. Safety and efficacy of the rapid four-step technique for cricothyrotomy using a Bair Claw. J Emerg Med 2000;19(2): 125–9.

80. Eisenburger P, Laczika K, List M, et al. Comparison of conventional surgical versus Seldinger technique emergency cricothyrotomy performed by inexperienced clinicians. Anesthesiology 2000;92(3):687–90.

81. DiGiacomo JC, Angus LD, Gelfand BJ, et al. Cricothyrotomy technique: standard versus the rapid four step technique. J Emerg Med 1999;17(6):1071–3.

82. Chan TC, Vilke GM, Bramwell KJ, et al. Comparison of wire-guided cricothyrotomy versus standard surgical cricothyrotomy technique. J Emerg Med 1999; 17(6):957–62.

83. Davis DP, Bramwell KJ, Vilke GM, et al. Cricothyrotomy technique: standard versus the rapid four-step technique. J Emerg Med 1999;17(1):17–21.

84. Brofeldt BT, Panacek EA, Richards JR. An easy cricothyrotomy approach: the rapid four-step technique. Acad Emerg Med 1996;3(11):1060–3.

85. Brimacombe J. Emergency cricothyrotomy. J Trauma 1995;39(2):395.

86. Hawkins ML, Shapiro MB, Cue JI, et al. Emergency cricothyrotomy: a reassessment. Am Surg 1995;61(1):52–5.

87. Linsdey D. Emergency cricothyrotomy. Am J Emerg Med 1994;12(1):124–5.

88. Erlandson MJ, Clinton JE, Ruiz E, et al. Cricothyrotomy in the emergency department revisited. J Emerg Med 1989;7(2):115–8.

89. Bagade A, Jefferson O, Ball DR. Retrograde tracheal intubation. Anaesthesia 2006;61(12):1223–4.

90. Lenfant F, Benkhadra M, Trouilloud P, et al. Comparison of two techniques for retrograde tracheal intubation in human fresh cadavers. Anesthesiology 2006; 104(1):48–51.

91. Rosenblatt WH, Wagner PJ, Ovassapian A, et al. Practice patterns in managing the difficult airway by anesthesiologists in the United States. Anesth Analg 1998; 87(1):153–7.

92. Dhara SS. Retrograde intubation—a facilitated approach. Br J Anaesth 1992; 69(6):631–3.

93. Stern Y, Spitzer T. Retrograde intubation of the trachea. J Laryngol Otol 1991; 105(9):746–7.

94. Barriot P, Riou B. Retrograde technique for tracheal intubation in trauma patients. Crit Care Med 1988;16(7):712–3.

95. McNamara RM. Retrograde intubation of the trachea. Ann Emerg Med 1987; 16(6):680–2.

96. Hung OR, al-Qatari M. Light-guided retrograde intubation. Can J Anaesth 1997; 44(8):877–82.

97. Chau-In W, Pongmetha S, Sumret K, et al. Translaryngeal retrograde wire-guided fiberoptic intubation for difficult airway: a case report. J Med Assoc Thai 2005;88(6):845–8.

98. Harrison WL, Bertrand ML, Andeweg SK, et al. Retrograde intubation around an in situ combitube: a difficult airway management strategy. Anesthesiology 2005; 102(5):1061–2.

99. Weksler N, Klein M, Weksler D, et al. Retrograde tracheal intubation: beyond fibreoptic endotracheal intubation. Acta Anaesthesiol Scand 2004;48(4):412–6.

100. Arima H, Sobue K, Tanaka S, et al. Difficult airway in a child with spinal muscular atrophy type I. Paediatr Anaesth 2003;13(4):342–4.

101. Arya VK, Dutta A, Chari P, et al. Difficult retrograde endotracheal intubation: the utility of a pharyngeal loop. Anesth Analg 2002;94(2):470–3 [table of contents].

102. Morais RJ, Kotsev SN, Hana SJ. Modified retrograde intubation in a patient with difficult airway. Saudi Med J 2000;21(5):490–2.

103. Simon HK, Sullivan F. Confidence in performance of pediatric emergency medicine procedures by community emergency practitioners. Pediatr Emerg Care 1996;12(5):336–9.

104. Borland LM, Swan DM, Leff S. Difficult pediatric endotracheal intubation: a new approach to the retrograde technique. Anesthesiology 1981;55(5):577–8.

105. Osborn IP, Cohen J, Soper RJ, et al. Laryngeal mask airway—a novel method of airway protection during ERCP: comparison with endotracheal intubation. Gastrointest Endosc 2002;56(1):122–8.

106. Butler FS, Cirillo AA. Retrograde tracheal intubation. Anesth Analg 1960;39: 333–8.

107. Waters DJ. Guided blind endotracheal intubation. For patients with deformities of the upper airway. Anaesthesia 1963;18:158–62.

108. Bourke D, Levesque PR. Modification of retrograde guide for endotracheal intubation. Anesth Analg 1974;53(6):1013–4.

109. Nadarajan SK. Improving the success of retrograde tracheal intubation. Anesthesiology 2006;105(4):855–6 [author reply 856].

110. Shantha TR. Retrograde intubation using the subcricoid region. Br J Anaesth 1992;68(1):109–12.

111. Harvey SC, Fishman RL, Edwards SM. Retrograde intubation through a laryngeal mask airway. Anesthesiology 1996;85(6):1503–4.

112. Rosenblatt WH, Angood PB, Maranets I, et al. Retrograde fiberoptic intubation. Anesth Analg 1997;84(5):1142–4.

113. Roberts KW, Solgonick RM. A modification of retrograde wire-guided, fiberoptic-assisted endotracheal intubation in a patient with ankylosing spondylitis. Anesth Analg 1996;82(6):1290–1.

114. Eidelman LA, Pizov R. A safer approach to retrograde-guided fiberoptic intubation. Anesth Analg 1996;82(5):1108.

115. Bissinger U, Guggenberger H, Lenz G. Retrograde-guided fiberoptic intubation in patients with laryngeal carcinoma. Anesth Analg 1995;81(2):408–10.

116. Audenaert SM, Montgomery CL, Stone B, et al. Retrograde-assisted fiberoptic tracheal intubation in children with difficult airways. Anesth Analg 1991;73(5): 660–4.

117. Gupta B, McDonald JS, Brooks JH, et al. Oral fiberoptic intubation over a retrograde guidewire. Anesth Analg 1989;68(4):517–9.
118. Lechman MJ, Donahoo JS, Macvaugh H III. Endotracheal intubation using percutaneous retrograde guidewire insertion followed by antegrade fiberoptic bronchoscopy. Crit Care Med 1986;14(6):589–90.
119. Smith CE, Dejoy SJ. New equipment and techniques for airway management in trauma. Curr Opin Anaesthesiol 2001;14(2):197–209.
120. Biswas BK, Bhattacharyya P, Joshi S, et al. Fluoroscope-aided retrograde placement of guidewire for tracheal intubation in patients with limited mouth opening. Br J Anaesth 2005;94(1):128–31.
121. Bhattacharya P, Biswas BK, Baniwal S. Retrieval of a retrograde catheter using suction, in patients who cannot open their mouths. Br J Anaesth 2004;92(6):888–901.
122. Bissinger U, Plinkert PK, Guggenberger H. Problematic intubation in the patient with laryngeal-hypopharyngeal carcinoma. Retrograde controlled fiber bronchoscopy technique. HNO 1998;46(7):666–71.

Challenges and Advances in Intubation: Rapid Sequence Intubation

Sharon Elizabeth Mace, MD, FACEP, FAAP[a,b,c,d],*

KEYWORDS

- Intubation • Rapid sequence intubation
- Endotracheal intubation

DEFINITION/OVERVIEW

Rapid sequence intubation (RSI) is a process whereby pharmacologic agents, specifically a sedative (eg, induction agent) and a neuromuscular blocking agent are administered in rapid succession to facilitate endotracheal intubation.[1]

RSI in the emergency department (ED) usually is conducted under less than optimal conditions and should be differentiated from rapid sequence induction (also often abbreviated RSI) as practiced by anesthesiologists in a more controlled environment in the operating room to induce anesthesia in patients requiring intubation.[2–6] RSI used to secure a definitive airway in the ED frequently involves uncooperative, nonfasted, unstable, critically ill patients. In anesthesia, the goal of rapid sequence induction is to induce anesthesia while using a rapid sequence approach to decrease the possibility of aspiration. With emergency RSI, the goal is to facilitate intubation with the additional benefit of decreasing the risk of aspiration.

Although there are no randomized, controlled trials documenting the benefits of RSI,[7] and there is controversy regarding various steps in RSI in adult and pediatric patients,[8–13] RSI has become standard of care in emergency medicine airway management[14–17] and has been advocated in the airway management of intensive care unit or critically ill patients.[18] RSI has also been used in the prehospital care setting,[14,19,20]

[a] Cleveland Clinic Lerner College of Medicine of Case Western Reserve, Cleveland, OH 44195, USA

[b] Observation Unit, Cleveland Clinic, 9500 Euclid Avenue, Cleveland, OH 44195, USA

[c] Emergency Services Institute, E19, Cleveland Clinic, 9500 Euclid Avenue, Cleveland, OH 44195, USA

[d] Case Western Reserve University, Metro Health Medical Center, 8500 Metro Health Drive, Cleveland, OH 44109, USA

* Emergency Services Institute, E19, Cleveland Clinic, 9500 Euclid Avenue, Cleveland, OH 44195.
E-mail address: maces@ccf.org

Emerg Med Clin N Am 26 (2008) 1043–1068
doi:10.1016/j.emc.2008.10.002
0733-8627/08/$ – see front matter © 2008 Elsevier Inc. All rights reserved.

emed.theclinics.com

although the results have been mixed, especially in trauma patients (most notably in traumatic brain injury patients), such that an expert panel found that "the existing literature regarding paramedic RSI was inconclusive."[20] Furthermore, training and experience "affect performance" and that a successful "paramedic RSI program is dependent on particular emergency medical services (EMS) and trauma system characteristics."[20]

ADVANTAGES AND DISADVANTAGES OF RAPID SEQUENCE INTUBATION

The purpose of RSI is to make emergent intubation easier and safer, thereby increasing the success rate of intubation and decreasing the complications of intubation. The rationale behind RSI is to prevent aspiration and its potential problems, including aspiration pneumonia, and to counteract the increase in systemic arterial blood pressure, heart rate, plasma catecholamine release, intracranial pressure (ICP), and intraocular pressure (IOP) that occurs with endotracheal intubation. Blunting the rise in ICP may be critical in patients with impaired cerebral antoregulation from central nervous system illness/injury. Similarly, avoiding an increase in IOP may be desirable in the patient with glaucoma or an acute eye injury. RSI eliminates the normal protective airway reflexes (such as coughing, gagging, increased secretions, and laryngospasm) that can make intubation more difficult. Use of RSI may limit cervical spine movement, thus, allowing for better control of the cervical spine during intubation with less potential for injury. RSI decreases the trauma to the airway that occurs with intubation. RSI should also decrease or eliminate the discomfort that occurs with intubation and the patient's recall of the intubation.[1]

Disadvantages of RSI are (1) the potential for side effects or complications related to the drugs administered for RSI, (2) prolonged intubation leading to hypoxia, and (3) "emergent" or a "crash" airway resulting in a cricothyroidotomy or other "emergent" airway procedure.[1]

RAPID SEQUENCE INTUBATION: THE PROCEDURE

RSI generally consists of seven steps: (1) preparation, (2) preoxygenation, (3) pretreatment, (4) paralysis with induction, (5) protection and positioning, (6) placement of the tube in the trachea, and (7) postintubation management.[1,17] These seven steps can be modified when appropriate to fit the clinical situation.[21]

Step 1—Preparation

Preparation involves having all the necessary equipment and supplies including medications that may be needed for an emergency intubation such as oxygen, suction, bag-valve mask (BVM), laryngoscope and blades, endotracheal (ET) tubes with a stylet with one size larger and smaller than the anticipated ET size, resuscitation equipment, and supplies for rescue maneuvers (eg, laryngeal mask airways [LMA] or cricothyrotomy) in case of a failed intubation according to the Can't Intubate, Can't Ventilate American Society of Anesthesiologists (ASA) guidelines.[22] The patient should have an intravenous line placed and be put on continuous monitoring to include vital signs (heart rate, respirations, blood pressure, pulse oximetry), cardiac rhythm monitoring, and, preferably, capnography.

The mnemonic "SOAPME" is one way to remember the essential equipment needed for intubation: Suction, Oxygen, Airway, Pharmacology, Monitoring, Equipment.[23] For the airway, include the ET tubes, laryngoscopes, blades, stylets, and BVM. For pharmacology, select, draw up, and label the appropriate medications (sedative, neuromuscular blocker, ancillary drugs) based on the history, physical examination, and equipment available. Monitoring should include pulse oximetry and cardiac monitoring at a minimum; also preferably with capnography.[24]

Assembling adequate personnel needed to assist in the procedure and assigning their roles is also a key component of the preparation phase. Patient assessment should be done at this time. A focused history and physical examination should be done to identify any condition, illnesses, or injuries that may negatively affect airway procedures/manipulations, medication administration, BVM ventilation, intubation, RSI, or rescue airway procedures.

The preparation step is used to "MAP" (*M*onitor, *A*ssemble, *P*atient assessment) out a treatment plan for intubation using RSI and a backup contingency plan in case of a failed intubation (can't ventilate, can't intubate scenario).[25]

Step 2—Preoxygenation

Preoxygenation should be occurring during the preparation step. The purpose of preoxygenation is to replace the nitrogen in the patient's functional residual capacity (FRC) with oxygen or "nitrogen wash-out oxygen wash-in." "Denitrogenation" can be accomplished in 3 to 5 minutes by having the patient breathe 100% oxygen via a tight-fitting facemask or, if time is an issue, with four vital capacity breaths. Depending on circumstances, as long a period of preoxygenation as possible, (up to 5 minutes) should be administered. Ideally, positive pressure ventilation should be avoided during the preoxygenation step because of a risk for gastric insufflation and possible regurgitation. Because effective ventilation by the patient is not feasible in many ED patients, BVM ventilation may be necessary in apneic patients or patients with ineffective spontaneous breathing. In these instances, use of the Sellick procedure with gentle cricoid pressure should be applied in an attempt to limit gastric distention and avoid aspiration during BVM ventilation.

In the preoxygenation phase, replacing the nitrogen reservoir in the lungs with oxygen allows 3 to 5 minutes of apnea without significant hypoxemia in the normoxic adult.[26] One caveat to remember is that certain patients have a lesser FRC (eg, infants and children and patients with an elevated diaphragm, specifically obese adults or pregnant patients). These patients will become hypoxic in a shorter time, eg, a normal child or an obese adult may start to desaturate within 2 minutes, while a normal adult may tolerate up to 5 minutes of apnea before they become significantly hypoxic.[26]

Step 3—Pretreatment

Ancillary medications are administered during the pretreatment step to mitigate the negative physiologic responses to intubation. For maximal efficacy, the pretreatment drugs should precede the induction agent by 3 minutes, although this is not always possible. The pretreatment phase and preoxygenation phase can (and usually) do occur simultaneously during most instances of RSI in the ED. Medications and their usual dosages that may be given during the pretreatment phase are lidocaine 1.5 mg/kg, fentanyl 2–3 mcg/kg, and atropine 0.02 mg/kg (minimum 0.1 mg, maximum 0.5 mg). The clinical indications for these drugs are (1) for patients with elevated ICP and impaired autoregulation: administer lidocaine and fentanyl, (2) patients with major vessel dissection or rupture or those with significant ischemic heart disease give fentanyl, (3) adults with significant reactive airway disease, premedicate with lidocaine, and (4) atropine is indicated for pediatric patients ≤ 10 years old and in patients with significant bradycardia if succinylcholine is given. One caveat to remember is to give fentanyl with caution to any patient in shock (whether compensated or uncompensated) who is dependent on sympathetic drive because of a potential decrease in blood pressure with fentanyl administration.

In patients who are receiving succinylcholine as their induction agent and who are at risk for increased ICP, one tenth of the normal paralyzing dose of a nondepolarizing (ND) neuromuscular blocking agent (NMB) can be given 3 minutes before receiving succinylcholine. The purpose of the defasciculating dose of the ND-NMB is to prevent the fasciculations (and therefore, the increase in ICP) that occurs with succinylcholine. For example, the dose would be 10% of the paralyzing dose of rocuronium (10% of 0.6 mg/kg = 0.06 mg/kg). The mnemonic "LOAD" has been used to indicate the pretreatment drugs for RSI: L = lidocaine, O = opioid (specifically, fentanyl), A = atropine, and D = defasciculation.[27]

Step 4—Paralysis with Induction

Paralysis with induction is achieved by the rapid intravenous administration in quick succession of the induction agent and the NMB. The selection of a specific sedative depends on multiple factors: the clinical scenario, which includes patient factors (includes cardiorespiratory and neurologic status, allergies, comorbidity) and the clinician's experience/training and institutional factors, as well as the characteristics of the sedative.[28] Sedatives commonly used for induction during RSI are barbiturates (pentobarbitol, thiopental, and methohexitol),[29] opioids (fentanyl),[1] dissociative anesthetics (ketamine),[30] and nonbarbiturate sedatives (etomidate,[31] propofol,[32] and the benzodiazepines).[21,33] The dosages and characteristics of these agents and are summarized in **Table 1**. One caveat to remember is that the induction dosages of these sedatives may be different (generally, slightly higher) than the dose used for sedation. For example, for etomidate the usual dose for procedural sedation is 0.2 mg/kg and for RSI is 0.3 mg/kg.[31]

Step 5—Protection and Positioning

Positioning of the head and neck is essential to achieve the best view of the glottic opening for conventional laryngoscopy by aligning the three axes: oral, pharyngeal, and laryngeal. This is achieved by extension and elevation of the neck to obtain the "sniffing the morning air" or the "sipping English tea" position, assuming there are no contraindications such as known or potential cervical spine injury.[1]

Protection refers to the use of maneuvers to prevent regurgitation of gastric contents with possible aspiration. This is achieved via the Sellick maneuver, which is the application of firm pressure on the cricoid cartilage to avoid passive regurgitation of gastric contents. The correct performance of the Sellick maneuver involves the use of the thumb and index or middle finger to apply firm downward pressure on the cricoid cartilage anteroposteriorly.

Several caveats regarding the proper technique need to be considered: location, timing, and amount of pressure. Cricoid pressure should be applied as soon as the patient starts to lose consciousness and should be maintained until the correct endotracheal position is verified. Pressure should be gentle but firm enough to compress the esophagus between the cricoid cartilage and the anterior surface of the vertebral body. The cricoid cartilage is opposite the C4–C5 vertebrae in an adult, and C3–C4 in an infant. Common mistakes include premature release of cricoid pressure, which puts the patient at risk for aspiration, especially if accidental esophageal intubation occurred; misplaced position (avoid applying pressure over the thyroid cartilage or entire larynx which may impede passage of the tube); and incorrect amount of cricoid pressure. The applied pressure should be graded and inversely related to the size of the patient with less force in smaller patients. One recommendation in smaller patients is placing the other hand under the neck to avoid changing the neck position while applying cricoid pressure (with the opposite hand), to avoid malpositioning the neck. This is assuming there are no contraindications such as cervical spine injury. Should vomiting occur, cricoid pressure should be released immediately because of possible esophageal rupture, although there are no data to substantiate this possible complication, and neuromuscular blockade eliminates the possibility of active vomiting.

Step 6—Placement of the Endotracheal Tube in the Trachea

When the jaw becomes flaccid from the paralytics, it is time to begin intubation by standard methods. ET tube placement should be confirmed by the usual techniques.

Step 7—Postintubation Management

After ET tube placement and confirmation, the ET tube must be secured. A chest radiograph is done not only to check for proper ET tube placement but also to evaluate the pulmonary status and to monitor for any complications of the intubation and RSI. Continued sedation and analgesia, sometimes with paralysis as well as cardiopulmonary monitoring, is indicated as long as the patient requires advanced airway support.

PHARMACOLOGY: SEDATIVE AGENTS FOR RAPID SEQUENCE INTUBATION

According to the National Emergency Airway Registry (NEAR) study, the most frequently used induction agents were etomidate (69%), midazolam (16%), fentanyl (6%), and ketamine (3%).[34] Considering just pediatric patients using the NEAR registry,[6] etomidate was the most commonly used induction agent but was used in less than half the patients (only 42% compared with 69% for all patients),[34] followed by thiopental (22%), midazolam (18%), and ketamine (7%).[6]

Etomidate

Etomidate, the most commonly used sedative for RSI in adults, can also be administered for pediatric RSI.[31] The usual dose is 0.3 mg/kg or 20 mg in a 70-kg adult. It often is used in trauma patients with known or potential bleeding, hypovolemic patients, and patients with limited cardiac reserve, because it does not have significant cardiovascular effects. Etomidate also decreases ICP and the cerebral metabolic rate, which suggests that it may have a neuroprotective effect. These features are why some clinicians consider it the sedative of choice in a patient who has multiple trauma with both a head injury and hemorrhage or shock.

Etomidate does inhibit 11-β-hydroxylase, an enzyme necessary for adrenal steroid production.[35] Transient adrenal suppression has been noted after a single dose of etomidate, although this is probably not clinically significant.[36] Some data indicate that etomidate has a negative impact on patient outcome in critically ill patients with sepsis and septic shock.[37–39] This has led to the suggestion that a corticosteroid be coadministered when etomidate is given for RSI.[38] Although either dexamethasone (0.1 mg/kg) or hydrocortisone (1–2 mg/kg) may be given, dexamethasone often is chosen because it does not interfere with the adrenocorticotropin hormone (ACTH) stimulation test, which may be needed to later test for adrenal insufficiency. In any case, infusions of etomidate for continued postintubation sedation are contraindicated.[39]

Myoclonus is another side effect of etomidate that may interfere with intubation if a paralytic is not used,[40] although this is not the situation with RSI in which a sedative and paralytic generally are coadministered in quick succession.

Barbiturates

Thiopental is the most commonly used barbiturate for pediatric RSI[6] and may be the most commonly used barbiturate for anesthesia induction.[41] However, it used is less

Table 1
Medications for rapid-sequence intubation

Sedatives	Dose (IV) (mg/kg) for Intubation	Indication	Side Effects	Precautions, Contraindication	Reversal Agent	Comment
Etomidate	0.3 (usual 70 kg Adult dose = 100 mg)	Induction agent (sedative). Often used in hypovolemic, hemorrhagic patients, and in trauma patients, especially if head injury and hemorrhage	Can cause myoclonic movements	Adrenal insufficiency. Use with caution if in septic shock and sepsis and consider giving corticosteroid	-	Myoclonic movements may make intubation difficult if NMB not given
Barbiturates, Thiopental	3–4	Induction agent (sedative). Used in patients with ↑ ICP if hemodynamically stable	Negative CV effects. Use low doses cautiously if CV disease, shock, hypovolemia	Porphyria	-	Avoid intra-arterial injection (can cause gangrene). Avoid extravasation; causes tissue necrosis
Barbiturate, Methohexital	1–1.5	Induction agent (sedative). Used in patients with ↑ ICP if hemodynamically stable	Causes histamine release	Use with cause in asthmatics or if hypotensive	-	Avoid intra-arterial injection (can cause gangrene). Avoid extravasation (causes tissue necrosis).

Drug	Dose	Type	Adverse effects	Precautions	Reversal	Comments
Ketamine	0.5–2.0 (↓ dose if used with benzodiazepine or thiopental)	Induction agent (sedative). Often used if hypovolemic, hemorrhage, shock	Sympathomimetic effects ↑ICP, ↑IOP, ↑BP, ↑HR	Consider alternatives if ↑ICP, ↑IOP may cause emergence reaction	-	Use with atropine if age ≤10 years or significant bradycardia
Benzodiazepine, Midazolam	0.5–1.5	Induction agent (sedative)	Respiratory depression, apnea, paradoxical agitation	Minimal CV effects unless hypovolemic	Flumazenil	Dose varies widely, ↓ dose if given with opioids, in elderly, renal failure, liver disease, significant CV disease
Propofol	1–2.5 (↓ dose with age)	Induction agent (sedative)	Hypotension, hypoxia, apnea, bradycardia. Use cautiously if volume depletion, hypotension, CV disease	Allergy to egg, soybean oil, EDTA	-	Ultra short acting. Negative CV effects limits its use in man ED-RSI patients

Abbreviation: CV, cardiovascular.

commonly than etomidate for ED RSI, at least partly because many ED RSI patients are hemodynamically unstable. Thiopental decreases both cerebral blood flow and the metabolic demands of the brain, which makes it an ideal sedative agent in patients with known increased ICP or patients with head injury who are hemodynamically stable. Thiopental has negative cardiovascular effects: myocardial depression and peripheral vasodilatation. Thus, hypotension with associated hypoperfusion can occur in patients who are hypovolemic or have myocardial depression. Generally, when hypotension occurs, there is a compensatory baroreceptor mediated reflex tachycardia. Unfortunately, patients who are hypovolemic or in shock or who are already tachycardic may not be capable of further compensatory heart rate increases and can experience a drop in blood pressure with thiopental administration. Similarly, patients with preexisting cardiovascular disease may also experience hypotension when given thiopental. The conclusion is to avoid using thiopental, if possible, in patients with underlying cardiovascular disease, hypovolemia, or shock or limit thiopental to small frequent doses (1–3 mg/kg) while carefully monitoring blood pressure.[29]

Thiopental has some respiratory side effects. It has a dose- and rate-related (eg, high dose, rapid administration) respiratory depression of the central nervous system (CNS) that can cause apnea, especially in head injured or hypovolemic patients. With "light" anesthesia, several untoward effects may occur, especially during airway manipulation: catecholamine release causing systemic or intracranial hypertension, laryngospasm, cough, and bronchospasm, especially in asthmatic patients.[41] To mitigate or avoid these negative effects, it has been recommended to coadminister an analgesic (such as fentanyl) especially in head-injured patients.[27]

Tissue necrosis can occur with intraarterial injection or extravasation, so it is critical that thiopental be given intravenously as a dilute solution while being careful to avoid any tissue infiltration.[29,41]

Ketamine

Ketamine, a dissociative anesthetic, exerts its effects by interrupting the connection between the thalamo-neocortical tracts and the limbic system. Unlike all the other sedatives, it has an additional advantage in that it also has analgesic properties.

Ketamine's sympathomimetic effects, acting via a centrally mediated mechanism, cause an increase in heart rate, blood pressure, and cardiac output. This makes ketamine an excellent sedative in patients who are hypotensive, especially if secondary to shock, hemorrhage, dehydration, pericarditis, or tamponade. However, these sympathomimetic effects are undesirable in patients who already have significant hypertension or tachycardia.[30]

Ketamine also causes an increase in ICP by both an increase in systemic blood pressure and cerebral vasodilatation and, therefore, is contraindicated in patients with ICP, an intracerebral hemorrhage, an intracranial mass, or head trauma; although a recent study has challenged this contraindication.[42] This French study compared the cerebral hemodynamics of ketamine combined with midazolam and found no significant difference in ICP or cerebral perfusion pressure when compared with midazolam-sufentanil.[42]

It has previously been thought that young age (eg, <6 months) was a contraindication to the use of ketamine. However, a recent study indicates that ketamine is safe and effective even in neonates.[43]

Ketamine is probably the sedative of choice for asthmatic patients for many reasons. Ketamine, through the release of endogenous catecholamines, relieves bronchospasm by dilating bronchial smooth muscle and stimulating the pulmonary β receptors. Ketamine increases tracheobronchial/oropharyngeal secretions. This may have a positive effect by decreasing mucus plugging in some cases. The excess secretions may, however, interfere with visualization of the airway during laryngoscopy. Fortunately, pretreatment with atropine (preferred for RSI) or glycopyrollate (preferred for sedation) prevents excess secretions.[27,44] The dose of atropine for RSI is 0.01 to 0.02 mg/kg intravenously with a minimum of 0.1 mg and a maximum of 0.5 to 1.0 mg.[1,2,27,44] Glycopyrollate is the antimuscarinic drug of choice for procedural sedation because it has a greater antisialagogue effect and fewer side effects (less tachycardia, fewer dysrhythmias, and no CNS side effects).[44] In addition, atropine crosses the blood–brain barrier (glycopyrollate does not so it has no CNS side effects) and may increase the incidence of emergence reactions.[44] Although the routine use of atropine has been questioned, the consensus is that it is still useful in selected patients.[1,27] Atropine is used for RSI because it causes an increase in heart rate, which is desirable when offsetting the bradycardic effects of succinylcholine during RSI.[27]

Ketamine has respiratory/cardiovascular stability and maintains airway reflexes. As with all sedatives, rare instances of apnea and laryngospasm have been reported. Ketamine, an analog of phencyclidine (PCP), is associated with an occasional emergence reaction, so its use should probably be avoided in psychotic patients. Small doses of midazolam have been given for the treatment of emergence reactions. Traditional teaching is that coadministration of a benzodiazepam (eg, midazolam) with ketamine will prevent emergence reactions. This teaching has been challenged recently by several studies that reported the prophylactic administration of benzodiazepine did not decrease the incidence of emergence reactions[28,45,46] but actually increased the risk of respiratory depression and prolonged recovery, while paradoxically increasing the incidence of emergence reactions in a subset of patients.[45]

Benzodiazepines

Midazolam is the most commonly used benzodiazepine for RSI and ED sedation primarily because it has a rapid onset and short duration.[33] Other advantages of midazolam versus diazepam include fewer adverse effects, better amnesia, and greater potency.[33]

All of the benzodiazepines, including midazolam, diazepam, and lorazepam, have sedative, hypnotic, amnestic, anxiolytic, muscle relaxant, and anticonvulsant properties. Benzodiazepines bind to a specific benzodiazepine receptor site on the GABA (gamma-aminobutyric acid) receptor. GABA is an inhibitory neurotransmitter. This opens a chloride channel causing hyperpolarization of the neuronal cell membrane, thereby blocking neuronal depolarization or activation.

The antagonist, flumazenil, can reverse the effects of the benzodiazepines. Advantages of the benzodiazepines include minimal cardiovascular effects (unless the patient is hypovolemic), can be used in patients with coronary artery disease, positive nitroglycerin-like effect in patients with heart failure (decreases the increased ventricular filling pressure), and seizure treatment. The main disadvantage of the benzodiazepines is that they can cause respiratory depression and apnea. Other uncommon side effects are paradoxical agitation, vomiting, coughing, and hiccups.

The benzodiazepine dosage for RSI and sedation varies widely and should be decreased when given along with opioids, in the elderly, patients with renal failure, or severe hepatic disease, or significant heart disease.[33]

Propofol

Propofol is an ultra–short-acting sedative hypnotic agent. It has no analgesic effects, and its amnestic effects are variable. The advantages of propofol are its very quick onset and short duration. It also has antiemetic properties, can be used in malignant hypothermia patients, and the dosage is unchanged for patients with renal or liver disease, although higher doses may be needed in pediatric patients and lower doses in geriatric patients.[32] Side effects include hypotension, bradycardia, hypoxia and apnea,[32] so it should be administered slowly. Propofol also has negative cardiovascular effects so it should be used with caution in patients with volume depletion, hypotension, or cardiovascular disease.[32] Because of these side effects/complications its use as a sedative for RSI is limited in many ED patients.[38]

PATHOPHYSIOLOGY

A discussion of the anatomy and physiology of the neuromuscular junction is valuable in understanding how the neuromuscular blockers work.

Anatomy

The neuromuscular or myoneural junction is the junction between the nerve fiber ending or nerve terminal, the muscle fiber including the muscle fiber membrane or sarcolemma, and the interposed synaptic cleft (synaptic space). The motor end plate refers to the complex of branching nerve terminals that invaginate into (but actually lie outside) the sarcolemma. (**Fig. 1**) Subneural clefts are folds of the muscle cell (myocyte) membrane, which markedly increase the surface area at which the synaptic neurotransmitter Ach can act (**Fig. 2**). A single terminal branch of the nerve axon lies in the synaptic gutter or synaptic trough, which is an invagination of the sarcolemma (see **Figs. 1** and **2**). Structures found in the nerve terminal include synaptic vesicles containing the neurotransmitter Ach, the dense bar areas (Ach from the vesicles is released into the synaptic cleft through the neural membrane adjacent to the dense bars), voltage gated calcium channels (which are protein particles that penetrate the neural membrane), and mitochondria (which supply the adenosine triphosphate [ATP]- that acts as the energy source for the synthesis of Ach) (**Fig. 3**).

The nicotinic receptor, a protein particle located on the postsynaptic myocyte membrane has two parts: a binding component and an ionophore component. The binding component projects outward from the postsynaptic myocyte membrane into the synaptic space where it binds the neurotransmitter Ach. The ionosphere component extends through the postsynaptic neural membrane to the interior of the postsynaptic membrane. The ionosphere may serve as an ion channel that permits the movement of ions (in this case primarily sodium ions, as well as other ions) through the membrane (**Fig. 4**).

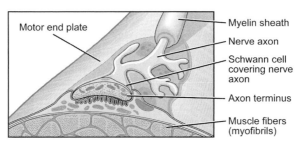

Fig. 1. Motor end plate of the neuromuscular junction. (*Courtesy of* Sharon E. Mace, MD, and Dave Schumick of the Cleveland Clinic Center for Medical Art and Photography, Cleveland, OH; with permission.)

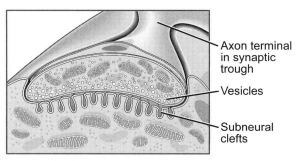

Fig. 2. Neuromuscular junction shows nerve axon terminal in synaptic trough, the sarcolemma with subneural clefts, and the interposed synaptic space. (*Courtesy of* Sharon E. Mace, MD, and Dave Schumick of the Cleveland Clinic Center for Medical Art and Photography, Cleveland, OH; with permission.)

Neurotransmitter: Acetylcholine

Acetylcholine (Ach), the neurotransmitter at cholinergic synapses, is released from the ending of preganglionic and postganglionic parasympathetic nerves and preganglionic sympathetic nerves. Ach is synthesized from choline and acetic acid in the nerve and packaged in vesicles. With nerve stimulation, the impulse reaches the nerve ending causing the Ach vesicles to travel to the nerve surface and rupture, thereby releasing Ach into the synaptic space (synaptic cleft). Exocytosis is the process whereby the Ach containing vesicles fuse with the nerve terminal membrane and release their Ach. When the action potential depolarizes the presynaptic membranes, the calcium ion channels open, increasing the neural membrane permeability to calcium, allowing calcium ions to stream into the presynaptic nerve ending. The calcium ions bind with "release sites" that are unique protein molecules on the inner surface of the presynaptic neural membranes. The coupling of the calcium ion to the specific protein molecule opens the release sites, which permits the vesicles to release the neurotransmitter Ach into the synaptic space (**Fig. 5**).

Ach then diffuses across the synaptic cleft to the motor endplate. Attachment of Ach to the nicotinic receptors on the skeletal muscle leads to a conformational change in the nicotinic receptor. This altered protein molecule on the nicotinic skeletal muscle receptor increases the permeability of the skeletal myocyte cell to various ions (sodium, potassium, chloride, and calcium) with an influx of sodium into the skeletal myocyte (see **Fig. 4**). This produces a large positive potential charge within the skeletal

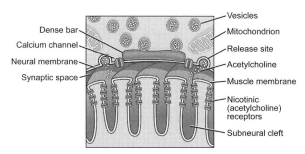

Fig. 3. Structures in the neromuscular junction. (*Courtesy of* Sharon E. Mace, MD, and Dave Schumick of the Cleveland Clinic Center for Medical Art and Photography, Cleveland, OH; with permission.)

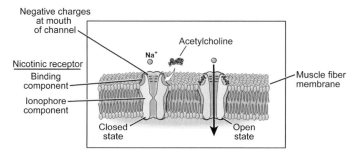

Fig. 4. Nicotinic receptors on the sarcolemma in the open and closed states. (*Courtesy of* Sharon E. Mace, MD, and Dave Schumick of the Cleveland Clinic Center for Medical Art and Photography, Cleveland, OH; with permission.)

myocyte, referred to as the "end plate potential." The end plate potential creates an action potential that travels along the skeletal myocyte membrane causing muscle contraction (**Fig. 6**).

The release of Ach from the nicotinic receptor on the skeletal myocyte ends depolarization. Ach can either diffuse back into the nerve ending or be broken down by the acetylcholinesterase enzyme into choline and acetic acid (see **Fig. 5**). Under normal circumstances, large amounts of the enzyme acetylcholinesterase are found in the synaptic space.

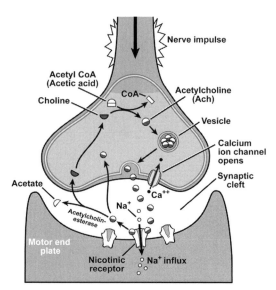

Fig. 5. Acetylcholine in the neuromuscular junction: synthesis, exocytosis, binding to the nicotinic receptor, release into synaptic space, and inactivation. (*Courtesy of* Sharon E. Mace, MD, and Dave Schumick of the Cleveland Clinic Center for Medical Art and Photography, Cleveland, OH; with permission.)

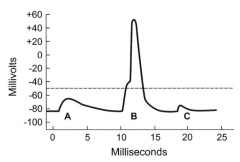

Fig. 6. Skeletal muscle end plate potential. The threshold potential of about −50 millivolts is indicated by the dashed line. (*A*) Effect of Curare. (*B*) Normal. (*C*) Effect of Botulinum toxin. (*Modified from* Guyton AG, editor. Textbook of physiology. 6th edition p. 139; with permission. *Courtesy of* Sharon E. Mace, MD, and Dave Schumick of the Cleveland Clinic Center for Medical Art and Photography, Cleveland, OH; with permission.)

The Flow of Ions and the Action Potential

Physiologically, an abrupt increase of greater than 20 to 30 millivolts causes further opening of additional sodium channels, allowing for an action potential in the skeletal muscle fiber membrane. A weak local end plate potential, less than 20 to 30 millivolts, will be insufficient to cause an action potential in the skeletal muscle fiber membrane. This is what happens with various drugs or toxins. For example, the drug curare competes with Ach for the nicotinic receptor sites on the skeletal muscle, which results in blocking the action of Ach in opening the sodium ion channels. The botulinum toxin prevents depolarization by decreasing the amount of Ach released by the nerve terminals. The flow of ions is important, because decreasing the resting membrane potential voltage to a less negative value increases neural excitability leading to depolarization when the threshold (about 50 millivolts in skeletal muscle) is reached, whereas conversely increasing the resting membrane potential to a more negative number makes the neuron less excitable (see **Fig. 6**).

NEUROMUSCULAR BLOCKERS
Definition

Neuromuscular blocking agents (NMBs) are substances that paralyze skeletal muscles by blocking nerve impulse transmission at the neuromuscular or myoneural (muscle-nerve) junction.

There are several critical factors to remember with RSI. First, a sedative is coadministered with the NMB. Patients given an NMB may be aware of their environment, including painful stimuli, even though they are unable to respond. Failure to sedate the patient allows the possibility of negative physiologic responses to airway manipulation such as increased ICP, hypertension, and tachycardia. In addition, the patient may be aware of and remember the intubation, which is considered inhumane. Concomitant sedative use limits or helps avoid these adverse physiologic responses to airway manipulation and may even result in a better view of the airway during laryngoscopy.

However, whenever an NMB is used, the physician must be prepared for a difficult or failed airway with the possibility that a surgical airway may be necessary if the patient cannot be oxygenated or ventilated adequately with a bag-valve mask or extraglottic device. Assessment of the airway, especially if there is the potential for a difficult or failed airway, should be done before administering an NMB.

NMBs are depolarizing or nondepolarizing. Depolarizing agents mimic the action of Ach. They case a sustained depolarization of the neuromuscular junction, which prevents muscle contraction. Nondepolarizing agents work by competitive inhibition to block Ach's action at the neuromuscular junction to prevent depolarization.

According to the NEAR registry, the most frequently used NMBs were succinylcholine (82%), rocuronium (12%), and vecuronium (5%).[34] For pediatric patients only, succinylcholine (90%) was also the most commonly used NMB, with vecuronium used in 7%, and rocuronium in 2%.[6]

Pharmacology

All NMBs are structurally similar to the neurotransmitter Ach. Ach and all NMBs are quaternary ammonium compounds; the positive charges of these compounds at the nitrogen atom account for their attraction to the cholinergic nicotinic (ionotropic) receptors at the neuromuscular junction and at other nicotinic receptor sites throughout the body. This nonspecific action at sites throughout the body, eg, nicotinic (ganglionic) and muscarinic autonomic sites, not just at the neuromuscular junction, helps explain some of their side effects.

DEPOLARIZING NEUROMUSCULAR BLOCKING AGENTS
Succinylcholine

Succinylcholine (Sch) is the only depolarizing agent currently available in the United States, has been used in innumerable patients since its introduction as an NMB in 1952, and is the most commonly used NMB for ED RSI.[6,34]

Sch is the prototype of the depolarizing agents. Because its chemical structure (eg, quaternary ammonium compound) is similar to that of Ach, it binds to the acetylcholine receptor (AchR) on the motor end plate and depolarizes the postjunctional neuromuscular membrane, resulting in continuous stimulation of the motor end plate AchRs. The neuromuscular block/motor paralysis is terminated when the NMB (eg, Sch) unbinds from the AchR and diffuses back into the circulation where it is hydrolyzed by plasma cholinesterase. Plasma cholinesterase (also referred to as "pseudocholinesterase" or "butylcholinesterase") rapidly hydrolyses Sch to succinylmonocholine (a very weak NMB) and choline. Sch's short duration of action is caused by the rapid hydrolysis by plasma cholinesterase both before Sch reaches and after Sch leaves the neuromuscular junction, because there is minimal if any pseudocholinesterase at the neuromuscular junction. Some Ach may diffuse back into the nerve terminal, although the majority of Ach is hydrolyzed by plasma cholinesterase. Muscle contraction will not reoccur until the neuromuscular junction returns to the resting state and then is depolarized again. Transient fasciculations (caused by initial depolarization) are followed by blockade of neuromuscular transmission with motor paralysis when Sch is given.

The major advantages of Sch are its rapid onset with complete motor paralysis occurring within 45 to 60 seconds and short duration of action lasting only 6 to 10 minutes when given in the recommended 1.5-mg/kg intravenous dose.

Dosing of Succinylcholine

There are some "pearls" regarding Sch dosing. Use the total body weight (not the lean weight) even in the morbidly obese or pregnant patient. Do not underdose the drug. It is preferable to overestimate rather than underestimate the dose because an insufficient dose may make it difficult to intubate if the patient is not adequately paralyzed. Thus, the preferred dose is 1.5 mg/kg (or about 100 mg in a 70-kg adult)[1] (some experts suggest 1.5 to 2.0 mg/kg in an adult)[47] and *not* 1 mg/kg as stated in some references. The recommended Sch dose in infants (including neonates) is 2 mg/kg based on their higher volume of distribution,[21,47] and some even recommend up to 3 mg/kg in newborns.[47] Administer Sch as a rapid bolus followed by a 20 to 30 cc saline flush to avoid incomplete paralysis. Sch has been given intramuscularly in a 3- to 4-mg/kg dose in a rare life-threatening situation in which there is inability to obtain venous access.[27]

Repeat doses or prolonged use of Sch is to be avoided for several reasons. Repeat dosing or prolonged use of Sch potentiates its effects at the sympathetic ganglia and vagal effects. The negative muscarinic effects from vagal stimulation may lead to bradycardia and hypotension even at recommended doses. This is one reason some experts recommend atropine pretreatment in infants/small children, anyone with significant bradycardia, and those receiving multiple doses of Sch. Desensitization blockage, whereby the neuromuscular membrane returns to the resting state and becomes resistant to further depolarization with Sch can also occur with repeat doses of Sch.

In patients with myasthenia gravis, there is a functional decrease in AchRs at the neuromuscular junction secondary to an antibody-mediated autoimmune destruction of the AchRs. Sch can be used in patients with myasthenia gravis, although the dose is increased to 2 mg/kg to reach and activate the remaining AchRs unaffected by the disease.

Be careful to check the expiration date on the drug vial, especially if the drug is not refrigerated, because Sch degrades gradually at room temperature. Refrigeration lowers the drug's degradation rate so that it maintains 90% activity for up to 90 days.

Succinylcholine Contraindications

The absolute contraindications to Sch are (1) a history of malignant hyperthermia in the patient or family and (2) patients at high risk of severe hyperkalemia.

Malignant Hypothermia

Malignant hyperthermia is a rare genetic myopathetic disorder precipitated by multiple drugs, especially certain inhalational anesthetics (such as halothane, sevoflurane, desiflurane, isoflurane) and Sch. It is thought to be caused by an abnormal ryanodine receptor causing marked leakage of calcium from the sarcoplasmic reticulum of skeletal muscle cells resulting in extremely high intracellular calcium levels.

Symptoms generally begin within an hour of the drug or anesthetic administration but may be delayed for hours. The clinical presentation generally includes muscle rigidity (especially masseter stiffness), increased CO_2 production, acidosis, sympathetic hyperactivity with hyperthermia (up to 113°F), and sinus tachycardia. Complications that can occur include rhabdomyolysis, electrolyte abnormalities, dysrhythmias, hypotension/shock, disseminated intravascular coagulation, and death. With intensive medical therapy including dantrolene sodium, the mortality rate has decreased from 70% to less than 10%. Thus, any history of malignant hyperthermia in the patient or any family member is an absolute contraindication to Sch. Unfortunately, with RSI in the ED, a history is often not available.

Hyperkalemia

Even in "normal" patients, Sch may increase the serum potassium up to 0.5 mEq/L because of depolarization of the myocytes (skeletal muscle cells). Generally, the rise has no clinical significance except in patients with a predisposition to hyperkalemia, such as a patient with rhabdomyolysis or patients with chronic skeletal muscle disease in whom there is "up-regulation" from increased sensitization of extrajunctional AchR in muscle. Such susceptibility is not present immediately after the onset of neuromuscular disease or after a traumatic injury but can develop within 4 to 5 days and last indefinitely.

Hyperkalemia can occur whenever there is massive tissue destruction or severe muscular wasting. The extrajunctional AchR sensitization becomes clinically significant 4 to 5 days after injury or illness onset, so the risk of life-threatening hyperkalemia does not start until days (usually 3–5 days) after the injury or illness onset. This is important because Sch can be used in the acute trauma patient, the acute stroke or head injured patient, or a patient with neuromuscular disease, immediately after their injury or disease onset. Patients with extensive muscle wasting from denervating neuromuscular diseases include patients with a spinal cord injury, multiple sclerosis, motor neuron injury, stroke, and muscular dystrophies, eg, Duchene muscular dystrophy or Becker muscular dystrophy.

With rhabdomyolysis, the destruction of myocytes secondary to tissue injury releases potassium from the cells causing the serum potassium level to increase. The second mechanism, up-regulation, causes hyperkalemia because the abnormal up-regulated AchRs have low conductance and prolonged ion channel opening times that lead to an increase in potassium. Up-regulation usually occurs within 3 to 5 days and lasts indefinitely, even years (3 or more years) after an acute injury or a progressive disease. Giving defasciculating doses of nonpolarizing NMBAs does not affect the hyperkalemic response. The hyperkalemic response to Sch has also been reported in patients in the intensive care unit with life-threatening infections, especially if there is disuse atrophy and chemical denervation of the Ach receptors. Sch also should not be used in patients with myopathies, including Duchene muscular dystrophy, because the Sch interacts with the unstable muscle membrane of the myopathic cells causing rhabomyolysis and hyperkalemia.

Although the longstanding tenet has been to avoid Sch in patients in chronic renal failure who have normokalemia, there is no supportive evidence for this.[47] In reality, most patients with renal failure undergo successful RSI with Sch without any untoward cardiovascular events.[47] However, Sch is *not* recommended for patients with known hyperkalemia because of concern that even the "usual" potassium increase of 0.5 mE/L may precipitate fatal dysrhythmias in a patient with existing significant hyperkalemia and acidosis. Thus, Sch should be avoided in patients with ECG changes of hyperkalemia.

Bradycardia

Bradycardia after Sch administration most frequently occurs in infants and children because of the vagal predominance of their autonomic nervous system but can also occur in patients of any age with repeated Sch doses. Pretreatment with atropine, 0.02 mg/kg, minimizes or eliminates this bradycardia response.

Prolonged Neuromuscular Blockade

Any factor that inhibits the breakdown of Sch will prolong neuromuscular blockade and paralysis. An abnormal form or a decrease in pseudocholinesterase (either acquired or congenital) leads to prolonged paralysis from delayed degradation of Sch. Various genetic variants of pseudocholinesterase exist including one disorder with defective pseudocholinesterase in which individuals receiving Sch remain paralyzed for up to 6 to 8 hours after a single dose of Sch. Decreased pseudocholinesterase levels can also occur secondary to various acquired disorders: liver disease, renal failure, anemia, pregnancy, chronic cocaine use, increased age, connective tissue disease, various malignancies, and organophosphate poisoning. However, this finding has little clinical significance because even large decreases in pseudocholinesterase activity cause small increments in the duration of neuromuscular paralysis after Sch administration because baseline pseudocholinesterase levels are quite high.

Increased Intracranial Pressure

The effect of Sch on ICP has been debated with various studies noting conflicting results. Some researches have noted small increases in ICP (range, 5–10 mm Hg), whereas other studies have shown no increase. More importantly, there has been no evidence of neurologic deterioration secondary to the transient ICP increase associated with Sch. Pretreatment with a nondepolarizing NMB prevents the increase in ICP, although the additional time and steps associated with such pretreatment may be impractical and time consuming in an airway emergency, and the suggested pretreatment dose of a nondepolarizing NMB may, by itself, cause some paralysis.

The extensive experience with Sch in the clinical setting of patients with acute intracerebral pathology documenting its safety and efficacy coupled with the dangers of a failed airway with secondary cerebral insult from hypoxia obviates against these theoretical, small, and likely clinically insignificant transient increases in ICP with Sch.[47]

Increased Intraocular Pressure

Sch can increase the IOP by 6 to 8 mm Hg. Sch has been used safely and effectively in patients with penetrating eye injuries during RSI anesthesia. Some experts have recommended the use of Sch even in patients with an open globe injury if there is a need for emergent securing of the airway, citing the greater risk from allowing the negative side effects of an uncontrolled intubation (including hypoxia and coughing or vomiting, which also likely results in a greater increase in IOP).

Trismus

Masseter muscle spasm (trismus) occurs in 0.001% to 0.1% of patients after Sch administration. It has been associated with malignant hyperthermia. However, it may occur in isolation. Management includes giving a standard dose of a ND-NMB, although a cricothyrotomy has been necessary in rare cases.[48,49]

Fasciculations

Fasciculations are involuntary, unsynchronized muscle contractions. They are caused by the depolarization of Ach receptors. This, in turn, initiates an action potential, which is propagated to all of the muscles supplied by the nerve. Fasciculations have various negative effects: myalgias, increased creatinine kinase, myoglobinemia, increased catecholamines (with secondary increased blood pressure and heart rate), and increased cardiac output (increased oxygen consumption and increased carbon dioxide production). The transient small increases in cerebral blood flow and ICP that occur with Sch may be caused by fasciculations. Defasciculation can be accomplished by pretreatment with lidocaine at 1.5 mg/kg or 10% of the intubating dose of a nondepolarizing NMB.

NONDEPOLARIZING NEUROMUSCULAR BLOCKING AGENTS

Nondepolarizing (ND) NMBs competitively block Ach transmission at the postjunctional cholinergic nicotinic receptors. Unlike Sch, which causes a conformational change in the AchR receptor resulting in depolarizination of the neuromuscular junction, the nondepolarizing NMB prevents Ach from access to the nicotinic receptor, thereby preventing muscle contraction. Fasciculations do not occur with the ND-NMBs.

Some ultra short ND NMBs are undergoing research, but they are not yet clinically available.[50] Currently, the only ultra short NMB available in the United States is the depolarizing NMB, Sch. However, doubling the dose of rocuronium from 0.6 mg/kg to 1.2 mg/kg shortens the onset of complete neuromuscular blockade from about 1.5 minutes (mean, 89 seconds) to 1 minute (mean, 55 seconds).[50] If Sch cannot be used and intubation in less than 90 seconds is needed, then the higher doses of the ND-NMB can be used.[50] The high dose regimen for RSI is preferred over the "priming technique," whereby a small subparalyzing dose of the ND-NMB (eg, 10% of the intubating dose) is given 2 to 4 minutes before the second large dose for tracheal intubation for several reasons: intubating conditions are less optimal than with Sch, priming has risks (including aspiration), and there are side effects.[50]

Indications for Nondepolarizing Neuromuscular Blocking Agents

The ND-NMBs are used: 1) for muscle relaxation if Sch is contraindicated or unavailable, 2) to maintain postintubation paralysis (remember that repeated doses of Sch should be avoided, if possible), and 3) as a pretreatment agent to lessen or eliminate the fasciculations and their side effects (eg, myalgias and increased IOP, ICP, intragastric pressure [IGP]) associated with Sch use.

The contraindication for the use of ND-NMBs is the same as for a depolarizing NMB, inability to secure the airway with the possibility of a difficult or failed airway.

Specific Nondepolarizing Neuromuscular Blocking Agents

The medical use of ND-NMBs originated from the use of curare as the poison in the arrows of South American Indians. Some of the ND-NMBs, such as d-tubocurarine, were originally isolated from various naturally occurring sources, especially various plants growing in several jungle regions throughout the world. Most ND-NMBs are classified according to chemical class: steroids (aminosteroids), benzylisoquinolinium, or others; or according to onset or duration of action: ultra short acting, short acting, intermediate, or long acting.[50]

The clinical duration (in minutes) for the NMB are ultra short acting, less than 10, short acting, 10 to 20; intermediate, 20 to 50; and long acting, greater than 50. Currently, there are no clinically approved ultra–short-acting ND-NMB blockers, although several ND-NMBs are being developed and tested. Short-acting ND-NMBs include rapacuronium and mivacurium; intermediate acting include vecuronium, rocuronium, atracurium, and cisatracurium; and long-acting include pancuronium, pipecuronium, d-tubocurarine, metacurine, doxacurium, alcuronium, and gallamine. The doses and classes of some of the commonly used ND-NMBs are given in **Table 2**. The older NMBs such as tubocurarine have a higher incidence of hypotension and cardiovascular side effects secondary to histamine release than the newer NMBs (for example, rocuronium, vecuronium, and cisatracurium), which are preferred.

Nondepolarizing Versus Depolarizing Agent for Rapid Sequence Intubation

Sch is still the most commonly used NMB in ED-RSI[6,34] and is the drug of choice for RSI in the ED[1] and anesthesia.[50] Of the ND-NMBs, rocuronium (0.6–1.2 mg/kg dose) is the most commonly used paralytic agents for RSI because of its rapid onset and short duration with vecuronium (0.15 mg/kg/dose) as a second choice.[34] Sch's advantages include rapid onset and offset (eg, short duration of action), profound depth of neuromuscular blockade, and better intubating conditions.

Comparative trials of Sch with rocuronium found that Sch (1 mg/kg) resulted in superior intubation conditions when compared with rocuronium (0.6 mg/kg).[51,52] However, a low dose of rocuronium was used.[51,52] Another recent study also noted similar results with Sch (1 mg/kg) providing superior intubation conditions when compared with rocuronium (again, a lower dose 0.6 mg/kg was used) with no difference in the incidence of adverse airway effects.[53] A Cochrane meta-analysis concluded "succinylcholine created superior intubation conditions to rocuronium when comparing both excellent and clinically acceptable intubating conditions."[54]

Use of Nondepolarizing Neuromuscular Blocking Agents as Pretreatment

The ND-NMBs in a dose that is approximately 10% of the intubating dose can be used as a pretreatment for Sch to prevent fasciculations and their side effects. Rocuronium is the most commonly used ND-NMB because of its rapid onset, and it can be given 1.5 to 3 minutes before the induction of anesthesia.

In clinical practice, the ND-NMB is generally administered 2 minutes before giving the intubating dose of Sch. Although defasciculation is achieved, there are several confounding issues to consider. Giving ND-NMB increases the muscle's resistance to Sch's action such that increasing the Sch dose by 50% is recommended. Use of a ND-NMB may result in less favorable conditions for tracheal intubation and slow the onset of Sch. Perhaps, more importantly, for the emergent intubation in the ED is the extra time (about 2 or more minutes) added to the procedure before intubation occurs. Some clinicians also use fasciculations as a clue to when neuromuscular blockade has occurred, and conditions are ready for ET tube placement. Use of a defasciculating dose of ND-NMB adds another drug to RSI (with the additional risk of possible side effects/complications and drug errors), another step, and additional time to the process.[21] Timing or the use of a small subparalyzing dose of a ND-NMB has several problems as well. There is a danger of aspiration, difficulty swallowing, and uncomfortable visual disturbances for the patient with partial neuromuscular block.[50]

A drug familiar to emergency medicine, lidocaine, can be used as an alternative to ND-NMB for priming before Sch administration. Lidocaine is effective in minimizing or preventing the fasciculations with their side effects that occur after Sch administration. The dose is 1.5 mg/kg of lidocaine.

The Future of Rapid-Sequence Intubation

There is a new reversal agent, sugammadex, which is anticipated to be clinically available (eg, approved by the US Food and Drug Administration) in the near future.[55–57] Some experts anticipate that the availability of a reversal agent for the ND-NMB will expand the use of nondepolarizing NMBs, specifically rocuronium (in a 1.2 mg/kg dose) for RSI,[57] and overall greatly decrease the use of Sch.[58] There is also a newer sedative, dexmedetomidine, which has been used in the operating room, but there are no data available regarding its use for RSI in the ED.[59] Esmolol has also been used as a preinduction agent for RSI. It most often is used for neurosurgical patients with an increase intracranial pressure and is synergistic with fentanyl. Currently, there are limited data regarding its use for RSI in the ED.

MODIFICATION OF RAPID-SEQUENCE INTUBATION

"Facilitated intubation" refers to the use of a sedative only (without a paralytic) to pharmacologically assist with intubation. Facilitated intubation, also referred to as "pharmacologically assisted intubation," has been recommended by some clinicians in specific circumstances because it does not involve neuromuscular blockade. Some advocate the avoidance of a neuromuscular paralysis and the use of sedation alone ("facilitated intubation") in clinical scenarios in which a difficult airway is anticipated.[21]

Table 2
Additional medications for rapid sequence intubation

Drug (Pretreatment Drugs)	Dose (IV) (mg/kg)* for Intubation	Indication	Side Effects	Precautions Contraindications	Reversal Agent	Comments
Lidocaine[a]	1.5	↑ ICP, adults with reactive airway disease	May cause hypotension	Allergy		Often used with fentanyl for ↑ICP
Fentanyl[a] (an opioid)	2–3 mcg/kg	↑ ICP, major vessel dissection/rupture, CAD	May cause hypotension	Avoid bolus injection to avoid chest wall/ masseter rigidity, bradycardia; Allergy	Naloxone, Naltrexone	Often used with lidocaine for ↑ ICP
Atropine	0.02 Minimum 0.1 mg Maximum 0.5 mg	Pediatric patients ≤10 yrs, Patients with significant bradycardia	May cause tachycardia, hypertension	Avoid if patient has significant tachycardia or hypertension		
Rocuronium (Defasculating dose of ND-NMB)[b]	0.06 (1/10th of paralyzing dose)	↑ ICP ↑ IOP	May cause incomplete paralysis	Avoid doses >0.06 (may cause paralysis), Allergy	Sugammadex (not yet available)[c]	

Neuromuscular Blocking Agents				Mechanism of Action, Reversal Agents	
Succinylcholine	Adult 1.5 (some recommend 2 in adults); ↑ dose to 2 myasthenia gravis patients, Infants 2, Newborns 3, Avoid repeat doses/prolonged use	Depolarizing neuromuscular blocker, Short acting	Bradycardia in children (pretreat with atropine) use with caution if ↑ ICP/IOP/IGP, patients with pseudocholinesterase inhibitors	Contraindication malignant hyperthermia, patients with known severe hyperkalemia, nonacute (>4–5 days) burn patients or neuromuscular disease patients (may cause hyperkalemia), Allergy	Depolarization of motor end plate at myoneural junction, No reversal agent	Use with atropine if age ≤10 years or significant bradycardia, Onset 30–60 sec, Duration 6–10 minutes
Rocuronium	0.6–1.0 1.2 high dose	Nondepolarizing neuromuscular block, Intermediate acting	High dose, 1.2 mg/kg has a shortened onset but long duration	Allergy	Blocks acetylcholine from binding to receptors, Sugammadex, (not yet available)[c]	Onset high dose 1 min, Low dose 1½ min, Duration 20 min

(continued on next page)

Table 2
(continued)

Drug (Neuromuscular Blocking Agents)	Dose (IV) (mg/kg)* for Intubation	Indication	Side Effects	Precautions Contraindications	Reversal Agent	Comments
Vecuronium[d]	0.1	Nondepolarizing neuromuscular blocker, Intermediate acting	Onset 2.5–3 min. Duration, 20–40 min.	Allergy	Blocks acetylcholine from binding to receptors, Sugammadex, (not yet available)[c]	Slow onset, Long duration
Pancuronium[d]	0.1	Nondepolarizing neuromuscular blocker, Long acting	Onset 2–3 min, Duration 60–100 min.	Allergy	Blocks acetylcholine from binding to receptors, Sugammadex (not yet available)[c]	Slow onset, Long duration

Note: Doses are in mg/kg except for fentanyl, which is in mcg/kg; doses for intubation are generally higher than for procedural sedation. Not all the available drugs are listed, but the more commonly used drugs are given.

Abbreviations: ICP, intracranial pressure; IOP, intraocular pressure; IGP, intragastric pressure; CAD, coronary artery disease; CV, cardiovascular; ND, nondepolarizing; NMB, neuromuscular blocker; BP, blood pressure; HR, heart rate.

[a] Coadministration of lidocaine and fentanyl may have a synergistic effect.
[b] Lidocaine also prevents fasciculations with succinylcholine so a defasciculating dose of ND-NMB may be unnecessary if lidocaine is given.
[c] Sugammadex is a new reversal agent, anticipated to be available in the near future, which can reverse the ND-NMBs.
[d] The ND-NMBs that have a longer duration (specifically, vecuronium and pancuronium) are not commonly used for RSI in the ED because of their long duration.

For facilitated intubation, the most common sedative used has been etomidate, although midazolam has also bee used.[60–62] Proponents of facilitated intubation suggest that there may be clinical scenarios in which paralysis is not an option.

A study in the prehospital air medical setting, using 0.3 mg/kg of etomidate as their sedative without any NMB reported an 89% rate of successful intubation, difficult intubation in 16%, and episodes of clenched jaws and orofacial muscle spasm.[60] A later study from the same investigators (an air medical transport service) prospectively compared facilitated intubation using etomidate versus RSI using etomidate and succinylcholine. The results were: 63% (15 of 24) of the facilitated intubation (etomidate only) group received additional medications versus 4% (1 of 25) in the RSI group, and laryngoscopic conditions using several scoring systems was significantly more difficult for the facilitated intubation (etomidate only) versus RSI.[61] The conclusion was that facilitated intubation (etomidate only) had a decreased rate of success when compared with RSI (etomidate + succinylcholine). A prehospital study of facilitated intubation using midazolam alone noted a successful intubation rate of only 62.5%, which is less than the usual success rate for prehospital RSI.[62] When comparing successful rates of intubation, based on these studies, RSI has higher success rates than facilitated intubation.

For ED intubations, the results of the NEAR studies confirm the superiority of RSI over facilitated intubation.[6,34] The successful intubation rate for first attempt was RSI = 85%, and sedative only (no NMB) = 76%. The successful rate for first intubation was RSI = 91%, and sedative only (no NMB) = 88%.[34] For pediatric patients, the first attempt intubation success rates were RSI, 78%; sedative only, 44%; and no medication 47%.[6]

SUMMARY

RSI is the process involving administration of a sedative (eg, induction agent) followed almost immediately by a NMB to facilitate endotracheal intubation. The procedure of RSI generally consists of seven steps: preparation, preoxygenation, pretreatment, paralysis with induction, protection and positioning, placement of the endotracheal tube, and post intubation management. The purpose of RSI is to make emergent intubation easier and safer, thereby increasing the success rate of intubation while decreasing the complications. Possible disadvantages are complications from the additional drugs, prolonged intubation with hypoxia, and precipitating an emergent or crash airway. Controversy has arisen regarding various steps in RSI; however, RSI remains the standard of care in emergency medicine airway management.

REFERENCES

1. Murphy MF, Walls RM. Rapid sequence intubation. In: Mace SE, Ducharme J, Murphy MF, editors. Pain management and sedation emergency department management. New York: McGraw-Hill Co.; 2006. p. 211–8 [Chapter 28].
2. Hopson LR, Dronen SC. Pharmacologic adjuncts to intubation. In: Roberts JR, Hedges JR, editors. Clinical procedures in emergency medicine. 4th edition. Philadelphia: Saunder; 2004. p. 100–14 [Chapter 5].
3. Taryle DA, Chandler JE, Good JT Jr, et al. Emergency room intubations - complications and survival. Chest 1979;75:541–3.
4. Kovacs G, MacQuarrie K, Campbell S. Pretreatment in rapid sequence intubation: indicated or contraindicated? CJEM 2006;8(4):243–4.
5. Bledsoe GH, Schrexnayder SM. Pediatric rapid sequence intubation: a review. Pediatr Emerg Care 2004;20(5):339–44.

6. Sagarin MJ, Chiang V, Sakles JC, et al. Rapid sequence intubation for pediatric emergency airway management. Pediatr Emerg Care 2002;18(6):417–23.

7. Weiss M, Gerber AC. Rapid sequence induction in children - it's not a matter of time. Paediatr Anaesth 2008;18:97–9.

8. Brimacombe JR, Berry AM. Cricoid pressure. Can J Anaesth 1997;44(11):1219.

9. Jackson SH. Efficacy and safety of cricoid pressure needs scientific validation. Anesthesiology 1996;84(3):751–2.

10. Ellis DY, Harris T, Zideman DH. Cricoid pressure in emergency department rapid sequence tracheal intubations: a risk-benefit analysis. Ann Emerg Med 2007; 50(6):653–65.

11. Salhi B, Stettner E. In defense of the use of lidocaine in rapid sequence intuba-tion. In: Mower III WR, Knopp RK, editors. Clinical controversies: lidocaine admin-istration before rapid sequence intubation in patients with traumatic brain injuries. Ann Emerg Med 2007;49(1):84–6.

12. Vaillancourt C, Kapur AK. Opposition to the use of lidocaine in rapid sequence intubation. In: Mower III WR, Knopp RK, editors. Clinical controversies lidocaine administration before rapid sequence intubation in patients with traumatic brain injuries. Ann Emerg Med 2007;49(1):86–7.

13. Zelicof-Paul A, Smith-Lockridge A, Schnadower D, et al. Controversies in rapid sequence intubation in children. Curr Opin Pediatr 2005;17:355–62.

14. Wang HE, Davis DP, Wayne MA, et al. Prehospital rapid-sequence intubation - what does the evidence show? Prehosp Emerg Care 2004;8(4):366–77.

15. Kovacs G, Law JA, Ross J, et al. Acute airway management in the emergency department by non-anesthesiologists. Can J Anaesth 2004;51(2):177–80.

16. ACEP Policy Statement. Rapid-sequence intubation. Approved by ACEP Board of Directors - October 2006, Available at: www.ACEP.org Accessed 7/02/08.

17. Walls RM. Rapid sequence intubation. In: Walls RM, Murphy MF, Luten RC, Schneider RE, editors. Manual of emergency airway management. Philadelphia: Lippincott Williams and Wilkins; 2004. p. 22–32 [Chapter 3].

18. Reynolds SF, Heffner J. Airway management of the critically ill patient. Chest 2005;127(4):1397–412.

19. Alves DW, Lawner B. Should RSI be performed in the prehospital setting? Prac-tical Summaries in Acute Care 2006;1(6):45–52.

20. Davis DP, Fakhry SM, Wang HE, et al. Paramedic rapid sequence intubation for severe traumatic brain injury: perspectives from an expert panel. Prehosp Emerg Care 2007;11(1):1–8.

21. Decker JM, Lowe DA. Rapid sequence induction. In: Henretig FM, King C, edi-tors. Textbook of pediatric emergency procedures. Baltimore (MD): Williams & Wilkins; 1997. p. 141–59.

22. Caplan RA, Benumof JL, Berry FA, et al. Practice guidelines for the management of the difficult airway: an updated report by the American Society of Anesthesiol-ogists Task Force on Management of the Difficult Airway. Anesthesiology 2003; 98:1269–77.

23. Gerardi MJ, et al. Evaluation and management of the multiple trauma patients. In: Strange GR, Ahrens WR, Lelyveld S, et al, editors. Pediatric emergency medi-cine. New York: McGraw-Hill; 1996. p. 37–57 [Chapter 8].

24. Murphy MF. Preprocedural patient assessment and intraprocedural monitoring. In: Mace SE, Ducharme J, Murphy MF, editors. Pain management and sedation emergency department management. New York: McGraw-Hill; 2006. p. 47–53 [Chapter 8].

25. Murphy MF, Doyle DJ. Airway evaluation. In: Hung OR, Murphy MF, editors. Management of the difficult and failed airway. New York: McGraw-Hill; 2008 [Chapter 1].

26. Benumof JL, Dagg R, Benumof R. Critical hemoglobin desaturation will occur before return to an unparalyzed state following 1 mg/kg intravenous succinylcholine. Anesthesiology 1997;87(4):979–82.

27. Schneider RE, Caro DA. Pretreatment agents. In: Walls RM, Murphy MF, editors. Manual of emergency airway management. 2nd edition. Philadelphia: Lippincott, Williams & Wilkins; 2004. p. 183–8 [Chapter 16].

28. Mace SE, et al. Clinical policy: evidence based approach to pharmacologic agents used in pediatric sedation and analgesia in the emergency department. Ann Emerg Med 2004;44(4):342–77.

29. Mace SE. Barbituartes. In: Mace SE, Ducharme J, Murphy M, editors. Pain management and sedation: emergency department management. New York: McGraw Hill; 2006. p. 125–31 [Chapter 19].

30. Mace SE. Ketamine. In: Mace SE, Ducharme J, Murphy M, editors. Pain management and sedation. New York: McGraw Hill; 2006. p. 132–8 [Chapter 20].

31. Mace SE. Etomidate. In: Mace SE, Ducharme J, Murphy M, editors. Pain management. New York: McGraw Hill; 2006. p. 121–4 [Chapter 18].

32. Mace SE. Propofol. In: Mace SE, Ducharme J, Murphy M, editors. Pain management and sedation: emergency department management. New York: McGraw Hill; 2006. p. 114–20 [Chapter 17].

33. Mace SE. Benzodiazepines. In: Mace SE, Ducharme J, Murphy M, editors. Pain management and sedation: emergency department management. New York: McGraw Hill; 2006. p. 139–47 [Chapter 21].

34. Sagarin MJ, Barton ED, Chung YM, et al. Airway management by US and Canadian emergency medicine residents: a multicenter analysis of more than 6,000 endotracheal intubation attempts. Ann Emerg Med 2005;46(4):328–36.

35. Bergen JM, Smith DC. A review of etomidate for rapid sequence intubation in the emergency department. J Emerg Med 1997;35(2):221–30.

36. Schenarts CL, Burton JH, Riker RR. Adrenocortical dysfunction following etomidate induction in emergency department patients. Acad Emerg Med 2001;8(1):1–7.

37. Jackson WL. Should we use etomidate as an induction agent for endotracheal intubation in patients with septic shock? A critical appraisal. Chest 2005;127:1031–8.

38. Walz JM, Zayaruzny M, Heard SO. Airway management in critical illness. Chest 2007;131(2):608–20.

39. Bloomfield R. Etomidate and fatal outcome-even a single bolus dose may be detrimental for some patients. Br J Anaesth 2006;97(1):116–7.

40. Kociszewski C, Thomas SH, Harrison T, et al. Etomidate vs. succinylcholine for intubation in air medical setting. Am J Emerg Med 2000;18:757–63.

41. Reves JG, Glass PSA, Lubarsky DA, et al. Intravenous nonopioid anesthetics: barbiturates. In: Miller RD, editor. Miller's anesthesia. 6th edition. Philadelphia: Elsevier Churchill Livingstone; 2005. p. 326–33 [Chapter 10].

42. Bourgoin A, Albanese J, Wereszcynski N, et al. Safety of sedation with ketamine in severe head injury patients: comparison with sufentanil. Crit Care Med 2003; 31:711–7.

43. Berkenbosch JW, Graff GR, Stark JM. Safety and efficacy of ketamine sedation for infant flexible fiberoptic bronchoscopy. Chest 2004;125(3):1132–7.

44. Mace SE. Adjunctive medications: atropine and glycopyrrolate. In: Mace SE, Ducharme J, Murphy M, editors. Pain management and sedation: emergency department management. New York: McGraw Hill; 2006. p. 101–9 [Chapter 15].

45. Wathen JE, Roback MG, Mackenzie T, et al. Does midazolam alter the clinical effects of intravenous ketamine sedation in children? A double-blind, randomized, controlled, emergency department trial. Ann Emerg Med 2000;36:579–88.

46. Sherwin TS, Green SM, Khan A, et al. Does adjunctive midazolam reduce recovery agitation after ketamine sedation for pediatric procedures? A randomized, double-blind, placebo-controlled trial. Ann Emerg Med 2000;35:229–38.

47. Schneider RE, Caro DA. Neuromuscular blocking agents. In: Walls RW, Murphy MF, editors. Manual of airway management. 2nd edition. Philadelphia: Lippincott, Williams & Wilkins; 2004. p. 200–11 [Chapter 18].

48. Bauer SJ, Orio K, Adams BD. Succinylcholine induced masseter spasm during rapid sequence intubation may require a surgical airway: case report. Emerg Med J 2005;22:456–8.

49. Gill M, Graeme K, Guenterberg K. Masseter spasm after succinylcholine administration. J Emerg Med 2005;29(2):167–71.

50. Naguib M, Lien CA. Pharmacology of muscle relaxants and their antagonists. In: Miller RD, editor. Miller's anesthesia. 6th edition. Philadelphia: Elsevier Churchill Livingstone; 2005. p. 482–572 [Chapter 13].

51. Sluga M, Ummenhofer W, Studer W, et al. Rocuronium versus succinylcholine for rapid sequence induction of anesthesia and endotracheal intubation: a prospective, randomized trial in emergent cases. Anesth Analg 2005;101:1356–61.

52. Andrews JL, Kumar N, Van Den Brom RHG, et al. A large simple randomized trial of rocuronium versus succinylcholine in rapid-sequence induction of anaesthesia along with propofol. Acta Anaesthesiol Scand 1999;43:4–8.

53. Mencke T, Knoll H, Schrieber JU, et al. Rocuronium is not associated with more vocal cord injuries than succinylcholine after rapid-sequence induction: a randomized, prospective, controlled trial. Anesth Analg 2006;102:943–9.

54. Perry J, Lee J, Sillberg VAH, et al. Rocuronium bersus succinylcholine for rapid sequence induction intubation. (database online). Cochrane Database Syst Rev 2008;(2):CD002788.

55. deBoer HD, Driessen JJ, Marcus MA, et al. Reversal of rocuronium induced (1.2 mg/kg) profound neuromuscular block by suggammadex: a multicenter dose-finding and safety study. Anesthesiology 2007;107(2):239–44.

56. Puhringer FK, Rex C, Sielenkamper AW, et al. Reversal of profound, high-dose rocuronium induced neuromuscular blockade by sugammadex at two different time points. Anesthesiology 2008;109:188–97.

57. Naguib M. Sugammadex: another milestone in clinical neuromuscular pharmacology. Anesth Analg 2007;104(3):575–81.

58. Cook DR. Can succinylcholine be abandoned? Anesth Analg 2000;90(Suppl 55): S24–8.

59. Reves JG, Glass PSA, Lubarsky DA, et al. Intravenous nonopioid anesthetics. In: Miller RD, editor. Miller's anesthesia. 6th edition. Philadelphia: Elsevier Churchill Livingstone; 2006. p. 317–78 [Chapter 10].

60. Bozeman WP. Etomidate as a sole agent for endotracheal intubation in the prehospital air medical setting. Air Med J 2002;21(4):32–6.

61. Bozeman WP. A comparison of rapid sequence intubation and etomidate only intubation in the prehospital air medical setting. Prehosp Emerg Care 2000;4(1): 14–8.

62. Wang HE, O'Connor RE, Megargel RE, et al. The utilization of midazolam as a pharmacologic adjunct to endotracheal intubation by paramedics. Prehosp Emerg Care 2000;4:14–8.

The Laryngeal Mask Airway: Prehospital and Emergency Department Use

Isabel Barata, MD[a,b,*]

KEYWORDS

- Laryngeal mask airway • Pediatrics • Neonate
- Children • Adult • Difficult airway • Indications
- Complications • Use

HISTORICAL ASPECTS

The laryngeal mask airway (LMA) is a supraglottic airway device that is designed to provide and maintain a seal around the laryngeal inlet for spontaneous ventilation and allow controlled ventilation at modest levels (≤ 15 cm H_2O) of positive pressure.[1,2] The LMA was designed by Dr. Archie I.J. Brain[3] between 1981 and 1988. Its original purpose was to reduce the need for more invasive methods of airway management while offering a more reliable alternative to the face mask. This article addresses characteristics of the LMA, indications and contraindications for its use (because these are applicable to all ages in the prehospital and emergency department setting), and potential complications arising from its use.

CHARACTERISTICS OF THE LARYNGEAL MASK AIRWAY

All LMA airway devices have three main components: mask, airway tube, and inflation line (**Fig. 1**).[2] The LMA is composed of a small "mask" designed to sit in the hypopharynx, with an anterior surface aperture overlying the laryngeal opening (**Fig. 2**).[2] The rim of the mask is composed of an inflatable silicone cuff that fills the hypopharyngeal space, creating a seal that allows positive-pressure ventilation with pressure up to 20 cm H_2O.[4] When fully inserted, the distal tip of the LMA cuff presses against the upper esophageal sphincter.[3] Its sides face into the pyriform fossae, and the upper border rests against the base of the tongue (**Fig. 3**).[2] The adequacy of the seal depends on correct placement and appropriate size. It is depends less on the cuff

[a] Department of Emergency Medicine, North Shore University Hospital, Manhasset, NY, USA
[b] New York University School of Medicine, New York, NY, USA
* Department of Emergency Medicine, North Shore University Hospital, Manhasset, NY

Emerg Med Clin N Am 26 (2008) 1069–1083
doi:10.1016/j.emc.2008.07.006
0733-8627/08/$ – see front matter © 2008 Elsevier Inc. All rights reserved.

emed.theclinics.com

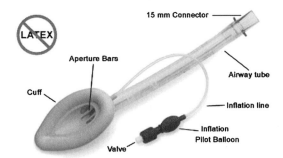

Fig. 1. The LMA Classic. (*Courtesy of* LMA North America, Inc., San Diego, CA; with permission.)

filling pressure or volume. Attached to the posterior surface of the mask is a barrel (airway tube) that extends from the mask's central aperture through the mouth and can be connected to an bag valve mask, ventilator, or anesthesia circuit. The aperture bars are designed to prevent the epiglottis from obstructing the LMA barrel. The airway tube of the LMA varies in length and diameter. Several different types of LMAs have been developed over the years to accommodate varying needs, including facilitating endotracheal intubation (ETI) (**Table 1**).[2]

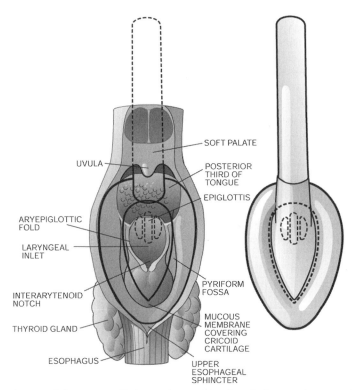

Fig. 2. Dorsal view of the LMA cuff shows the position in relation to pharyngeal anatomy. (*Courtesy of* LMA North America, Inc., San Diego, CA; with permission.)

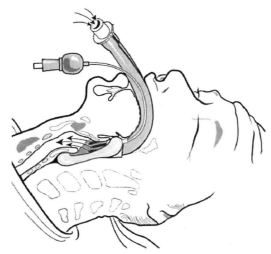

Fig. 3. Schematic of a properly positioned LMA. (*Courtesy of* LMA North America, Inc., San Diego, CA; with permission.)

INDICATIONS FOR USE OF THE LARYNGEAL MASK AIRWAY IN THE PREHOSPITAL AND EMERGENCY DEPARTMENT SETTING

The LMA is indicated in the known or difficult airway situation.[2,5–7] The American Society of Anesthesia (ASA) algorithm stands as a model for the approach to the difficult airway for nurse anesthetists, emergency medicine physicians, and prehospital personnel, in addition to anesthesiologists. **Fig. 4** depicts the ASA difficult airway algorithm, and **Fig. 5** depicts five places where the LMA fits into the ASA difficult airway algorithm.[5–7] The clinical record of LMA use in "cannot ventilate, cannot intubate" situations has been excellent. In patients whose lungs cannot be ventilated because of supraglottic obstruction and whose trachea cannot be intubated because of unfavorable anatomy airway abnormalities[8,9] (but not periglottic pathologic findings), the LMA should be immediately available and considered as the first treatment choice.[5] The LMA can serve as a bridge to secure airway management. It has an important role as an alternative airway when intubation is impossible. No prospective controlled studies of the risk-to-benefit ratio of LMA use in the management of patients with difficult airways exist. There are numerous reports confirming the excellent rating of LMA safety and reliability in difficult airway situations, however.

The LMA is also indicated as a method of establishing a clear airway during resuscitation in the profoundly unconscious patient with absent glossopharyngeal and laryngeal reflexes who may need ventilation. LMAs are an important adjunct for advanced life support and, as such, should be regarded as a device providing temporary airway support rather than a replacement for a tracheal tube. They are an acceptable alternative when used by experienced providers, however.[10,11]

Pediatric respiratory arrest is a technically challenging scenario infrequently faced by prehospital providers. Pediatric prehospital ETI is a complex procedure, and one study showed that it may result in worse neurologic outcome in these patients.[12] Alternatives to ETI include bag-valve-mask (BVM) ventilation and the LMA. This study[13] showed that LMAs may play a role in the prehospital setting when the benefits of ease of training, success and speed of insertion, and no need for direct visualization

Table 1
Laryngeal mask airway summary

LMA Airway	Primary Use	PPV	Spontaneous Breathing	Reusable	Adult Sizes	Pediatric Sizes	Ease of Intubation	Use with MRI
LMA Classic	Routine general anesthesia cases	Up to 20 cm H_2O	+++	Y	4, 5, 6	1, 1½, 2, 2½, 3	++	++
LMA ProSeal	Cases needing higher seal pressures; gastrointestinal tract access needed	Up to 30 cm H_2O	++	Y	4, 5	1, 1½, 2, 2½, 3	+	+
LMA Flexible	Head and neck cases	Up to 20 cm H_2O	+	Y	4, 5, 6	2, 2½, 3	−	+
Single-use LMA Flexible	Head and neck cases	Up to 20 cm H_2O	+	N	4, 5	2, 2½, 3	−	+
LMA Unique	Routine general anesthesia; stock crash carts for rescue airway	Up to 20 cm H2O	+++	N	4, 5	2, 2½, 3	++	++
LMA Fast Track	Facilitates intubation	Up to 20 cm H_2O	++	Y	4, 5	3	+++	−

Abbreviations: PPV, positive-pressure ventilation; +, compatible; ++, recommended; +++, optimal; (−), not compatible.
Courtesy of LMA North America, Inc., San Diego, CA; with permission.

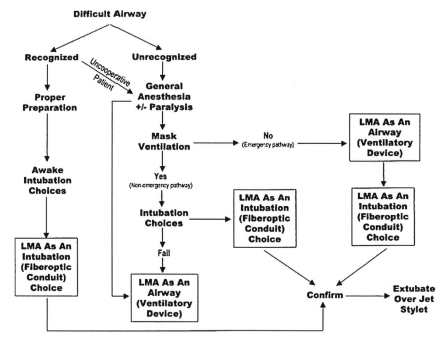

Fig. 4. ASA difficult airway algorithm.

of laryngeal structures, in addition to the lesser need for ancillary equipment, are important factors.

ADVANTAGES AND DISADVANTAGES OF USING THE LARYNGEAL MASK AIRWAY

To determine if the LMA offered any advantages over other forms of airway management, Brimacombe[14] performed a meta-analysis of randomized prospective trials comparing the LMA with the endotracheal tube (ETT) and face mask. Of the 858 LMA publications identified to December 1994, 52 publications met the criteria for the analysis.[14] Thirty-two different issues were tested using Fisher's method for combining the P values.[14] Results are summarized in **Tables 2** and **3**.

When an LMA is used, the provider's hands are free, the patient can produce an effective cough, and spontaneous ventilation is possible. Even when the LMA is malpositioned, ventilation may be adequate. One definition of the appropriate position of the LMA consists of the epiglottis and esophagus outside the rim of the LMA and the laryngeal opening within the rim of the LMA.[5] This is obtained only 45% to 60% of the time; however, in 94% to 99% of adult and pediatric patients, there is no difficulty with ventilation and the airway is ultimately judged to be clinically acceptable.[5]

CONTRAINDICATIONS TO LARYNGEAL MASK AIRWAY USE

The primary contraindication to elective use of the LMA is a risk for gastric contents aspiration (eg, full stomach, hiatus hernia with significant gastroesophageal reflux, morbid obesity, intestinal obstruction, delayed gastric emptying, unknown fasting status).

The LMA should not be used as a substitute for an ETT because of the potential risk for regurgitation and aspiration in some patients undergoing elective procedures or in

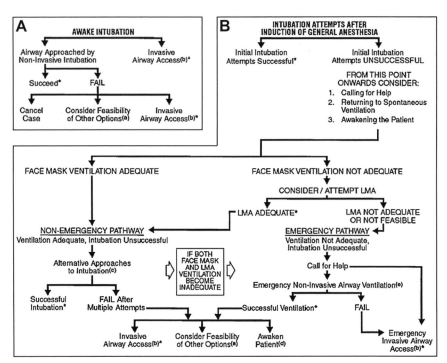

Fig. 5. The LMA fits into the ASA algorithm on the management of the difficult airway in five places, as an airway (ventilatory device) or a conduit for a fiberscope. (*From* Benumof JL. Laryngeal mask airway and the ASA difficult airway algorithm. Anesthesiology 1996;84:686; with permission.)

patients with a difficult airway on a nonemergency pathway (**Box 1**).[3] Obese patients may have an increased volume and acidity of stomach contents and frequently require high airway pressure ventilation. Some evidence indicates that the LMA may be useful in moderately obese patients if no symptoms of reflux are present, however.[15] Other contraindications include poor lung compliance or high airway resistance. Because the LMA forms a low-pressure seal around the larynx, it should be avoided in patients with a fixed decreased pulmonary compliance, such as patients who have pulmonary fibrosis. In addition, the LMA is contraindicated in patients with subglottic airway obstruction and limited mouth opening (<1.5 mm).[15]

If dealing with a difficult airway on the emergency pathway "cannot intubate, cannot ventilate" or with a profoundly unresponsive patient in need of resuscitation, the risk for regurgitation and aspiration must be weighed against the potential benefit of establishing an airway.

PRINCIPLES OF LARYNGEAL MASK AIRWAY USE
Types and Size Selection

LMAs are designed for different purposes (see **Table 1**).[2] For example, the LMA Unique (LMA North America, Inc., San Diego, California) is designed for single use and is ideal for crash carts for rescue airway. LMAs are also available in different sizes for neonates, infants, young children, older children, and adults (two sizes). Not every type of LMA is available in all different sizes, however. As with adults, when using the LMA in pediatric

Table 2
Advantages and disadvantages of the laryngeal face mask compared with the endotracheal tube

Advantages	Disadvantages
Increased speed and ease of placement by inexperienced personnel	Lower seal pressure
Increased speed of placement by anesthetists	Higher frequency of gastric insufflation
Improved hemodynamic stability at induction and during emergence	
Minimal increase in intraocular pressure after insertion	
Reduced anesthetic requirements for airway tolerance	
Lower frequency of coughing during emergence	
Improved oxygen saturation during emergence	
Lower incidence of sore throats in adults	

Modified from Brimacombe JR. The advantages of the LMA over the tracheal tube or facemask: a meta-analysis. Can J Anesth 1995;42:1020; with permission.

patients, size selection is critical to its successful use and to the avoidance of minor and significant complications. Size selection is weight based; however, in pediatrics, if the patient is approaching the upper weight limit for one size, the next larger size is recommended (**Table 4**).[16] The manufacturer recommends that the clinician choose the largest size that comfortably fits in the oral cavity and then inflate to the minimum pressure that allows ventilation to 20 cm H_2O without an air leak.[2]

Preinsertion Preparation

Prepare the LMA by verifying the patency of the cuff and then deflating the cuff (**Fig. 6**).[2] The posterior tip of the deflated cuff should be lubricated to prevent trauma, rolling over of the mask tip, blockage of the aperture, and aspiration of lubricant.[2,17] The mask should be lubricated with a nonsilicone and nonlocal anesthetic-containing lubricant. Nonaqueous lubricants cause softening and swelling of the cuff and an unpleasant sensation in the pharynx.[2] Analgesic lubricants can cause an unpleasant sensation in the pharynx, an allergic reaction, and reduced laryngeal reflex competence.[2,17] An adequate level of anesthesia is necessary before attempting insertion.

Insertion Methods

After establishing an adequate depth of anesthesia and lubrication of the cuff, the appropriately sized LMA is inserted into the mouth, with the aperture facing the

Table 3
Advantages and disadvantages of the laryngeal face mask compared with the face mask

Advantages	Disadvantages
Easier placement by inexperienced personnel	Esophageal reflux is more likely
Improved oxygen saturation	
Less hand fatigue	
Improved operating conditions during minor pediatric otological surgery	

Modified from Brimacombe JR. The advantages of the LMA over the tracheal tube or facemask: a meta-analysis. Can J Anesth 1995;42:1020; with permission.

Box 1
Contraindications to laryngeal mask airway use

Nonfasted patients, including patients whose fasting cannot be confirmed

Grossly or morbidly obese patients

Patients who are more than 14 weeks' pregnant

Multiple or massive injury

Acute abdominal or thoracic injury

Any condition associated with delayed gastric emptying

Using opiate medication before fasting

Patients with a fixed decreased pulmonary compliance

Patients in whom the peak inspiratory pressures are anticipated to exceed 20 to 30 cm H_2O

Adult patients who are unable to understand instructions or cannot adequately answer questions regarding their medical history

Courtesy of LMA North America, Inc., San Diego, CA; with permission.

---

base of the tongue and the cuff tip pressed against the posterior pharyngeal wall. Although the standard method involves total cuff deflation to form a thin flat wedge shape, some clinicians prefer to insert the LMA with the cuff partially inflated. The ideal head position for LMA insertion is the sniffing position. The operator's nondominant hand is placed under the occiput to flex the neck on the thorax and extend the head at the atlanto-occipital joint (creating a space behind the larynx; this action also tends to open the mouth).[18] The index finger insertion technique and the thumb insertion technique are recommended techniques of insertion (**Figs. 7–9**).[2] The index finger of the dominant hand is used to guide the LMA into the hypopharynx until resistance is felt, and the cuff is then inflated with the appropriate volume of air. Resistance indicates that the cuff tip has reached the upper esophageal sphincter. The thumb insertion technique allows the operator to stand to one side of the patient, thus allowing insertion when access to the head end of the patient is not feasible.[17]

Table 4
Selection guidelines for the laryngeal face mask

Mask Size	Patient Size	Maximum Cuff Inflation Volume (Alr)	Maximum ETT ID
1	Neonates and infants up to 5 kg	Up to 4 mL	3.5 mm
1½	Infants 5–10 kg	Up to 7 mL	4.0 mm
2	Infants and children 10–20 kg	Up to 10 mL	4.5 mm
2½	Children 20–30 kg	Up to 24 mL	5.0 mm
3	Children 30–50 kg	Up to 20 mL	6.0 mm cuffed
4	Adults 50–70 kg	Up to 30 mL	6.0 mm cuffed
5	Adults 70–100 kg	Up to 40 mL	7.0 mm cuffed
6	Large adults greater than 100 kg	Up to 50 mL	7.0 mm cuffed

Abbreviation: ID, internal diameter.

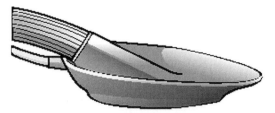

Fig. 6. LMA cuff properly deflated for insertion. (*Courtesy of* LMA North America, Inc., San Diego, CA; with permission.)

This technique can also be applied to insert the device emergently after an accidental tracheal extubation in a patient who is in the prone position.[17] The angled lateral approach is helpful in patients with a high arched palate.[17] As the tip of the mask passes the base of the tongue, the shaft can be slid back to midline. Laryngoscopy to hold the tongue out of the way can improve placement in patients who have gross tonsillar hypertrophy.[17] Partially or fully inflated insertion, however, can increase the possibility of malposition, because the tip of the mask travels in front of the arytenoids toward the larynx and may cause partial airway obstruction or lead to coughing or laryngospasm as a result of stimulation of protective airway reflexes.[17] This method of insertion with the cuff partially or fully inflated may cause the LMA to rest high in the pharynx, leaving the entrance to the esophagus exposed and therefore increasing the risk for regurgitation and aspiration.[17]

Insertion Problems

Problems that may lead to difficult LMA placement include inadequate depth of anesthesia, which may result in coughing or breath holding during insertion,[2] or the

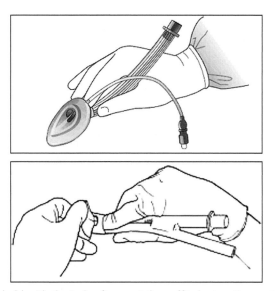

Fig. 7. LMA airway held with the index finger at the cuff/tube junction or in the LMA Proseal introducer strap. (*Courtesy of* LMA North America, Inc., San Diego, CA; with permission.)

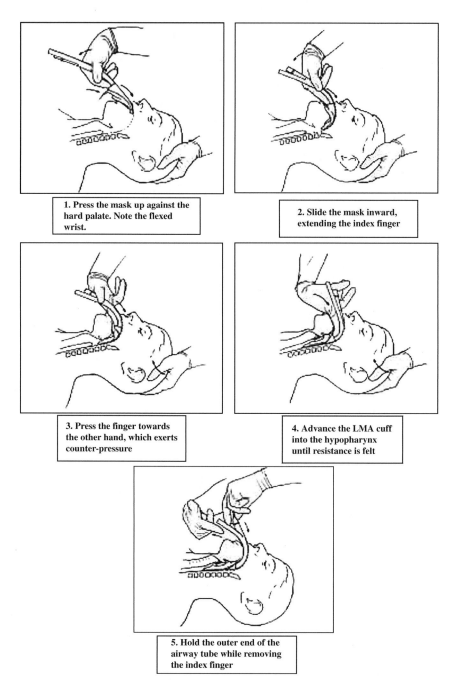

1. Press the mask up against the hard palate. Note the flexed wrist.

2. Slide the mask inward, extending the index finger

3. Press the finger towards the other hand, which exerts counter-pressure

4. Advance the LMA cuff into the hypopharynx until resistance is felt

5. Hold the outer end of the airway tube while removing the index finger

Fig. 8. Index finger insertion technique. (*Courtesy of* LMA North America, Inc., San Diego, CA; with permission.)

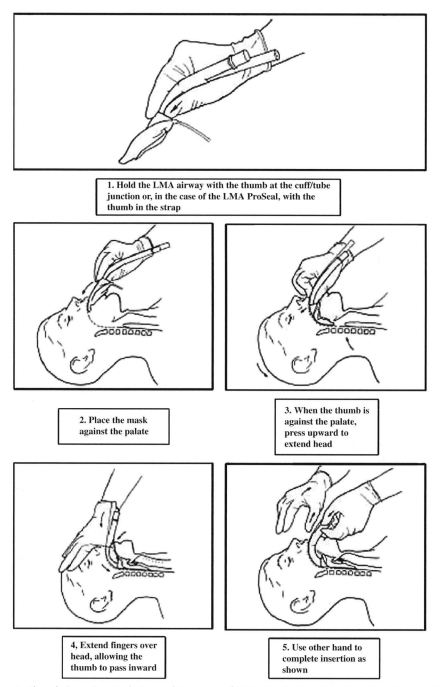

1. Hold the LMA airway with the thumb at the cuff/tube junction or, in the case of the LMA ProSeal, with the thumb in the strap

2. Place the mask against the palate

3. When the thumb is against the palate, press upward to extend head

4, Extend fingers over head, allowing the thumb to pass inward

5. Use other hand to complete insertion as shown

Fig. 9. Thumb insertion technique. (*Courtesy of* LMA North America, Inc., San Diego, CA; with permission.)

patient's mouth may not be able to be opened sufficiently to insert the mask. First, ensure adequate anesthesia, and then have an assistant pull the jaw down; once the mask has passed beyond the teeth, stop the jaw traction because this may allow the tongue and epiglottis to drop downward, blocking passage of the mask.[2] Also, if the cuff fails to flatten or begins to curl over as it is advanced, withdraw the mask and reinsert it. In the case of tonsillar obstruction, a diagonal shift of the mask is sometimes helpful.

Inflation

The inflation volumes listed on the chart (see **Fig. 4**) are the maximum and should not be considered the recommended inflation volumes;[2] frequently, only half of the maximum volume is sufficient to obtain a seal. It is important to note that with varying sizes, there are varying cuff inflation volumes to obtain a seal or achieve an intracuff pressure of 60 cm H_2O. When an adequate seal cannot be obtained with 60-cm H_2O cuff pressure, the LMA may be malpositioned or sizing should be re-evaluated. Light anesthesia may also contribute to poor seal or partial or complete laryngospasm. Excessive intracuff pressure can result in malposition and pharyngolaryngeal morbidity, including sore throat, dysphagia, and nerve injury.[2]

Signs of correct placement include slight outward movement of the tube on inflation, the presence of a smooth oval swelling in the neck around the thyroid and cricoid area, and no cuff visible in the oral cavity.[2] In addition, auscultate the neck area to check for abnormal sounds that might indicate mild laryngeal spasm or light anesthesia.

Securing

Once the LMA is checked for proper placement and adequate gas exchange is confirmed, a bite block should be placed, if not built in, before taping the device in place.[2] Bite block and taping stabilize the LMA and prevent potential occlusion of the tube. Gentle pressure to the outer end of the airway tube as it is fixed ensures that the tip of the mask is pressed securely against the upper esophageal sphincter.[2]

Suctioning

Avoid suctioning the airway tube once the LMA is in place because suctioning and physical stimulation may provoke laryngeal spasm if anesthesia is light. The inflated cuff should protect the larynx from oral secretions, and suctioning is not likely to be required.

Positive-Pressure Ventilation

When delivering positive-pressure ventilation by means of the LMA, ensure that tidal volumes are 6 to 8 mL/kg; keep peak inspiratory pressure less than 20 cm H_2O; and monitor continuously for airway integrity, any gas leak, and abdominal distention.[19]

Removal

Removing the LMA awake versus under anesthesia and removal with the cuff inflated versus deflated are both controversial issues, with various studies reporting differing results. The manufacturer advises removing the LMA with the cuff deflated and when the patient can open the mouth on command;[2] if the cuff is deflated before the return of effective swallowing and cough reflexes, secretions in the upper pharynx may enter the larynx, provoking coughing or laryngeal spasm.[2] Once airway patency and respiratory depth are verified, oral suctioning may be performed if required.

Overall, the incidence of complications after removal of the LMA is 10% to 13%, and complications include coughing, laryngospasm, retching, vomiting, breath holding, stridor, desaturation, and excessive salivation.[20–22] Removal of the LMA when inflated reduces the risk for aspiration of oropharyngeal secretions.[23]

COMPLICATIONS FROM LARYNGEAL MASK AIRWAY USE

Complications from LMA use can be categorized into mechanical, traumatic, and pathophysiologic.[24] Mechanical complications relate to the technical performance as an airway device and include failed insertion (0.3%–4%), ineffective seal (<5%), and malposition (20%–35%).[24] Traumatic complications relate to local tissue damage and include sore throat (10%, with ranges from 0%–70%),[24] dysphagia (4%–24%), and dysarthria (4%–47%).[24] The LMA may cause transient changes in vocal cord function.[25] Fourteen cases of nerve palsy have been reported: recurrent (7 cases), hypoglossal (5 cases), and lingual (2 cases).[26,27] Only 1 of these cases did not resolve spontaneously, and this case was possibly related to cuff overinflation. During the procedures, nitrous oxide was one of the inhalation agents, which can increase cuff pressures by 9% to 38%.[28] Pathophysiologic complications relate to the LMA's effects on the body and include coughing (<2%), vomiting (0.02%–5%), detectable regurgitation (0%–80%), and clinical regurgitation (0.1%).[24]

A predominant clinical perception is that the LMA does not protect the trachea from aspiration. Brimacombe and Berry[29] performed a meta-analysis of 101 publications on the LMA dating from 1988 to 1993 and concluded that pulmonary aspiration with the LMA is uncommon (2.3 per 10,000 cases). The overall incidence of perioperative aspiration ranges from 2.3 to 10.2 (children) per 10,000 cases.[30] Keller and colleagues[31] performed a Medline literature review of case reports of aspiration of gastric contents associated with the LMA and found just 23 cases of suspected pulmonary aspiration (with an estimated 200,000,000 uses of the LMA worldwide). Of these, only 13 cases were verified as true aspiration events, and none resulted in death, although five patients required positive-pressure ventilation. There is only one report in which aspiration occurred when the patient had no risk factors.[31] There were predisposing factors in most of the cases, including obesity, dementia, emergency surgery, upper abdominal surgery, Trendelenburg position, intraperitoneal insufflation, or a difficult airway.[32–37] Evidence suggests but does not prove that the correctly placed LMA Proseal (LMA North America, Inc., San Diego, California) reduces aspiration risk compared with the LMA Classic (LMA North America, Inc., San Diego, California).[38]

If pharyngeal regurgitation or pulmonary aspiration is suspected, the patient should be placed in the head-down position, 100% oxygen should be administered, anesthesia should be deepened, suctioning should be performed, and the severity of the regurgitation or aspiration event should be assessed fiberoptically.[39] The decision about whether to intubate the trachea or continue with the LMA depends on how well the LMA is functioning, the severity of the regurgitation or aspiration event, and the anticipated risk for further regurgitation or aspiration.[39] Because removal of the LMA or passing of a gastric tube may lead to further regurgitation, fiberoptic intubation through the LMA should be considered.[39]

SUMMARY

The LMA now has a well-established role in airway management. There are several different types of LMAs to accommodate many different patient needs. The LMA has become one of the most important and versatile tools in the management of patients with difficult airways. The LMA has many advantages over the ETT and face mask; however, because of the potential risk for regurgitation and aspiration, it is imperative to determine if LMA use is appropriate or not. When used properly the LMA is safe and represents an important advance in airway management.

REFERENCES

1. Available at: http://www.lmana.com/docs/LMA_Airways_Manual.pdf. Accessed January 2008.
2. LMA airway instructional manual. The Laryngeal Mask Company Limited; 2005.
3. Brain AIJ. Historical aspects and future directions. Int Anesthesiol Clin 1998;36: 1–18.
4. Keller C, Brimacombe J. Mucosal pressure, mechanism of seal, airway sealing pressure, and anatomic position for the disposable versus reusable laryngeal mask airways. Anesth Analg 1999;88:1418–20.
5. Benumof JL. Laryngeal mask airway and the ASA difficult airway algorithm. Anesthesiology 1996;84:685–99.
6. Bogetz MS. Using the laryngeal mask airway to manage the difficult airway. Anesthesiol Clin North America 2003;20:863–70.
7. Practice guidelines for management of the difficult airway. Anesthesiology 2003; 98:1269–77.
8. Selim M, Mowafi H, Al-Ghamdi A, et al. Intubation via LMA in pediatric patients with difficult airways. Can J Anaesth 1999;46(9):891–3.
9. Munro HM, Butler PJ, Washington EJ. Freeman-Sheldon (whistling face) syndrome. Anaesthetic and airway management. Paediatr Anaesth 1997;7(4):345–8.
10. 2005 American Heart Association (AHA) guidelines for cardiopulmonary resuscitation (CPR) and emergency cardiovascular care (ECC) of pediatric and neonatal patients: pediatric basic life support. Pediatrics 2006;117(5):e989–1004.
11. 2005 American Heart Association (AHA) guidelines for cardiopulmonary resuscitation (CPR) and emergency cardiovascular care (ECC) of pediatric and neonatal patients: pediatric basic life support. Circulation 2005;112(Suppl 24):IV1–203.
12. Gausche M, Lewis RJ, Stratton SJ, et al. Effect of out-of-hospital pediatric endotracheal intubation on survival and neurological outcome: a controlled clinical trial. J Am Med Assoc 2000;283:783–90.
13. Guyette FX, Roth KR, LaCovey DC, et al. Feasibility of laryngeal mask airway use by prehospital personnel in simulated pediatric respiratory arrest. Prehosp Emerg Care 2007;11(2):245–9.
14. Brimacombe JR. The advantages of the LMA over the tracheal tube or facemask: a meta-analysis. Can J Anaesth 1995;42:1017–23.
15. Brimacombe JR, Berry AM, White PF. The laryngeal mask airway: limitations and controversies. Int Anesthesiol Clin 1998;36:155–82.
16. Boehringer LA, Bennie RE. Laryngeal mask airway and the pediatric patient. Int Anesthesiol Clin 1998;36:45–60.
17. Ferson DZ. Laryngeal mask airway: preanesthetic evaluation and insertion techniques in adults. Int Anesthesiol Clin 1998;36:29–44.
18. Calder I, Picard J, Chapman M, et al. Mouth opening: a new angle. Anesthesiology 2003;99:799–801.
19. Komatsu H, Chujo K, Morita J, et al. Spontaneous breathing with the use of a laryngeal mask airway in children: comparison of sevoflurane and isoflurane. Paediatr Anaesth 1997;7:111–5.

20. Parry M, Glaisyer H, Bailey P. Removal of LMA in children. Br J Anaesth 1997;78: 337–44.
21. Splinter WM, Reid CW. Removal of the laryngeal mask airway in children: deep anesthesia versus awake. J Clin Anesth 1997;9(1):4–7.
22. Laffon M, Plaud P, Dubousset AM, et al. Removal of laryngeal mask airway: airway complications in children, anaesthetized versus awake. Paediatr Anaesth 1993;3:23–8.
23. Kitching AJ, Blogg CE. Removal of the laryngeal mask airway in children: anaesthetized compared with awake. Br J Anaesth 1996;76:874–6.
24. Brimacombe JR. Problems with the laryngeal mask airway: prevention and management. Int Anesthesiol Clin 1998;36:139–54.
25. Erskine RJ, Rabey PG. The laryngeal mask airway in recovery. Anaesthesia 1992; 47(4):354.
26. Lowinger D, Benjamin B, Gadd L. Recurrent laryngeal nerve injury caused by a laryngeal mask airway. Anaesth Intensive Care 1999;27:202–5.
27. Sommer M, Schuldt M, Runge U, et al. Bilateral hypoglossal nerve injury following the use of the laryngeal mask airway without the use of nitrous oxide. Acta Anaesthesiol Scand 2004;48:377–8.
28. Lumb AB, Wrigley MW. The effect of nitrous oxide on laryngeal mask cuff pressure: in vitro and in vivo studies. Anaesthesia 1992;47:320–3.
29. Brimacombe JR, Berry A. The incidence of aspiration associated with the laryngeal mask airway: a meta-analysis of published literature. J Clin Anesth 1995;7: 297–305.
30. Ng A, Smith G. Gastroesophageal reflux and aspiration of gastric contents in anesthetic practice. Anesth Analg 2001;93:494–513.
31. Keller C, Brimacombe J, Bittersohl J, et al. Aspiration and the laryngeal mask airway: three cases and a review of the literature. Br J Anaesth 2004;93:579–82.
32. Brain AI. The laryngeal mask and the oesophagus. Anaesthesia 1991;46(8): 701–2.
33. Wilkinson PA, Cyna AM, MacLeod DM, et al. The laryngeal mask: cautionary tales. Anaesthesia 1990;45(2):167–8.
34. Nanji GM, Maltby JR. Vomiting and aspiration pneumonitis with the laryngeal mask airway. Can J Anaesth 1992;38:69–70.
35. Brimacombe J, Berry A. Aspiration and the laryngeal mask airway—a survey of Australian intensive care units. Anaesth Intensive Care 1992;20(4):534–5.
36. Griffin RM, Hatcher IS. Aspiration pneumonia and the laryngeal mask airway. Anaesthesia 1990;45(12):1039–40.
37. Alexander R, Arrowsmith JE, Frossard JR. The laryngeal mask airway: safe in the x-ray department. Anaesthesia 1993;48(8):734.
38. Cook TM, Lee G, Nolan JP. The ProSeal laryngeal mask airway: a review of the literature. Can J Anaesth 2005;52:739–60.
39. Tournadre JP, Chassard D, Berrada KR, et al. Cricoid cartilage pressure decreases lower esophageal sphincter tone. Anesthesiology 1997;86:7–9.

Needle Cricothyrotomy

Sharon Elizabeth Mace, MD, FACEP, FAAP[a,b,c,d,*], Nazeema Khan, MD[e]

KEYWORDS

- Percutaneous translaryngeal jet ventilation
- Transtracheal jet ventilation • Complications
- Controversy • Benefits

DEFINITIONS

With cricothyrotomy, an opening is made in the cricothyroid membrane to establish an airway (**Fig. 1**).[1,2] Other terms for cricothyrotomy are *cricothyrostomy, coniotomy, laryngotomy,* and *laryngostomy*.[1] With needle cricothyrotomy, a needle or small cannula is passed percutaneously through the cricothyroid membrane to permit translaryngeal jet ventilation (TLJV),[1–3] whereas an *open,* or *surgical,* cricothyrotomy is the use of surgical means (eg, scalpel) to create the opening in the cricothyroid membrane,[1–4] and a *cricothyrotome* is a device or kit used to create a surgical airway without resorting to a formal open cricothyrotomy (**Figs. 2** and **3**).

Transtracheal jet ventilation (TTJV) or *percutaneous transtracheal jet ventilation* (PTJV) is the delivery of oxygen by way of a catheter inserted through the cricothyroid membrane using a needle cricothyrotomy.[2,3] In reality, the cricothyroid membrane is actually part of the larynx, whereas the trachea begins inferior to the cricoid cartilage; therefore TTJV or PTJV is actually a misnomer and TLJV, or percutaneous translaryngeal ventilation (PTLV), would be a more anatomically correct term.[2] Unfortunately, the term TTJV is widely used, but TLJV or PTLV are used in this article.

Surgical airway management according to some authors includes surgical (or open) cricothyrotomy,[4] use of a cricothyrotome, and needle cricothyrotomy with PTLV. Other textbooks consider *surgical airway management* to include a formal open cricothyrotomy, or a cricothyrotome, with needle cricothyrotomy considered another airway technique.[4] However, in this article, this definition of needle cricothyrotomy with PTLV is used as a unique procedure distinct from cricothyrotome or open cricothyrotomy, because the technique, contraindications, and complications differ

[a] Cleveland Clinic Lerner College of Medicine of Case Western Reserve, Cleveland, OH 44195, USA
[b] Observation Unit, Cleveland Clinic, 9500 Euclid Avenue, Cleveland, OH 44195, USA
[c] Emergency Services Institute, E19, Cleveland Clinic, 9500 Euclid Avenue, Cleveland, OH 44195, USA
[d] Case Western Reserve University, Metro Health Medical Center, 8500 Metro Health Drive, Cleveland, OH 44109, USA
[e] Joe DiMaggio Children's Hospital, Hollywood, FL, USA
* Corresponding author. Emergency Services Institute, E19, Cleveland Clinic, 9500 Euclid Avenue, Cleveland, OH 44195.
E-mail address: maces@ccf.org (S.E. Mace).

Emerg Med Clin N Am 26 (2008) 1085–1101
doi:10.1016/j.emc.2008.09.004
0733-8627/08/$ – see front matter © 2008 Elsevier Inc. All rights reserved.

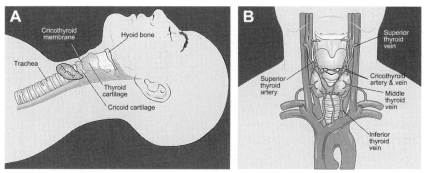

Fig. 1. Anatomy. (*A*) Side view. (*B*) Anterior view. (*Courtesy of* S.E. Mace, MD, and J. Loerch, Clinic Cleveland Center for Medical Art and Photography, Cleveland, OH; with permission.)

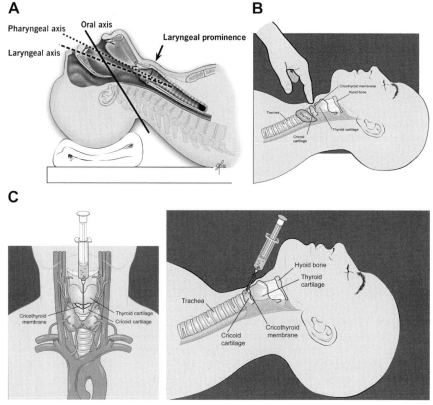

Fig. 2. Needle cricothyrotomy procedure. (*A*) Positioning (assuming no contraindications) to expose the external anatomy (eg, laryngeal prominence). (*B*) Locating the cricothyroid membrane (palpation of the cricothyroid membrane). (*C*) Needle puncture of the cricothyroid membrane (*anterior and side views*). (*D*) Seldinger (guidewire) technique for cricothyrotomy (*cutaway of side view* and *side view*) (*E*) Catheter secured and ventilation with bag-valve–mask. (*Courtesy of* S.E. Mace, MD, and J. Loerch, Clinic Cleveland Center for Medical Art and Photography, Cleveland, OH; with permission.)

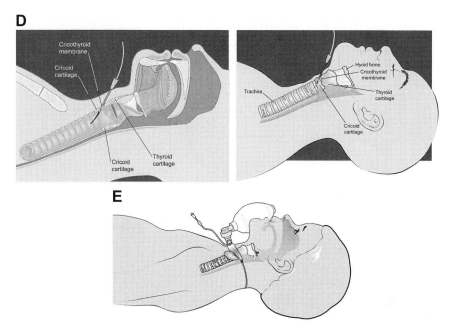

Fig. 2. (*continued*)

somewhat between a surgical cricothyrotomy (through a cricothyrotome or open) and a needle cricothyrotomy.

Jet ventilation implies that oxygen is administered through a small-caliber catheter rather than a larger tracheostomy tube as with open cricothyrotomy or a cricothyrotome.[2,3] Initially, continuous flow oxygen was delivered through the needle cricothyrotomy, which allowed adequate oxygenation but not ventilation. More recently, the technique involves supplying short bursts of oxygen followed by a longer passive exhalation phase to allow ventilation with both inhalation of oxygen and exhalation of carbon dioxide.[2]

INDICATIONS

The primary indication for needle cricothyrotomy is inability to secure the airway through other noninvasive methods (**Box 1**).[1–3] This inability usually signifies a failed airway as defined by any of the following: inability to maintain an oxygen saturation greater than 90%, inadequate ventilation (cyanosis, inadequate or absent breath sounds, hemodynamic instability) with bag-valve mask ventilation, and failed intubation.[5] Needle cricothyrotomy (unlike surgical cricothyrotomy) can be performed in patients of any age.[2,3]

CONTRAINDICATIONS

An absolute contraindication to cricothyrotomy (surgical or needle) is when endotracheal intubation can be accomplished easily and quickly with no contraindications. Two trauma scenarios also present contraindications: tracheal transaction with the distal end retracting into the mediastinum and significant cricoid cartilage/laryngeal injury (eg, a fractured larynx), because the airway must be secured below the injury.[1,2] Other conditions that make cricothyrotomy (surgical or needle) more difficult (thus, are

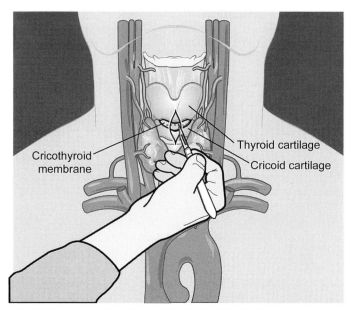

Cricothyroid
membrane

Thyroid cartilage

Cricoid cartilage

Fig. 3. Surgical cricothyrotomy. Use of a scalpel for the skin incision versus a needle puncture with needle cricothyrotomy. (*Courtesy of* S.E. Mace, MD, and J. Loerch, Clinic Cleveland Center for Medical Art and Photography, Cleveland, OH; with permission.)

relative conditions) are massive neck edema/anatomic distortion and acute laryngeal disease.[1,2] A modified technique for locating the cricothyroid membrane has been suggested in patients who have massive neck edema.[6,7] Another relative contraindication is a bleeding diathesis, which can be treated and is probably less concerning for a needle cricothyrotomy than for a surgical cricothyrotomy (see **Box 1**).

Complete upper airway obstruction has been listed as a contraindication to needle cricothyrotomy,[2,3] because of a concern for increased lung volumes with possible barotrauma if gases in the lung cannot escape.[8–11] Increased intrathoracic pressure and hypoxemia can also lead to ventricular dysfunction and decreased cardiac output with cardiovascular collapse. The tenet that complete upper airway obstruction is an absolute contraindication to PTLV has been questioned recently based on its successful use in multiple animal studies[12–16] and several case reports.[17,18] Some clinicians have suggested that altering the mode of oxygen delivery and allowing time for expiration may decrease the incidence of barotrauma, and that in an emergency PTLV could be used if other airway techniques have been unsuccessful if lower oxygen delivery pressure, large-than-usual catheters, and longer exhalation times are used.[3]

Because of anatomic differences between pediatric and adult patients, young age is a contraindication for surgical cricothyrotomy but not needle cricothyrotomy. In fact, needle cricothyrotomy is preferred, and surgical cricothyrotomy (open or with a cricothyrotome) is contraindicated in infants and young children because the cricothyroid membrane is too small to insert a tracheostomy tube and there is a greater risk for damage to surrounding structures. However, the exact age at which a needle cricothyrotomy rather than a surgical cricothyrotomy is indicated is a matter of debate. Experience with pediatric cricothyrotomy is limited,[3] although two small series have shown successful use of needle cricothyrostomy with PTLV in infants and children from aged 4 months to 11 years.[19,20] In view of the limited data on pediatric

---

Box 1
Indications and contraindications for cricothyrotomy

Indications

Inability to secure the airway by other noninvasive means[a]

Failed airway[a]

Inability to maintain oxygen saturation greater than 90% with bag-valve–mask ventilation[a]

Inadequate ventilation: cyanosis, absent breath sounds, hemodynamic instability with bag-valve–mask ventilation[a]

Failed intubation: three or more failed intubation attempts, failure to intubate after 10 minutes[a]

Aid to intubation in the difficult airway[b,c]

Absolute contraindications

When endotracheal intubation can be accomplished easily and quickly with no contraindications[a]

Tracheal transaction with the distal end retracting into the mediastinum[a]

Significant cricoid cartilage/laryngeal injury, such as fractured larynx[a]

Complete upper-airway obstruction[b,d]

Relative contraindications

Bleeding diathesis[a]

Massive neck edema/anatomic distortion[a]

[a] Needle or surgical cricothyrotomy (open or cricothyrotome).
[b] Needle cricothyrotomy only.
[c] Several reports suggest that PTLV may help in intubating patients who have a difficult/failed airway by lifting up the epiglottis and improving visualization of the glottis.
[d] Initially considered an absolute contraindication to needle cricothyrotomy; however, recent data suggest needle cricothyrotomy with PTLV can be performed with complete airway obstruction if lower oxygen delivery pressures are present, a larger cannula is used, and longer exhalation times are used, and therefore may be a relative contraindication.

---

cricothyrotomy, the marked individual variation for a given age, and the many factors involved (eg, size/weight, clinical state, comorbidity, acute illness/injury, anatomic variables, practitioner experience),[2,3] a precise evidence-based age cutoff may not be possible. Thus, depending on the author, the lower age limit (ranging from 5 to 10 to 12 years) at which surgical cricothyrotomy is contraindicated is somewhat arbitrary.[21–23]

ANATOMY OF THE LARYNX: PEDIATRIC VERSUS ADULT

Compared with the adult anatomy, the pediatric airway has a smaller (in absolute size and proportionally) cricothyroid membrane, greater overlap between the thyroid cartilage and cricoid cartilage with less accessibility to the narrower slit-like cricothyroid membrane, and smaller comparatively underdeveloped funnel or conical-shaped airway (verses the larger, more cylindric-shaped adult airway). Furthermore, in the pediatric larynx, the narrowest part of the airway is the cricoid cartilage (versus the vocal cords in the adult airway). The pediatric larynx also has a comparatively flat thyroid cartilage without a vertical midline prominence (compared with the adult's prominent Adam's [or Eve's] apple" where the two quadrilateral lamina of the thyroid cartilage meet), resulting in the standard landmarks for cricothyrotomy being difficult to show and not very prominent. In children, the larynx is located more rostral, or superior (opposite C2–C3 interspace in a young infant and C3–C4 interspace in an older infant, versus C4–C5 in an adult), making the cricothyroid membrane more difficult to access, and children have a more compliant (collapsible) airway. Because the laryngeal prominence is not fully developed until adolescence, other useful landmarks are the cricoid cartilage and the hyoid bone. The pediatric airway has a smaller diameter with greater resistance to gas flow according to the formula $R \propto 1 \div$ (lumen radius),[4] where R is airway resistance. Resistance to gas flow is inversely proportional to the fourth power of the radius of the airway lumen, meaning that small decreases in the luminal diameter cause large increases in the airway resistance (**Box 2**; **Fig. 4**).

COMPLICATIONS

Most cricothyrotomy series report on surgical cricothyrotomies[24–28] and not needle cricothyrotomies with PTLV. For surgical cricothyrotomy in the emergency department, acute complication rates from 8.7% to 40% have been reported, with bleeding and misplacement of the tube the most common complications. Acute complications with either surgical or needle cricothyrotomy include incorrect or unsuccessful placement, subcutaneous emphysema, barotrauma with pneumothorax/pneumomediastinum, obstruction, prolonged procedure time, and injury to surrounding structures, including vocal cord injury and damage to the laryngeal cartilages (eg, thyroid cartilage and cricoid cartilage). Possible late complications are infection, voice changes, and dysphasia/swallowing difficulty (**Box 3**).

Some complications noted with surgical cricothyrotomy (eg, barotrauma, infection, perforation of the trachea) may also occur with needle cricothyrotomy with PTLV. However, other complications may be less frequent. Theoretically, some complications, such as damage to the laryngeal cartilage and subglottic stenosis,

---

Box 2
Pediatric larynx anatomy versus adult

Smaller size of cricothyroid membrane (absolute size and proportional)

Slit-like shape of cricothyroid membrane (versus rectangular shape in adults)

Overlapping thyroid cartilage and cricoid cartilage

Rostrally located cricothyroid membrane (opposite C3/C4 in infant, opposite C4/C5 in adult)

Less accessibility to cricothyroid membrane because of greater overlap of thyroid cartilage and cricothyroid cartilage and more rostral (superior) location of larynx

Small funnel (conical)-shaped airway (large cylindric-shaped adult airway)

Landmarks are not prominent and are difficult to see because of flat thyroid cartilage without vertical midline prominence (adults have a prominent "Adam's/Eve's apple")

More compliant collapsible airway

Cricoid cartilage is narrowest part of airway (vocal cords are narrowest part of airway in adult)

Smaller diameter airway with increased resistance to flow

Airway resistance (R) is inversely proportional to the fourth power of the radius of the airway lumen ($R \propto 1 \div$ [lumen radius]^4)

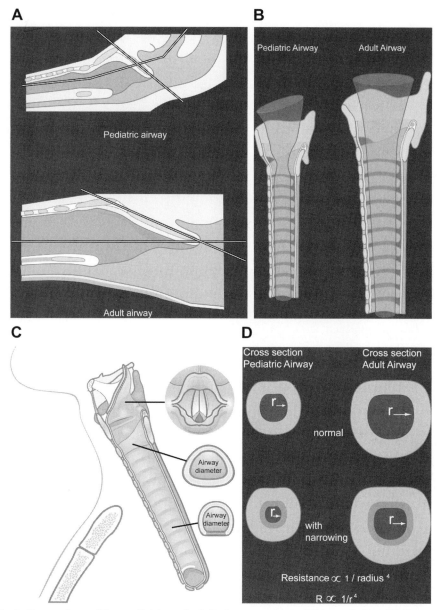

Fig. 4. Comparison of the pediatric and adult airway anatomy. (*A*) Lateral view. (*B*) Shape of the pediatric and adult larynx. (*C*) Airway diameter. (*D*) Airway resistance as affected by the radius of the airway. (*Courtesy of* S.E. Mace, MD, and J Loerch, Clinic Cleveland Center for Medical Art and Photography, Cleveland, OH; with permission.)

would seem less likely to occur with a smaller cannula than the larger tracheostomy tube.

Subcutaneous emphysema and barotrauma (eg, pneumothorax, pneumomediastinum) and catheter-related problems (eg, obstruction/blockage of the catheter, kinking

---

Box 3
Complications of needle cricothyrotomy with percutaneous translaryngeal ventilation

Catheter-related

    Catheter misplacement (unsuccessful or incorrect placement)

    Blockage/obstruction of catheter

    Kinking of the catheter

    Dislodgement of catheter

Barotrauma-related

    Subcutaneous emphysema

    Pneumothorax

    Pneumomediastinum

    Pneumatocele

Stimulation of airway reflexes

    Laryngospasm

    Coughing

Damage to surrounding structures

    Tracheal perforation

    Esophageal perforation

    Mediastinal perforation

    Dysphonia/voices changes (caused by vocal cord injury, laryngeal fracture, or damage to laryngeal cartilage)

    Persistent stoma

    Feeling of "a lump in the throat"

Other

    Bleeding, hematoma

    Infection

    Aspiration[a]

[a] Some data suggest that TTJV may decrease the frequency of aspiration.

---

of the catheter, catheter displacement, misplaced or unsuccessful needle or catheter placement) seem to be the most common complications of needle cricothyrotomy with PTLV (**Box 3**).[10,11,29–33]

In a series of emergency PTLV for acute respiratory failure, successful cannulation of the cricothyroid membrane occurred in 79.3% (23/29 patients) and no immediate fatalities occurred from PTLV.[30] Reasons for unsuccessful cannulation were poor landmarks, catheter kinking, and catheter misplacement. Reported complications included subcutaneous emphysema and pneumomediastinum requiring chest tube placement.[30] No major bleeding episodes or infections occurred at the puncture site and the subcutaneous emphysema resolved without intervention.[30]

A series of patients undergoing PTLV for elective endoscopic laryngeal surgery reported a 7.5% (20/265) incidence of complications.[31] Minor complications (6.4%) included hemodynamic instability (which resolved spontaneously), cervical emphysema, failure of cannula insertion/ventilation, hypoxemia, laryngospasm, mucosal damage, and myocardial ischemia. Major complications (1.1%) were tension pneumothorax, pneumothorax, and cervicomediastinal emphysema.[31]

Theoretically, needle cricothyrotomy should create less trauma to the skin, cricothyroid membrane, and contiguous structures. However, some force is necessary to puncture the cricothyroid membrane, and therefore a risk for perforating the posterior trachea and esophagus still exists, and use of larger needles is associated with a greater risk for perforating the esophagus.[34]

NEEDLE CRICOTHYROTOMY WITH TRANSLARYNGEAL JET VENTILATION: EQUIPMENT

Equipment that should be immediately available before performing the needle cricothyrotomy with PTLV include large-bore needle with an overlying catheter, syringe, local anesthetic, "standard prep and drape" (eg, sterile drapes, gloves), antiseptic solution, trach tape or suture material to secure the catheter, oxygen source, high-pressure oxygen tubing, jet ventilator device, and three-way stopcock or Luer lock (**Box 4**).

Box 4
Equipment for needle cricothyrotomy and translaryngeal jet ventilation

Needle cricothyrotomy

Standard preparation and draping: sterile drapes/gloves/other setup, antiseptic solution

Needle with overlying cannula[a]

    Adult 12 or 14 g

    Child 16 or 18 g

3- or 5-mL syringe containing local anesthetic (eg, lidocaine with epinephrine)

Luer lock or three-way stopcock to attach the catheter to the distal end of the high-pressure oxygen tubing

Trach tape or suture material to secure catheter

Ventilation

Oxygen

Deliver 100% oxygen

High-pressure oxygen source

50 psi for adults and adolescents (directly from oxygen wall outlet)

25 to 35 psi for children (from a standard regulator set at 10–12 L/min)[b]

Manual jet ventilator device

    Push button device, Y connector, or three-way stopcock or Luer lock to allow for inhalation and exhalation (usual I:E is 1:4 or 1:5)

High-pressure tubing, attached to oxygen at one end and cannula/catheter at other with manual jet ventilator device in middle

[a] Alternatively, a commercially available kit can be used.
[b] See text for additional settings.

Originally, a 12- or 14-gauge angiocatheter was used. Commercial PTLV catheters have recently become available, which are designed to result in less kinking (stiffer material), are curved for easier placement and less chance (at least theoretically) of perforating the posterior wall, and have distal side holes and at the tip to allow a wider dispersion of the delivered gas (eg, oxygen). Most reports have used 12- to 16-gauge catheters (2.5–2.8 mm internal diameter) in adults and 16- to 18-gauge in children. Oxygen flow is a function of the catheter size, and therefore larger catheter diameter allows greater oxygen flow.[35] Various commercial kits are now available, with some using a Seldinger technique to gain access to the larynx or trachea.

The needle/catheter should be attached to a 3- or 5-mL syringe that contains several milliliters of sterile normal saline or, preferably, local anesthetic (eg, lidocaine with epinephrine). A Luer lock or three-way stopcock is used to attach the catheter to the distal end of the high-pressure oxygen tubing.

The high-pressure oxygen tubing is connected to the oxygen source at one end and the Luer lock or three-way stopcock at the other, with a manual on/off device (valve, tubing with a hole in the side, or other setup) that allows for exhalation and inhalation (**Fig. 5**). Commercial devices are available, such as the Enk oxygen flow modulator set by Cook Critical Care (Bloomington, Indiana). Other devices have a pressure gauge connected to a hand-triggered push button–type jet injector, which can control the amount of air pressure reaching the catheter.[36] There are commercially prepared kits that are preassembled for use, containing a manual jet ventilator, pressure gauge, adapter, 14-gauge angiocatheter, and trach tie (eg, PTLV kits can be obtained from Life-Assist, Inc., Rancho Cordova, California, or from Instrumentation Industries, Inc, Bethel, Pennsylvania). This equipment should be setup in advance of any airway emergency and placed in an emergency airway cart or box in the emergency department for easy and immediate access.

Two early methods for delivering oxygen use a standard ventilation bag attached to the catheter with a 3.5-mm pediatric endotracheal (ET) tube adapter (**Fig. 6**A) or 7.0-mm adult ET tube adapter connected to the back of a plungerless 3-mL syringe[37]

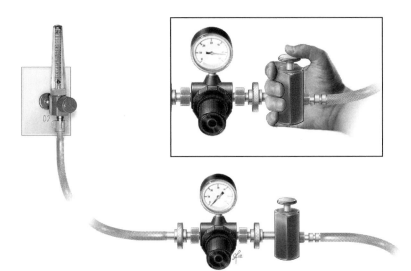

Fig. 5. Manual on-off device for transtracheal jet ventilation. (*Courtesy of* S.E. Mace, MD, and J. Loerch, Clinic Cleveland Center for Medical Art and Photography, Cleveland, OH; with permission.)

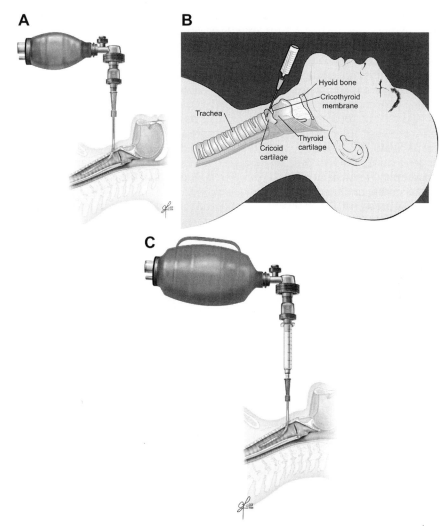

Fig. 6. Ventilation using a standard ventilation bag (*A*) using a 3.5-mm pediatric endotracheal tube (ET) adapter; (*B*) using a 7.0-mm adult ET adapter connected to a plungerless 3 mm syringe without a bag-valve–mask attached; and (*C*) using a 7.0-mm adult ET adapter connected to a plungerless 3-mm syringe with a bag-valve–mask attached. (*Courtesy of* S.E. Mace, MD, and J. Loerch, Clinic Cleveland Center for Medical Art and Photography, Cleveland, OH; with permission.)

(**Fig. 6**B,C). Because this setup using a standard ventilation bag is rigid, and therefore slight movements of the bag may dislodge the catheter, it has been modified by connecting one end of standard intravenous tubing to the PTLV catheter and the other distal cut end to a 2.5-mm ET tube, which is then attached to the bag.

A ventilation bag setup is not recommended for adults because of difficulty in technically providing an adequate tidal volume while allowing sufficient time for exhalation.[38,39] A recent study measuring flow rates found that resuscitation bags (whether pediatric or adult) do not provide adequate ventilation in adults.[40] The investigators' recommendation was, instead of using resuscitation bags for adults needing PTTV, use an unregulated oxygen source of at least 50 psi.[40] Thus, the preferred method for adults and older adolescents is to supply oxygen through a standard 50-psi wall source rather than with a resuscitation bag.

Unfortunately, similar studies applicable to pediatric patients are unavailable. For children, some experts have suggested using 25 to 35 psi.[3] Another author lists the following PSI and estimated tidal volume (TV) parameters for PTLV: 30 to 50 psi with TV of 700 to 1000 cm^3 for adults; 10 to 25 psi with TV of 340 to 625 for children 8 years of age or older (older school-aged children and adolescents); 5 to 10 psi with TV of 240–340 for children aged 5 to 8 years; and 5 psi with TV of 100 for children younger than 5 years.[41] Others suggest that in young children, particularly those younger than 5 years, a resuscitation bag can be used because of their smaller lung capacities, and therefore smaller tidal volumes.[3] Using a 50-psi oxygen source, flow rates based on catheter size are 1300 mL/s for 13-gauge and 1200 mL/s for 14-gauge,[42] although another source gives a flow rate of 1600 mL/s for a 14-gauge.[2] Clinical experience with PTJV is limited, which may explain the variation in recommended settings.

A technologic advancement with PTLV is the use of pressure monitoring during jet ventilation.[9] However, this technique requires special equipment.[9] Using pressure monitoring during PTLV has been suggested as a way to decrease the incidence of barotrauma with PTLV.[9]

NEEDLE CRICOTHYROTOMY WITH PERCUTANEOUS TRANSLARYNGEAL VENTILATION: THE PROCEDURE ITSELF

The patient should be positioned supine with the neck exposed. Hyperextension of the neck (eg, with a "sniffing the morning air" or "sipping English tea" positioning for intubation) may help expose the laryngeal prominence (superior notch of the thyroid cartilage) if no contraindication is present, such as cervical spine injury see **Fig. 2**A. Clinicians should move their finger down the thyroid cartilage in the midline into a small depression above the cricoid cartilage to locate the cricothyroid membrane (see **Fig. 2**B). In adults, four fingerbreadths above the sternal notch or 2 to 3 cm below the laryngeal prominence is the approximate location of the cricothyroid membrane (**Box 5**).

The individual performing the procedure, if right-handed, should be positioned to the patient's left toward the head of the bed. If time allows, the anterior neck should be sterilely prepared and draped. A syringe containing several 3 to 5 mL of lidocaine, with epinephrine or lidocaine on the needle, should be placed. Some clinicians prefer lidocaine with epinephrine because it may decrease bleeding and results in higher levels of lidocaine (and presumably provides better anesthesia) with the same volume (mL) of local anesthetic. Again, if time allows and the patient is awake or responsive, the site should be infiltrated with local anesthetic. Some lidocaine should be left in the syringe for two purposes: (1) it can be injected into the airway for a local anesthetic and may decrease or avoid unwanted airway reflexes, including coughing and laryngospasm, and (2) the needle can be confirmed to be in the airway by having the clinician withdraw on the syringe to determine if air bubbles enter the fluid in the syringe. If lidocaine cannot be used (eg, because of allergy), then normal saline can be used to show bubbles in the syringe.

After locating the cricothyroid membrane (the small depression between the cricoid cartilage inferiorly and the thyroid cartilage superiorly) with the nondominant hand (see **Fig. 2**B), the clinician should insert the needle (with the syringe containing lidocaine with epinephrine attached) at a 30° to 45° angle caudally through the skin,

---

Box 5
Needle cricothyrotomy with percutaneous translaryngeal ventilation

Positioning

   Position the patient so that the neck is hyperextended to expose the laryngeal prominence

   The practitioner, if right-handed, stands to the patient's left toward the head of the bed

Preparation

   All equipment available and assembled

   Sterile preparation and draping

   Anesthetize the area with lidocaine with epinephrine if time permits

   Syringe containing lidocaine with epinephrine attached to needle/catheter

Procedure: placement of catheter

   Locate cricothyroid membrane

   Hold trachea in place while providing tension on the skin with the thumb and middle finger of nondominant hand

   Direct needle caudally at 30° to 45° while pulling back on syringe; the presence of air bubbles signifies entry into the trachea

   Slide catheter over needle until the catheter hub fits securely (snugly) on the skin surface

   Remove needle and syringe as a unit

Postprocedure management

   Connect catheter to high-pressure oxygen tubing with other end of tubing attached to wall oxygen (with manual jet ventilator device in between both ends of the high-pressure tubing)

   Give a gentle burst of oxygen (test dose) to check for correct placement

   Secure catheter with trach tie or suture in place

   Ventilate (usual I:E is 1:4 or 1:5)

---

subcutaneous tissue, and cricothyroid membrane. A small nick in the skin surface may be made with a scalpel before the needle insertion to help puncture the skin if much skin resistance is anticipated. Ideally, the needle puncture should be in the lower (inferior) part the cricothyroid membrane to avoid the cricothyroid artery and vein that course across the upper part of the cricothyroid membrane. The syringe should be aspirated when the needle is advanced. Bubbles in the fluid or increased ease of aspiring air signifies that the needle has traversed the cricothyroid membrane and is now in the airway (see **Fig. 2C**).

While holding the needle in place, the clinician should advance the catheter to the hub and then remove the needle (see **Fig. 2D**). The catheter should be held in place by hand until its placement is confirmed and it is connected to the oxygen source. One person should be designated to hold the hub of the catheter in place until it is secured with suturing or a trach tie to prevent dislodgement or subcutaneous emphysema (see **Fig. 2E**). Before the catheter is secured, the hub should be held flush against the skin to avoid any air leaks.

The usual inhalation–exhalation ratio (I:E ratio) is 1:4 or 1:5, or 1 second for inhalation of oxygen and 4 or 5 seconds for passive exhalation, to provide for ventilation.[3] In patients who have a partial upper-airway obstruction, an I:E of 1:9 has been recommended to decrease risk for barotrauma.[3] As with endotracheal intubation, placement should be verified using the usual means, including end tidal carbon dioxide changes, chest rise, and oxygenation improvement. Placing the catheter in the subcutaneous tissue can cause massive subcutaneous emphysema, and therefore some clinicians suggest performing a test of oxygen with a resuscitation bag or a low psi before administering the full 50 psi (in an adult) or 25 to 35 psi (in a pediatric patient) to determine if the catheter is incorrectly placed and limit the amount of subcutaneous emphysema.

The catheter can also be misplaced into the airway in the trachea or larynx in an area other than through the cricothyroid membrane. In this case, if the oxygenation and clinical condition improves, leaving the misplaced tube temporarily in the airway until another airway can be secured may be best. If the catheter cannot be placed in the cricothyroid membrane (eg, because of injury to the cricoid cartilage), then the catheter may be inserted between two adjacent tracheal rings. However, the clinician should try to avoid the region of tracheal rings two to four, because the isthmus of the thyroid gland usually lies anterior to these rings. During PTLV, oropharyngeal secretions may be expelled through the patient's nose and mouth, and therefore proper barrier precautions (eg, gown, gloves, masks) should be taken.

CONTROVERSY ASSOCIATED WITH PERCUTANEOUS TRANSLARYNGEAL VENTILATION

The long-standing tenet has been that PTLV is only a temporizing measure and cannot provide ventilation for an extended period. Previous teaching has been that oxygenation is adequate with PTLV, but hypercarbia and respiratory acidosis occur because of inadequate ventilation, and therefore PTLV can only be used for approximately 30 to 45 minutes in an adult.[43] Early methods of PTLV used continuous low-flow oxygen (*apneic oxygenation*) without allowing for exhalation.[44]

However, numerous studies have documented adequate ventilation with a normal arterial pCO_2 and pH with PTLV for periods longer than 20 minutes.[42,45–50] Furthermore, transtracheal or transglottal jet ventilation is commonly used for anesthesia during laryngeal surgeries for controlled mechanical ventilation.[31–33,51,52] Allowing for ventilation, not just oxygenation, with adequate expiratory time and using a high-flow oxygen source are variables shown to improve PTLV, and is a practice that challenges the previously held maxim.[12,16] However, further studies evaluating more prolonged ventilatory times with PTLV are needed.

ADDITIONAL BENEFITS OF PERCUTANEOUS TRANSLARYNGEAL VENTILATION

Several case reports suggest that PTLV may help in difficult or failed intubations. In patients for whom intubation failed, PTLV was performed to obtain an airway. However, once PTLV was used, intubating patients became easier. The high intratracheal pressure from PTLV seemed to lift the epiglottis and open the glottis, allowing visualization of the vocal cords and making intubation easier. The escape of gas under high pressure caused the edges of the glottis to flutter, allowing recognition of the glottis and thereby assisting in intubation.[17,18]

PTLV may also have a benefit in preventing aspiration. Several animal studies have shown that PTLV may prevent aspiration.[53–55] Whether this capability is secondary to the escaping pressure forcing secretions out of the airway or another mechanism remains to be determined. Similarly, experts have also suggested that the escaping pressure from PTLV may help expel a foreign body in the upper airway.

SUMMARY

Needle cricothyrotomy with PTLV can be a life-saving procedure when an emergency airway is needed. Needle cricothyrotomy is preferred over surgical cricothyrotomy in infants and young children. Appropriate ventilatory parameters using a high-flow oxygen source and an adequate expiratory time (I:E ratio) may limit the complications of barotrauma and allow for a more extended time of ventilation. Preliminary reports suggest that PTLV may be also useful in the endotracheal intubation of patients who have a difficult or failed airway and may help prevent aspiration, although further studies are needed. Emergency physicians should be familiar with the indications, contraindications, complications, and procedure of this type of rescue airway, which is also used to ventilate patients during elective laryngeal surgery.

REFERENCES

1. Mace SE. Cricothyrotomy. J Emerg Med 1988;6:309–19.
2. Hebert RB, Bose S, Mace SE. Cricothyrotomy and transtracheal jet ventilation. In: Roberts JR, Hedges JR, editors. Procedures in emergency medicine. Philadelphia: Elsevier Publishing Co; 2008, Chapter 6.
3. Greenfield RH. Percutaneous transtracheal ventilation. In: Henritg FM, King C , editors. Textbook of pediatric emergency procedures. Baltimore (MD): Williams and Wilkins; 1997. p. 239–49, Chapter. 17.
4. Launcelot GO, Johnson LB. Surgical airway. In: Hung OR, Murphy MF, editors. Management of the difficult and failed airway. New York: McGraw-Hill; 2008. p. 191–202, Chapter 12.
5. American Society of Anesthesiologists Task Force on Management of the Difficult Airway. Practice guidelines for management of the difficult airway. Anesthesiology 2003;98(5):1269–77.
6. Simon RR, Brenner BE. Emergency cricothyrotomy in the patient with massive neck swelling. I. Anatomical aspects. Crit Care Med 1983;11:114–8.
7. Simon RR, Brenner BE. Emergency cricothyrotomy in the patient with massive neck swelling. II. Clinical aspects. Crit Care Med 1983;11:119–23.
8. Jorden RC, Moore EE, Marx JA, et al. A comparison of PTV and endotracheal ventilation in an acute trauma model. J Trauma 1985;25:978–83.
9. Carl ML, Rhee KJ, Schelagle ES, et al. Effects of graded upper-airway obstruction on pulmonary mechanics during transtracheal jet ventilation in dogs. Ann Emerg Med 1994;24:1137.
10. Nunn C, Uffman J, Bhananker SM. Bilateral tension pneumothoraxes following jet ventilation via an airway exchange catheter. J Anesth 2007;21:76–9.
11. Cook TM, Bigwood B, Cranshaw J. A complication of transtracheal jet ventilation and use of the Aintree intubation catheter during airway resuscitation. Anaesthesia 2006;61:692–7.
12. Stothert JC, Stout MJ, Lewis LM, et al. High-pressure percutaneous transtracheal ventilation: the use of large gauge intravenous type catheters in the totally obstructed airway. Am J Emerg Med 1990;8(3):184–9.
13. Campbell CT, Harris RC, Cook MH, et al. A new device for emergency percutaneous transtracheal ventilation in partial and complete airway obstruction. Ann Emerg Med 1988;17:927–31.
14. Frame SB, Timerlake GA, Kerstein MD, et al. Transtracheal needle catheter ventilation in complete airway obstruction: an animal model. Ann Emerg Med 1989;18:127–33.
15. Neff CC, Pfister RC, vanSonnenberg E. Percutaneous transtracheal ventilation: experimental and practical aspects. J Trauma 1983;23:84–90.

16. Frame SB, Simon JM, Kerstein MD, et al. Percutaneous transtracheal catheter ventilation (PTCV) in complete airway obstruction–a canine model. J Trauma 1989;29:774–81.

17. Chandradeva K, Palin C, Ghosh SM, et al. Percutaneous transtracheal jet ventilation as a guide to tracheal intubation in severe upper airway obstruction from supraglottic edema. Br J Anaesth 2005;94(5):683–6.

18. McLeod AD, Turner MW, Torlot KJ. Safety of transtracheal jet ventilation upper airway obstruction. Br J Anaesth 2005;95(4):560–1.

19. Smith RB, Myers N, Sherman H. Transtracheal ventilation in paediatric patients: case reports. Br J Anaesth 1974;46:313–4.

20. Ravussin P, Bayer-Berger M, Monnier P, et al. Percutaneous transtracheal ventilation for laser endoscopic procedures infants and small children with laryngeal obstruction: report of two cases. Can J Anaesth 1987;34:83–6.

21. Strange GR, Niederman LG. Surgical cricothyrotomy. In: Henretiz FM, King C, editors. Textbook of pediatric emergency procedures. Baltimore(MD): MD. Williams and Wilkins; 1997. p. 351–6, Chapter 25.

22. Gens DR. Surgical airway management. In: Tintinalli JE, Kelen GD, Stapczynski JS, editors. Emergency medicine: a comprehensive study guide. 6th edition. New York: McGraw-Hill; 2004. p. 119–24, Chapter 20.

23. Walls RM. Airway. In: Marx JA, Hockberger ES, Walls RM, editors. 6th edition, Rosen's emergency medicine: concepts and clinical practice, vol. 1. Philadelphia: Mosby Elsevier; 2006. p. 2–25, Chapter 1.

24. Isaacs JH Jr, Pedersen AD. Emergency cricothyrotomy. Am Surg 1997;63(4):346–9.

25. Gerich TG, Schmidt U, et al. Prehospital airway management in the acutely injured patient. The role of surgical cricothyrotomy revisited. J Trauma 1998;45: 312–4.

26. Boyle MF, Hatton D, Sheets C. Surgical cricothyrotomy performed by air ambulance flight nurses: a 5-year experience. J Emerg Med 1993;11:41–5.

27. Spaite DW, Joseph M. Prehospital cricothyrotomy: an investigation of indications, technique, complications, and patient outcome. Ann Emerg Med 1990;19: 279–85.

28. Nugent WL, Rhee KJ, Wisner DH. Can nurses perform surgical cricothyrotomy with acceptable success and complication rates? Ann Emerg Med 1991;20: 367–70.

29. Swartzman S, Wilson MA. Percutaneous transtracheal jet ventilation for cardiopulmonary resuscitation: evaluation of a new jet ventilator. Crit Care Med 1984;12: 8–13.

30. Patel RG. Percutaneous transtracheal jet ventilation. Chest 1999;116:1689–94.

31. Yves Jacquet, Monnier P, VanMelle G, et al. Complications of different ventilation strategies in endoscopic laryngeal surgery. Anesthesiology 2006;104:52–9.

32. Russell WC, Maguire AM, Jones GW. Cricothyroidotomy and transtracheal high frequency jet ventilation for elective laryngeal surgery. An audit of 90 cases. Anaesth Intensive Care 2000;28:62–7.

33. Weymuller EA, Pavlin EG, Paugh D, et al. Management of difficult airway problems with percutaneous transtracheal ventilation. Ann Otol Rhinol Laryngol 1987;96:34–7.

34. Abbrecht PH, Kyle RR, Reams WH, et al. Insertion forces and risk of complications. J Emerg Med 1992;10:417–26.

35. Marr JK, Yamamoto LG. Gas flow rates through transtracheal ventilation catheters. Am J Emerg Med 2004;22:264–6.

36. Yildiz Y, Preussier NP. Percutaneous transtracheal emergency ventilation during respiratory arrest: comparison of the oxygen flow modulator with a hand

triggered emergency jet injector in an animal model. Am J Emerg Med 2006;24: 455–9.

37. Chong CF, Wang TL, Chang H. Percutaneous transtracheal ventilation without a jet ventilator. Am J Emerg Med 2003;21:507–8.

38. Yealy DM, Plewa MC, Stewart RD. An evaluation of cannula and oxygen sources for pediatric jet ventilation. Am J Emerg Med 1991;9:20–3.

39. Yealy DM, Stewart RD, Kaplan RM. Myths and pitfalls in emergency translaryngeal ventilation: correcting misimpressions. Ann Emerg Med 1988;17:690–2.

40. Hooker EA, Danzl DF, O'Brien D, et al. Percutaneous transtracheal ventilation: resuscitation bags do not provide adequate ventilation. Prehospital Disaster Med 2006;21(6):431–5.

41. Gerardi MJ. Evaluation and management of the multiple trauma patients. In: Strange GR, Ahrens WR, Lelyveld S, et al, editors. Pediatric emergency medicine. New York: McGraw Hill 2002. p. 55–73. Chapter 10.

42. Stewart RD. Manual translaryngeal jet ventilation. Emerg Med Clin North Am 1989;7:155–64.

43. Airway and Ventilatory Management. Advanced Trauma Life Support (ATLS). 7th edition. Chicago: American College of Surgeons; 2004. p. 48–9.

44. Okamoto K, Morioka T. Transtracheal O_2 insufflation (TOI) as an alternative method of ventilation during cardiopulmonary resuscitation. Resuscitation 1990; 20:253–62.

45. Manoach S, Corinaldi C, Paladine L, et al. Percutaneous transcricoid jet ventilation compared with surgical cricothyrotomy in a sheep airway salvage model. Resuscitation 2004;62(1):79–87.

46. Tran TP, Rhee KJ, Schultz HD, et al. Gas exchange and lung mechanics during percutaneous transtracheal ventilation in an unparalyzed canine model. Acad Emerg Med 1998;5:320–4.

47. Carl ME, Rhee KJ, Schelegle ES, et al. Pulmonary mechanics of dogs during transtracheal jet ventilation. Ann Emerg Med 1994;24:1126–36.

48. Cote CJ, Eavey RD, Todres ID, et al. Cricothyroid membrane puncture: oxygenation and ventilation in a dog model using an intravenous catheter. Crit Care Med 1988;16:615–9.

49. Scuderi PE, McLeskey CH, Comer PB. Emergency percutaneous transtracheal ventilation during anaesthesia using readily available equipment. Anesth and Analgesia 1982;61(10):867–70.

50. Ward KR, Menegazzi JJ. Translaryngeal jet ventilation and end-tidal pCO_2 monitoring during various degrees of upper airway obstruction. Ann Emerg Med 1991;20(11):1193–7.

51. Gulleth Y, Spiro J. Percutaneous transtracheal jet ventilation in head and neck surgery. Arch Otolaryngol Head Neck Surg 2005;131(10):886–90.

52. Monnier PH, Ravussin P, Savarx M, et al. Percutaneous transtracheal ventilation for laser endoscopic treatment of laryngeal and subglottic lesions. Clinical Otolaryngology and Allied Sciences 1988;13(3):209–17.

53. Yealy DM, Plewa MC. Manual translaryngeal jet ventilation and the risk of aspiration in a canine model. Ann Emerg Med 1990;19(11):1238–41.

54. Jawan B, Cheung HK, Chong ZK, et al. Aspiration and transtracheal jet ventilation with different pressures and depths of chest compression. Crit Care Med 1999; 27(1):142–5.

55. Jawan B, Cheung HK, Chong ZK, et al. Aspiration in transtracheal oxygen insufflation with different insufflation flow rates during cardiopulmonary resuscitation in dogs. Anesth Analg 2000;91:1431–5.

Index

Note: Page numbers of article titles are in **boldface** type.

Emerg Med Clin N Am 26 (2008) 1103–1110
doi:10.1016/S0733-8627(08)00110-7
0733-8627/08/$ – see front matter © 2008 Elsevier Inc. All rights reserved.

emed.theclinics.com

Moving?

Make sure your subscription moves with you!

To notify us of your new address, find your **Clinics Account Number** (located on your mailing label above your name), and contact customer service at:

E-mail: elspcs@elsevier.com

800-654-2452 (subscribers in the U.S. & Canada)
314-453-7041 (subscribers outside of the U.S. & Canada)

Fax number: 314-523-5170

Elsevier Periodicals Customer Service
11830 Westline Industrial Drive
St. Louis, MO 63146

*To ensure uninterrupted delivery of your subscription, please notify us at least 4 weeks in advance of move.